AF688043

Physical Activity, Exercise and Diet: Pediatrics Essentials

Physical Activity, Exercise and Diet: Pediatrics Essentials

Editor: Duncan Bayer

FOSTER ACADEMICS
www.fosteracademics.com

www.fosteracademics.com

FOSTER ACADEMICS

Cataloging-in-Publication Data

Physical activity, exercise and diet : pediatrics essentials / edited by Duncan Bayer.
p. cm.
Includes bibliographical references and index.
ISBN 978-1-64646-622-1
1. Children--Health and hygiene. 2. Pediatrics. 3. Exercise for children. 4. Children--Nutrition.
5. Diet. 6. Physical fitness for children. I. Bayer, Duncan.
RJ101 .P49 2023
618.92--dc23

© Foster Academics, 2023

Foster Academics,
118-35 Queens Blvd., Suite 400,
Forest Hills, NY 11375, USA

ISBN 978-1-64646-622-1 (Hardback)

This book contains information obtained from authentic and highly regarded sources. Copyright for all individual chapters remain with the respective authors as indicated. All chapters are published with permission under the Creative Commons Attribution License or equivalent. A wide variety of references are listed. Permission and sources are indicated; for detailed attributions, please refer to the permissions page and list of contributors. Reasonable efforts have been made to publish reliable data and information, but the authors, editors and publisher cannot assume any responsibility for the validity of all materials or the consequences of their use.

Trademark Notice: Registered trademark of products or corporate names are used only for explanation and identification without intent to infringe.

Contents

Preface

Physical activity and diet is crucial throughout childhood for maintaining body mass index (BMI), maintaining optimum body composition and lowering the risk of diet-related chronic diseases later in life. Children require a nutritious, well-balanced diet that includes foods from every food category in order to receive a variety of nutrients for good health. Milk and dairy products, grains, oils and fats, beans, meat, as well as vegetables and fruits are important food items for children. Physical activity is necessary for the healthy development and growth of children, as it benefits their minds and bodies. The amount of physical activity required by children varies according to their age. Exercise helps to manage and prevent non-communicable diseases, like diabetes, cancer, and cardiovascular disease. The symptoms of anxiety and depression are also decreased by exercise. This book covers the role of physical activity, exercise and diet in pediatrics. It will prove to be immensely beneficial to students and researchers in this field.

This book is a result of research of several months to collate the most relevant data in the field.

When I was approached with the idea of this book and the proposal to edit it, I was overwhelmed. It gave me an opportunity to reach out to all those who share a common interest with me in this field. I had 3 main parameters for editing this text:

1. Accuracy – The data and information provided in this book should be up-to-date and valuable to the readers.

2. Structure – The data must be presented in a structured format for easy understanding and better grasping of the readers.

3. Universal Approach – This book not only targets students but also experts and innovators in the field, thus my aim was to present topics which are of use to all.

Thus, it took me a couple of months to finish the editing of this book.

I would like to make a special mention of my publisher who considered me worthy of this opportunity and also supported me throughout the editing process. I would also like to thank the editing team at the back-end who extended their help whenever required.

Editor

1

Diet-Related Behaviors and Diet Quality among School-Aged Adolescents Living in Greece

Vassiliki Benetou [1,*], Afroditi Kanellopoulou [1,2], Eleftheria Kanavou [3], Anastasios Fotiou [3], Myrto Stavrou [3], Clive Richardson [4], Philippos Orfanos [1] and Anna Kokkevi [3]

1 Department of Hygiene, Epidemiology and Medical Statistics, School of Medicine, National and Kapodistrian University of Athens, 115-27 Athens, Greece; afkanellopoulou@gmail.com (A.K.); phorfanos@med.uoa.gr (P.O.)
2 Department of Hygiene and Epidemiology, School of Medicine, University of Ioannina, 451-10 Ioannina, Greece
3 University Mental Health, Neurosciences, & Precision Medicine Research Institute "Costas Stefanis" (UMHRI), 115-27 Athens, Greece; erevna.HBSC@epipsi.gr (E.K.); afotiou@med.uoa.gr (A.F.); erevna.hbsc@epipsi.gr (M.S.); akokkevi@med.uoa.gr (A.K.)
4 Department of Economic and Regional Development, Panteion University of Social and Political Sciences, 176-71 Athens, Greece; crichard@panteion.gr
* Correspondence: vbenetou@med.uoa.gr;

Abstract: Prevalence of diet-related behaviors (i.e., breakfast consumption, eating with the family) and their association with a 17-point diet quality score, constructed on the basis of reported frequency (in days/week) of vegetable, fruit, sweets and sugar-sweetened beverages consumption, was investigated among 3525 adolescents (51.5% girls) aged 11, 13 and 15 years, who were participants in the Greek arm of the international Health Behaviour in School-Aged Children (HBSC) cross-sectional study, during 2018. Almost one-third (32.9%) of the sample had breakfast ≤1 day/weekdays, 20.2% rarely ate with the family, 26.1% had a meal while watching TV ≥5 days/week, 31.7% had a snack in front of a screen ≥5 days/week and 24.1% ate in fast-food restaurants at least once/week. Multivariable ordinal logistic regression revealed that eating breakfast ≤1 day/weekdays compared to 4–5 days/weekdays (Odds ratio (OR): 1.56, 95% con-fidence interval (CI): 1.34–1.82), eating rarely with the family compared to almost every day (OR: 1.35, 95% CI: 1.13–1.60) and eating in fast-food restaurants ≥2 times/week vs. rarely (OR: 4.59, 95% CI: 3.14–6.70) were associated with higher odds of having poor diet quality. High frequency of having meals/snacks in front of a screen/TV was also associated with poor diet quality. Efforts to prevent or modify these behaviors during adolescence may contribute to healthier diet.

Keywords: diet quality; adolescents; diet-related behaviors; cross-sectional study; breakfast; fast-foods; family

1. Introduction

Nutrition plays a fundamental role in the development of each child's full potential and influences their later susceptibility to chronic diseases [1,2]. Especially during adolescence, the second fastest growth period after infancy, adequate nutrition in terms of quantity and quality is essential in order to meet the increased demands of pubertal growth and development and achieve optimal physical, cognitive and mental health [3]. Furthermore, as dietary habits and diet-related behaviors are formed and established during this period, adolescence offers a unique opportunity to develop and promote healthy dietary habits and behaviors [4]. Family and peers, school, mass media and advertising, as well as the socio-economic and cultural environment are among the contributing factors in the formation of diet-related behaviors and food choices [5].

Skipping breakfast, snacking in front of a screen, eating in fast-food restaurants and eating infrequently with the family are, in general, highly prevalent behaviors among adolescents and have been linked to both unhealthy diets and adverse health outcomes [6–14]. Skipping breakfast has been associated with excess adiposity, worse blood lipid profile and blood pressure levels, insulin-resistance and metabolic syndrome, whereas regular breakfast consumption has been associated with better diet quality and improved cognitive and academic performance among school-aged children and adolescents [6,8–10]. Excessive time spent in front of a screen (e.g., smartphones, tablets, computers and TV) has been associated with increased intake of sugar-sweetened beverages, fast-foods, sweets and salty snacks as well as higher total energy intake and higher risk of childhood obesity [7]. Regular fast-food consumption has been associated with regular consumption of sweets/candies and sugar-sweetened beverages, as well as higher total energy intake and poorer diet quality [11–13]. On the other hand, having frequent family meals has been associated with consumption of healthy food groups and better diet quality [14–16].

Existing data on the prevalence of the above-mentioned diet-related behaviors among children and adolescents in Greece are relatively old, while research has focused more on associations with obesity and relevant biomarkers and less on associations with dietary factors or diet quality [17–21]. Findings based on the most recent study conducted during 2015 among 177,091 students aged 8–17 years living in Greece revealed that skipping breakfast reached 22.4% and 23.1% among boys and girls, respectively, and was associated with poor diet as assessed by the Mediterranean Diet Quality Index for children and adolescents [17]. In the same study, 23.0% of boys and 16.0% of girls reported consuming fast-foods more than once/week, whereas frequent fast-food consumption was strongly correlated with unhealthy dietary habits such as consuming sweets/candy regularly [19]. Furthermore, increased screen time was also associated with lower adherence to the Mediterranean diet [20].

Based on the above, the aim of this study was to provide more recent data on the prevalence of important diet-related behaviors, in particular eating breakfast, eating with the family, snacking or having a meal in front of the TV or a screen and eating in fast-food restaurants, in a representative sample of school-aged adolescents living in Greece and to explore further how these behaviors are linked to consumption of key food groups and beverages for adolescent diet, such as vegetables, fruits, sweets and sugar-sweetened beverages, incorporated in an index that could partly reflect the quality of their diet. We hypothesized that specific diet-related behaviors would be associated with less favorable dietary choices and poorer diet quality, as expressed by the above index, among adolescents.

2. Material and Methods

2.1. Study Population

Data on eating habits were derived from the 2018 Greek arm of the international Health Behaviour in School-aged Children (HBSC) study [22], a nationally representative survey of 11, 13 and 15-year-old students conducted by the University Mental Health, Neurosciences and Precision Medicine Research Institute quadrennially since 1998. The survey received ethical approval from the Ministry of Education. The study protocol required active parental consent. Prior to survey administration students were informed orally that their participation was voluntary and that they could opt out of filling the survey.

Trained assistants group-administered anonymous questionnaires to 6th, 8th and 10th grade students in the classroom during two consecutive regular class periods. In line with HBSC's study protocol, a multistage stratified random cluster sampling procedure with the school class as the sampling unit was employed to secure the nationwide sample of students in each year. Stratification was based on (a) administrative region (Nomenclature for territorial units of statistics, 2nd level in the European Union's classification) (10 out of Greece's 13 regions, excluding the Ionian and North and South Aegean islands for logistical reasons) and (b) school type (comprehensive/technical/private).

The response rate of schools was 93%, while the response rate of students from participating schools was 87%; about 6% of the registered students were absent on the day of administration and 7% of students who were present refused (their parents or themselves) to fill in the questionnaire. Excluding about 8% of the filled-in student questionnaires due to a high proportion of missing values or being outside the age limits imposed by the HBSC survey methodology, the final number of students was 3863 (50.1% girls), of whom 32.0% were 11 years old, 34.0% 13 years old and 34.1% 15 years old, from 238 schools.

2.2. *Food Consumption and Construction of a Diet Quality Score*

A standardized questionnaire with core and optional questions used across the HBSC participating countries included a section for recording food consumption. Specifically, students were asked to assess their frequency of consumption during a typical week for the following food groups and beverages: (a) fruits, (b) vegetables/salads, (c) sweets (including chocolates and candies), (d) sugar-sweetened beverages, (e) coffee, and (f) energy drinks (the last two being national items). The available responses were seven ranging from "never" to "more than once a day, every day".

We further combined the information on the consumption of four food groups/items: vegetables/salads, fruits, sweets and sugar-sweetened beverages, to construct a diet quality score, which has the simplicity of expressing several dietary exposures through one variable. The rational of the specific diet score was based on the food-based dietary recommendations included in the Greek National Dietary Guidelines for children and adolescents [23]. Thus, for groups/items that are recommended as part of a healthy everyday diet and in particular vegetables/salads and fruits, the scoring took the values of 0–4, with higher values depicting more frequent consumption (in days/week) and better diet quality as follows: (i) ≤1 day/week = 0; (ii) 2–4 days/week = 1; (iii) 5–6 days/week = 2; (iv) 7 days/week = 3 and (v) >once/day = 4. For food groups/items that are not recommended as part of a healthy everyday diet, that is consumption of sweets and sugar-sweetened beverages, the scoring took the values of 0–4, with higher values depicting less frequent consumption and better diet quality as follows: (i) ≤1 day/week = 4; (ii) 2–4 days/week = 3; (iii) 5–6 days/week = 2; (iv) 7 days/week = 1; (v) >once/day = 0. The total score could take values from 0 to 16, where zero corresponds to the worst possible combination of the four food groups/items, and thus the worst diet quality (i.e., once a week or less often consumption of fruits and vegetables/salads and more than once daily sweets and sugar-sweetened beverages) and 16 corresponds to the best possible combination and the best diet quality (i.e., once a week or less often consumption of sweets and sugar-sweetened beverages and more than once daily consumption of fruits and vegetables/salads). Thus, the higher the diet score, the better the quality of the diet.

2.3. *Diet-Related Behaviors*

Students were also asked to report their frequency of adopting the following diet-related behaviors: (a) eating snacks while watching TV (or DVD/video), (b) eating snacks while sitting in front of a screen for homework or games, (c) eating meals while watching TV, (d) eating in fast-food restaurants, (e) eating meals with their family and (f) eating breakfast, defined as more than a glass of milk or fruit juice (asked separately for schooldays and weekends). The available responses with respect to the first three questions (eating snacks/meals while in front of TV/screen) were six ranging from "never" to "every day". The available responses with respect to eating with the family were five, ranging from "every day" to "never" and with respect to eating in fast-food restaurants were seven, ranging from "never" to "five or more days/week". For breakfast, the question about the schooldays was used for this analysis with six available responses (from "never" to "all five days"). The reported responses were further grouped into fewer categories.

2.4. *Other Covariates*

Socio-demographic characteristics were recorded. Students were asked to report the year and month they were born and age groups were computed. They further reported their gender and their country of birth, including those of each of their parents. A family affluence scale (FAS) score was computed using a six-item assessment of common material assets or activities; responses were scored and summed to form an HBSC FAS summary score, which was then used to identify groups of young people in the lowest 20% (low affluence), middle 60% (medium affluence) and highest 20% (high affluence) [24].

With respect to physical activity, students were asked to report the number of days over the past week during which they were physically active for a total of at least 60 minutes. Physical activity was defined as any activity that increases the heart rate and makes the person get out of breath some of the time, with examples provided. There were eight response options, ranging from "none" to "7 days". Height in centimeters (without shoes) and weight in kilograms (without clothes) were self-reported and body mass index (BMI) was calculated as the ratio of weight in kilograms divided by the square of height in meters (kg/m^2).

2.5. *Statistical Analysis*

Participants' data were summarized by mean and standard deviation or median and interquartile range for continuous variables, and by frequencies and percentages for categorical variables. For continuous variables, differences between boys and girls (in total and by age group) were assessed via two-sample *t*-test and differences between age groups via one-way ANOVA. For categorical variables, relevant differences were assessed by Pearson's chi-square test.

The diet quality score was used as a categorical variable divided into three categories: good, moderate and poor. These categories corresponded to the dietary score's distribution tertiles as follows: poor: 0–9, moderate: 10–12 and good: 13–16.

In order to assess the association of diet quality score with diet-related behaviors ordinal logistic regression was applied. Unadjusted and adjusted odds ratios (OR) (obtained from univariable and multivariable regression analyses, respectively) and their 95% confidence intervals (CI) were computed using as reference category the good diet quality category. This was decided in order to identify behaviors associated with increased odds of not having a good diet quality score, as more easily interpretable and transferable to public health messages. In all models, standard errors were computed allowing for intragroup correlation (Clustered Sandwich Estimator) since non-independence of participants resulting from cluster sampling was suspected. Additional variables included in the final multivariable ordinal logistic regression model were gender, age group, and physical activity in the past 7 days (number of days), as well as place of birth, and family affluence which had been found to be associated (with $p < 0.20$) with diet quality in the univariable analyses. To further evaluate whether the association varied by gender we stratified the final multivariable analysis by gender. In order to assess the possible influence of BMI in our final multivariable model, we also ran an analysis on the sample of 3386 students with available data on BMI. All statistical analyses were conducted using STATA v13.1 (STATA Corporation, College Station, TX, USA).

3. Results

From the initial sample of 3863 school-aged adolescents who participated in the 2018 survey, 338 were excluded due to missing values in one or more variables of interest. Thus, the final sample consisted of 3525 adolescents, 1708 boys and 1817 girls, evenly distributed across predefined age groups (Table 1). Half of the participants came from the two prefectures where the largest cities of Greece are situated (37.7% from Attica where Athens/Piraeus is located, 14.7% from Thessaloniki prefecture where Thessaloniki is located). The vast majority (96.6%) were born in Greece, while more than 80% had both parents of Greek origin.

Table 1. Socio-demographic and baseline characteristics of 3525 participants in the 2018 Greek arm of the Health Behaviour of School-Aged Children Study.

Characteristics	*n* (%)
Gender	
Boys	1708 (48.5)
Girls	1817 (51.5)
Age group	
11-year olds	1085 (30.8)
13-year olds	1220 (34.6)
15-year olds	1220 (34.6)
Grade	
6th	1106 (31.4)
8th	1228 (34.8)
10th	1191 (33.8)
Region/municipality	
Attica	1328 (37.7)
Thessaloniki	519 (14.7)
Other	1678 (47.6)
Place of birth	
Greece	3404 (96.6)
Other	121 (3.4)
Mother's place of birth [a]	
Greece	2817 (80.2)
Other	694 (19.8)
Father's place of birth [a]	
Greece	2940 (83.8)
Other	568 (16.2)
Body mass index [b], kg/m^2, mean (sd)	20.3 (3.5)
Physical activity in the past 7 days, days, mean (sd)	4.0 (2.0)
Family affluence scale (FAS) score [c]	
Low 20% affluent	504 (14.3)
Middle 60% affluent	2258 (64.1)
High 20% affluent	763 (21.6)

Abbreviation: standard deviation (sd). [a] Number of students does not add up to 3525, due to missing values. [b] Available data for 3386 students. [c] Quantiles were calculated based on FAS score distribution of FAS score by gender and age group.

In Table 2, diet-related and lifestyle behaviors are presented in the total sample and by gender in the total sample and among 11-, 13- and 15-years old samples. More than half of the sample (52.5%) had breakfast almost every weekday, but 32.9% had it just one weekday or less often. The frequency of eating breakfast on weekdays differed by gender in the total sample ($p = 0.001$) and among the 15-year old sample ($p = 0.006$), with girls skipping breakfast (defined here as eating breakfast ≤1 day/week) more often than boys (34.6% vs. 31.1% in the total sample, 34.7% vs. 29.1% among the 15-year old sample). Eating with the family almost every day was a frequent habit reaching 79.8% for the total sample, 82.0% for boys and 77.7% for girls. The frequency of eating with the family differed significantly by gender among the total population ($p = 0.001$) and among the 13-year old ($p = 0.007$) and 15-year old students ($p = 0.001$), with fewer girls eating almost every day with their family compared to boys (75.0% vs. 81.4% in the 13-year olds and 72.7% vs. 80.8% in the 15-year olds).

Table 2. Diet-related and lifestyle behaviors and characteristics of 3525 participants in the 2018 Greek arm of the Health Behaviour of School-Aged Children Study for the total sample and by age group and gender.

Behaviors Characteristics	Total	All Ages (n = 3525)			11-Year Olds (n = 1085)			13-Year Olds (n = 1220)			15-Year Olds (n = 1220)		
		Boys (n = 1708)	Girls (n = 1817)	p-Value +	Boys (n = 523)	Girls (n = 562)	p-Value +	Boys (n = 591)	Girls (n = 629)	p-Value +	Boys (n = 594)	Girls (n = 626)	p-Value +
Eating breakfast on weekdays, days/week, n (%)				0.001			0.306			0.197			0.006
≤1	1160 (32.9)	531 (31.1)	629 (34.6)		167 (31.9)	187 (33.3)		191 (32.3)	225 (35.8)		173 (29.1)	217 (34.7)	
2–3	516 (14.6)	227 (13.3)	289 (15.9)		59 (11.3)	78 (13.9)		82 (13.9)	98 (15.6)		86 (14.5)	113 (18.1)	
4–5	1849 (52.5)	950 (55.6)	899 (49.5)		297 (56.8)	297 (52.8)		318 (53.8)	306 (48.6)		335 (56.4)	296 (47.3)	
Eating with family, n (%)				0.001			0.357			0.007			0.001
Rarely	713 (20.2)	307 (18.0)	406 (22.3)		83 (15.9)	78 (13.9)		110 (18.6)	157 (25.0)		114 (19.2)	171 (27.3)	
Almost everyday	2812 (79.8)	1401 (82.0)	1411 (77.7)		440 (84.1)	484 (86.1)		481 (81.4)	472 (75.0)		480 (80.8)	455 (72.7)	
Eating snacks while watching TV, days/week, n (%)				0.050			0.604			0.056			0.361
<1	1214 (34.4)	580 (34.0)	634 (34.9)		158 (30.2)	183 (32.6)		208 (35.2)	215 (34.2)		214 (36.0)	236 (37.7)	
1–2	948 (26.9)	434 (25.4)	514 (28.3)		140 (26.8)	144 (25.6)		136 (23.0)	185 (29.4)		158 (26.6)	185 (29.6)	
3–4	598 (17.0)	316 (18.5)	282 (15.5)		104 (19.9)	97 (17.3)		108 (18.3)	93 (14.8)		104 (17.5)	92 (14.7)	
≥5	765 (21.7)	378 (22.1)	387 (21.3)		121 (23.1)	138 (24.6)		139 (23.5)	136 (21.6)		118 (19.9)	113 (18.1)	
Eating snacks in front of PC/tablet/laptop, days/week, n (%)				<0.001			<0.001			<0.001			<0.001
<1	1219 (34.6)	479 (28)	740 (40.7)		152 (29.1)	239 (42.5)		162 (27.4)	246 (39.1)		165 (27.8)	255 (40.7)	
1–2	661 (18.8)	292 (17.1)	369 (20.3)		105 (20.1)	126 (22.4)		94 (15.9)	114 (18.1)		93 (15.7)	129 (20.6)	
3–4	527 (15.0)	292 (17.1)	235 (12.9)		96 (18.4)	76 (13.5)		93 (15.7)	70 (11.1)		103 (17.3)	89 (14.2)	
≥5	1118 (31.7)	645 (37.8)	473 (26.0)		170 (32.5)	121 (21.5)		242 (40.9)	199 (31.6)		233 (39.2)	153 (24.4)	
Eating meals while watching TV, days/week, n (%)				0.155			0.915			0.271			0.601
<1	1288 (36.5)	594 (34.8)	694 (38.2)		185 (35.4)	208 (37.0)		197 (33.3)	239 (38.0)		212 (35.7)	247 (39.5)	
1–2	754 (21.4)	383 (22.4)	371 (20.4)		133 (25.4)	135 (24.0)		139 (23.5)	126 (20.0)		111 (18.7)	110 (17.6)	
3–4	563 (16.0)	272 (15.9)	291 (16.0)		84 (16.1)	93 (16.5)		94 (15.9)	103 (16.4)		94 (15.8)	95 (15.2)	
≥5	920 (26.1)	459 (26.9)	461 (25.4)		121 (23.1)	126 (22.4)		161 (27.2)	161 (25.6)		177 (29.8)	174 (27.8)	

Table 2. *Cont.*

Behaviors Characteristics	Total	All Ages ($n = 3525$)			11-Year Olds ($n = 1085$)			13-Year Olds ($n = 1220$)			15-Year Olds ($n = 1220$)		
		Boys ($n = 1708$)	Girls ($n = 1817$)	p-Value [+]	Boys ($n = 523$)	Girls ($n = 562$)	p-Value [+]	Boys ($n = 591$)	Girls ($n = 629$)	p-Value [+]	Boys ($n = 594$)	Girls ($n = 626$)	p-Value [+]
Eating in fast-food restaurants, n (%)				<0.001			0.448			0.049			<0.001
Rarely	1171 (33.2)	547 (32.0)	624 (34.3)		225 (43.0)	250 (44.5)		175 (29.6)	199 (31.6)		147 (24.7)	175 (28)	
1–3 days per month	1505 (42.7)	693 (40.6)	812 (44.7)		216 (41.3)	242 (43.1)		261 (44.2)	284 (45.2)		216 (36.4)	286 (45.7)	
Once per week	617 (17.5)	320 (18.7)	297 (16.3)		60 (11.5)	54 (9.6)		107 (18.1)	119 (18.9)		153 (25.8)	124 (19.8)	
At least twice per week	232 (6.6)	148 (8.7)	84 (4.6)		22 (4.2)	16 (2.8)		48 (8.1)	27 (4.3)		78 (13.1)	41 (6.5)	
Family affluence scale (FAS) score [a], n (%)				0.228			0.737			0.398			0.211
Least (20%) affluent	504 (14.3)	245 (14.3)	259 (14.3)		71 (13.6)	83 (14.8)		95 (16.1)	87 (13.8)		79 (13.3)	89 (14.2)	
Middle (60%) affluent	2258 (64.1)	1073 (62.8)	1185 (65.2)		325 (62.1)	352 (62.6)		357 (60.4)	402 (63.9)		391 (65.8)	431 (68.8)	
Highest (20%) affluent	763 (21.6)	390 (22.8)	373 (20.5)		127 (24.3)	127 (22.6)		139 (23.5)	140 (22.3)		124 (20.9)	106 (16.9)	
Physical activity in the past 7 days, days, mean (sd)	4.0 (2.0)	4.3 (2.0)	3.7 (2.0)	<0.001	4.6 (2.0)	4.3 (1.8)	0.005	4.4 (2.0)	3.6 (2.0)	<0.001	4.0 (2.1)	3.4 (2.0)	<0.001

Abbreviation: standard deviation (sd). [a] Quantiles were calculated based on FAS score distribution of FAS score by gender and age group. [+] p-values from Pearson's X^2-test for categorical variables and two-sample t-test for continuous variables.

A total of 26.1% of the adolescents ate a meal and a total of 21.7% ate a snack almost every day while watching TV. Almost one-third (31.7%) of the sample reported eating snacks in front of a PC/tablet/laptop 5 or more days per week, with boys reporting this behavior in higher percentages than girls in all age groups. Eating in fast-food restaurants at least twice per week was reported by 6.6% of the total sample, with more boys than girls in all age groups except for the 11-year olds ($p = 0.448$). Physical activity in the past 7 days was also higher among boys compared to girls in the total population and across the age groups.

When differences between the age groups were studied, eating rarely with the family, eating in fast-food restaurants at least once per week and eating meals while watching TV almost every day were all more prevalent among the 15-year-olds compared to the other two younger groups (Supplementary Table S1). Eating frequently snacks in front of a PC/tablet was more prevalent among the 13-year olds whereas eating frequently snacks while watching TV more prevalent among the 11-year olds. Skipping breakfast did not differ across the age-groups. The 15-year olds had lower physical activity levels in comparison to 11- and 13-year olds (Supplementary Table S1).

In Table 3, frequency of consumption of specific food items, components of the diet quality score, as well as the diet quality score in the whole population, and by gender among 11-, 13- and 15-year olds is presented. The majority of the total population did not consume fruits (69.3%) or vegetables (66.3%) every day and boys reported eating fruits and vegetables less often compared to girls ($p = 0.001$). With respect to consumption of sweets and sugar-sweetened beverages, daily consumption reached 15.3% for sweets and 5.7% for the sugar-sweetened beverages, in the total population. More girls than boys reported frequent consumption of sweets, although only in the 15-year old group ($p = 0.025$), whereas boys consumed more sugar-sweetened beverages than girls in all age-groups. Overall, 17.9% of the population was classified in the good diet quality category, 39.4% in the moderate and 42.7% in the poor diet quality category. Girls had a statistically significantly better diet quality than boys in all age groups. When differences between the age groups were studied, consumption of fruits and vegetables was lower and consumption of sweets and sugar-sweetened beverages was higher in the 13- and 15-year old age groups compared to the 11-year olds. Consequently, the 15-year-old adolescents had worse diet quality compared to the younger age groups ($p < 0.001$) (Supplementary Table S2).

In Table 4 odds ratios and 95% confidence intervals, derived from the multivariable ordinal logistic regression, assessing the association of diet-related behaviors and other characteristics with diet quality score (using the good diet quality as a reference), are presented.

Table 3. Frequency of consumption of specific food items, mean diet quality score and categories of diet quality score of 3525 participants in the 2018 Greek arm of the Health Behaviour of School-Aged Children Study for the total sample and by age group and gender.

Food Items/Diet Quality Score	Total	All Ages (n = 3525)			11-Year Olds (n = 1085)			13-Year Olds (n = 1220)			15-Year Olds (n = 1220)		
		Boys (n = 1708)	Girls (n = 1817)	p-Value +	Boys (n = 523)	Girls (n = 562)	p-Value +	Boys (n = 591)	Girls (n = 629)	p-Value +	Boys (n = 594)	Girls (n = 626)	p-Value +
Fruits intake, days/week, n (%)				0.001			0.779			0.006			0.023
≤1	690 (19.6)	317 (18.6)	373 (20.5)		73 (14.0)	83 (14.8)		110 (18.6)	134 (21.3)		134 (22.6)	156 (24.9)	
2–4	1186 (33.6)	595 (34.8)	591 (32.5)		161 (30.8)	157 (27.9)		211 (35.7)	211 (33.5)		223 (37.5)	223 (35.6)	
5–6	566 (16.1)	307 (18.0)	259 (14.3)		90 (17.2)	98 (17.4)		111 (18.8)	76 (12.1)		106 (17.8)	85 (13.6)	
7	679 (19.3)	294 (17.2)	385 (21.2)		114 (21.8)	137 (24.4)		112 (19.0)	143 (22.7)		68 (11.4)	105 (16.8)	
>once daily	404 (11.5)	195 (11.4)	209 (11.5)		85 (16.3)	87 (15.5)		47 (8.0)	65 (10.3)		63 (10.6)	57 (9.1)	
Vegetables intake, days/week, n (%)				<0.001			0.049			0.001			0.226
≤1	679 (19.3)	377 (22.1)	302 (16.6)		129 (24.7)	99 (17.6)		124 (21.0)	96 (15.3)		124 (20.9)	107 (17.1)	
2–4	913 (25.9)	459 (26.9)	454 (25.0)		119 (22.8)	128 (22.8)		163 (27.6)	155 (24.6)		177 (29.8)	171 (27.3)	
5–6	743 (21.1)	358 (21.0)	385 (21.2)		95 (18.2)	106 (18.9)		135 (22.8)	126 (20.0)		128 (21.5)	153 (24.4)	
7	813 (23.1)	353 (20.7)	460 (25.3)		122 (23.3)	160 (28.5)		119 (20.1)	174 (27.7)		112 (18.9)	126 (20.1)	
>once daily	377 (10.7)	161 (9.4)	216 (11.9)		58 (11.1)	69 (12.3)		50 (8.5)	78 (12.4)		53 (8.9)	69 (11.0)	
Sweets intake, days/week, n (%)				0.086			0.428			0.155			0.025
≤1	1350 (38.3)	667 (39.1)	683 (37.6)		249 (47.6)	274 (48.8)		219 (37.1)	220 (35.0)		199 (33.5)	189 (30.2)	
2–4	1178 (33.4)	564 (33.0)	614 (33.8)		167 (31.9)	164 (29.2)		191 (32.3)	210 (33.4)		206 (34.7)	240 (38.3)	
5–6	455 (12.9)	234 (13.7)	221 (12.2)		41 (7.8)	61 (10.9)		93 (15.7)	79 (12.6)		100 (16.8)	81 (12.9)	
7	319 (9.0)	133 (7.8)	186 (10.2)		41 (7.8)	40 (7.1)		47 (8.0)	72 (11.4)		45 (7.6)	74 (11.8)	
>once daily	223 (6.3)	110 (6.4)	113 (6.2)		25 (4.8)	23 (4.1)		41 (6.9)	48 (7.6)		44 (7.4)	42 (6.7)	
Sugar-sweetened beverage intake, days/week, n (%)				<0.001			0.009			<0.001			<0.001
≤1	2477 (70.3)	1078 (63.1)	1399 (77.0)		394 (75.3)	470 (83.6)		355 (60.1)	455 (72.3)		329 (55.4)	474 (75.7)	
2–4	679 (19.3)	416 (24.4)	263 (14.5)		81 (15.5)	55 (9.8)		160 (27.1)	106 (16.9)		175 (29.5)	102 (16.3)	
5–6	168 (4.8)	104 (6.1)	64 (3.5)		25 (4.8)	14 (2.5)		30 (5.1)	30 (4.8)		49 (8.2)	20 (3.2)	
7	111 (3.1)	60 (3.5)	51 (2.8)		13 (2.5)	12 (2.1)		28 (4.7)	23 (3.7)		19 (3.2)	16 (2.6)	
>once daily	90 (2.6)	50 (2.9)	40 (2.2)		10 (1.9)	11 (2.0)		18 (3.0)	15 (2.4)		22 (3.7)	14 (2.2)	
Diet quality score [a], mean (sd)	9.9 (2.9)	9.7 (2.8)	10.1 (2.9)	<0.001	10.4 (2.7)	10.7 (2.7)	0.026	9.5 (2.8)	9.9 (2.8)	0.007	9.2 (2.9)	9.6 (3.0)	0.016
Diet quality groups [b], n (%)				<0.001			0.014			0.007			0.018
Poor	1504 (42.7)	773 (45.3)	731 (40.2)		184 (35.2)	176 (31.3)		262 (44.3)	261 (41.5)		327 (55.1)	294 (47.0)	
Moderate	1389 (39.4)	676 (39.6)	713 (39.2)		230 (44.0)	226 (40.2)		260 (44.0)	254 (40.4)		186 (31.3)	233 (37.2)	
Good	632 (17.9)	259 (15.2)	373 (20.5)		109 (20.8)	160 (28.5)		69 (11.7)	114 (18.1)		81 (13.6)	99 (15.8)	

Abbreviation: standard deviation (sd). [a] Values range from 0 to 16. Zero corresponds to the worst possible diet quality score (once a week or less often fruits and vegetables/salads and more than once daily sweets and sugar-sweetened beverages) and 16 to the best possible diet quality score (once a week or less often sweets and sugar-sweetened beverages and more than once daily fruits and vegetables/salads). [b] Calculated using dietary score's tertiles. Poor includes dietary scores from 0 to 9, moderate includes scores from 10 to 12 and good includes scores from 13 to 16. + p-values from Pearson's X^2-test for categorical variables and two-sample t-test for continuous variables.

Table 4. Adjusted odds ratios (OR) and associated 95% confidence intervals (CI) from multivariable ordinal logistic regression model for the association between diet-related behaviors and other characteristics and diet quality score † among 3525 participants in the 2018 Greek arm of the Health Behaviour of School-Aged Children Study.

Behaviors/Characteristics	**Diet Quality Score †**	
	OR (95% CI)	***p*-Value**
Gender		
Boys	1.37 (1.20–1.56)	<0.001
Girls	Ref.	
Age group		
11-year olds	Ref.	
13-year olds	1.31 (1.10–1.55)	0.002
15-year olds	1.53 (1.27–1.83)	<0.001
Place of birth		
Greece	Ref.	
Other	1.32 (0.90–1.93)	0.159
Physical activity in the past 7 days, days	0.80 (0.77–0.83)	<0.001
Eating breakfast on weekdays, days/week		
≤1	1.56 (1.34–1.82)	<0.001
2–3	1.17 (0.97–1.42)	0.108
4–5	Ref.	
Eating with family		
Rarely	1.35 (1.13–1.60)	0.001
Almost everyday	Ref.	
Eating snacks while watching TV, days/week		
<1	Ref.	
1–2	1.24 (1.03–1.50)	0.022
3–4	1.45 (1.18–1.78)	<0.001
≥5	1.42 (1.14–1.75)	0.001
Eating snacks in front of PC/laptop/tablet, days/week		
<1	Ref.	
1–2	1.15 (0.96–1.38)	0.136
3–4	1.48 (1.19–1.83)	<0.001
≥5	1.85 (1.55–2.21)	<0.001
Eating meals while watching TV, days/week		
<1	Ref.	
1–2	1.14 (0.96–1.35)	0.136
3–4	1.47 (1.19–1.80)	<0.001
≥5	1.45 (1.21–1.75)	<0.001
Eating in fast-food restaurants		
Rarely	Ref.	
1–3 days per month	1.52 (1.30–1.78)	<0.001
Once per week	2.16 (1.74–2.70)	<0.001
At least twice per week	4.59 (3.14–6.70)	<0.001
Family affluence scale (FAS) score [a]		
Least affluent 20%	Ref.	
Middle affluent 60%	0.84 (0.70–1.00)	0.056
Highest affluent 20%	0.65 (0.53–0.80)	<0.001

Abbreviation: Reference (Ref.); Odd Ratio (OR); Confidence Interval (CI). [a] Quantiles calculated based on FAS score distribution of FAS score by gender and age group. † Diet quality score (ranging from 0 to 16) is the outcome variable which is divided into three categories: good, moderate and poor. These categories are dietary score's tertiles calculated as follows; poor: dietary score from 0 to 9, moderate: dietary scores from 10 to 12, good: dietary scores from 13 to 16. Good diet quality category is the reference category in order to identify behaviors associated with increased odds of not having a good diet quality score.

Boys had 37% higher odds of having moderate or poor diet quality compared to girls (OR:1.37, 95% CI: 1.20–1.56) and the 15-year olds had 53% higher odds of having moderate or poor diet quality compared to the 11-year olds (OR:1.53, 95% CI: 1.27–1.83). Having breakfast once or less often during the weekdays compared to almost every weekday was associated with 56% higher odds of having worse diet quality (≤1 day/weekdays vs. 4–5 days, OR:1.56, 95% CI: 1.34–1.82). Similarly, eating rarely with the family compared to almost every day, was associated with higher odds of having worse diet quality (OR: 1.35, 95% CI: 1.13–1.60). The frequency of eating snacks or meals while watching TV was positively associated with poorer diet quality, as well as eating snacks in front of a PC, tablet or laptop. Eating in fast-food restaurants 1–3 days per month was associated with higher odds of having a moderate or poor diet quality compared to eating rarely. Notably, adolescents eating in fast-food restaurants at least twice per week had almost 4.6 times higher odds of exhibiting a moderate or poor diet quality compared to those eating rarely in fast food restaurants (OR: 4.59, 95% CI: 3.14–6.70). When data were stratified by gender, eating rarely with the family and eating snacks while watching TV were associated with worse diet quality only among girls (Supplementary Table S3). All other associations remained significant in boys and girls, whereas eating in fast-food restaurants was associated with much higher odds of having a worse diet quality (OR: 8.12, 95% CI: 4.34–15.18) in girls compared to boys (OR: 3.41, 95% CI: 2.15–5.41). The results from the multivariable analysis for the association between diet-related behaviors and other characteristics and diet quality score after including BMI in the model were practically identical (Supplementary Table S4).

4. Discussion

In this large sample of school-aged adolescents living in Greece, relatively high proportions, ranging from 20.2% to 32.9%, were regularly skipping breakfast, were frequently eating in front of a screen and in fast-food restaurants, and rarely eating with the family. Differences between boys and girls and across the age-groups were evident in some of the studied diet-related behaviors. Skipping breakfast, eating frequently in front of a screen and in fast-food restaurants, and eating rarely with the family were all independently associated with worse diet quality, assessed by a diet score incorporating frequency of fruit, vegetables, sweets and sugar-sweetened beverages consumption. Associations remain unchanged after controlling for important possible confounders such as physical activity, family affluence and body mass index.

Almost one-third of this sample, more girls than boys, had breakfast only once, or less often, during the week. Skipping breakfast is a frequent finding in similar studies conducted in Greece and around the world [8,17,18]. In a systematic review collecting data from 286,804 children and adolescents living in 33 countries during 2008–2018, most studies reported that at least 10–30% of children and adolescents never eat breakfast, with an increasing trend in adolescents and mostly in girls [8]. The main reasons that have been proposed are the lack of time and not feeling hungry in the morning, as well as the effort to control body weight, the latter especially among girls. It should be noted that skipping breakfast has been defined differently across the studies, an issue that adds complexity to the comparisons among studies and the interpretation of the results. In this study, adolescents skipping regular breakfast consumption (defined as eating something more than one glass of milk or juice in the morning), had worse diet quality in comparison to those eating regularly breakfast during the week. There is consistent evidence that breakfast forms an integral part of a healthy diet that positively impacts health and well-being in children [6,8–10,25,26] and in adults [27]. In a cross-sectional study from Belgium with 341 adolescents 13–18 years old, consumers of a good-quality breakfast had a better overall dietary pattern, both on a nutrient and food group level, in comparison to consumers of a low-quality breakfast [25]. In a representative sample of 4200 children, 2–18 years old, from the National Health and Nutrition Examination Survey in US during 2001–2008, consumers of most breakfast patterns had higher intakes of key nutrients (dietary fiber, vitamin D, calcium and potassium), as well as better diet quality indexes compared to breakfast skippers [26]. The importance of consuming a healthy breakfast every day is stressed in the Greek National Dietary Guidelines for infants, children and adolescents established in 2014 [23]. According to these guidelines, breakfast comprises one of the most important meals of the day and children are recommended to consume foods from the following three food groups at minimum: dairy products, cereals (preferably whole grain) and fruits or vegetables.

In this study, a relatively high proportion of adolescents (26.1%) had a meal while watching TV and 31.7%, more boys than girls, had a snack in front of a screen, five or more days per week. Furthermore, frequency of eating snacks in front of a screen (PC, tablet or laptop) or meals while watching TV was positively associated with poorer diet quality. In the context of the Greek arm of the HBSC study conducted 20 years ago (1997–1998), in a sample of 4211 students, TV viewing was positively associated with consumption of sodas, crisps, cakes, pastries, sweets and chocolates at least once a day, but negatively associated with consumption of fruits [21]. Other studies have also reported an association between high screen time and less healthy dietary patterns, such as less fruit and vegetable consumption and greater consumption of energy-dense snacks and sugar-sweetened beverages in all age groups [28–30].

Frequency of eating in fast-food restaurants at least once a week among this study sample was high (24.1%), with more boys than girls and more 15-year olds reporting this behavior. Furthermore, eating frequently in fast-food restaurants was the behavior with the highest odds of having poor diet quality, especially among girls, compared to other studied behaviors. Previous studies investigating fast-food consumption in relation to diet quality among adolescents in Greece, and elsewhere, have reported similar associations [11–13,19]. In most studies, fast-food consumption has been associated with higher availability and intake of sugar-sweetened beverages and French fries and lower intake of milk, fruit and vegetables, as well as a lower likelihood of being served vegetables or milk with home meals [13]. Consumption of fast-foods may also be a surrogate marker for other unhealthy behaviors associated with poor diet quality and dietary choices [31].

A high proportion of participants in this sample, reaching 80%, had a family meal almost every day, while 20% rarely had a family meal. Eating rarely with the family was associated with worse diet quality, a consistent finding across similar studies [14–16]. The healthier food choices associated with eating with the family are possibly due to the consumption of higher quality of foods, as well as increased opportunity to have family discussions about healthy eating and dietary choices [32]. A large proportion of the adolescents in this sample, more than 60%, did not adhere to the daily consumption of fruits and vegetables recommended by the Greek food-based dietary guidelines for children and adolescents. According to these guidelines, consumption of a variety of fruits and vegetables several times per day in every main meal is recommended [23]. Frequent fruit and vegetable consumption is essential during childhood and beyond, contributing to optimal diet and nutritional status, lowering risk of chronic diseases and promoting long-term health [33]. On the other hand, the proportion of adolescents who reported daily consumption of sweets and sugar-sweetened beverages was not negligible. Consumption of added sugars, including sweetened beverages and soft drinks, is associated with an increased risk of dental caries and childhood overweight/obesity. According to the national guidelines for children and adolescents, sweets should be consumed in moderation and during special occasions, whereas sugar-sweetened beverages should be avoided [23]. Based on the diet quality index and its three categories constructed by us, the majority of adolescents (82.0%) were classified in the moderate and poor diet quality categories with girls scoring better than boys in the younger age groups. Older adolescents had a worse diet quality compared to their younger counterparts. In the previous analysis of the Greek segment of the HBSC study in 1997–1998, similar results were found with respect to diet quality [21]. Girls had better diet quality compared to boys and older age was positively correlated with poor diet quality. Nevertheless, the diet quality index used in that study was defined differently, with more food groups available to combine in the index.

Our study has several limitations. First, the cross-sectional design of the study did not allow inference of causal associations between diet-related behaviors and diet quality. Second, information about diet was assessed through a non-quantitative food frequency questionnaire, which formed part of the HSBC questionnaire, with a limited number of food items, not allowing a comprehensive study of diet, both in terms of quantity as well as in terms of quality. In that respect, we could not use any of the existing validated diet quality scores for children and adolescents, and instead, we have tried to construct a diet quality score to capture adherence to a healthy dietary pattern combining in one variable, the frequent consumption of fruit and vegetables and the less frequent consumption of sweets and sugar-sweetened beverages. Nevertheless, this diet quality score was neither an established, nor a validated diet quality index and it was based on a limited number of items. All information collected was self-reported by adolescents, introducing a degree of information bias into the study. Residual confounding is also possible since variables that have not been collected or not adequately measured, were not accounted for in the analysis. On the other hand, advantages of our study are the large sample size, the standardized methodology in the context of an established multinational survey allowing comparisons to other participating countries, and the random sampling allowing generalizing our findings to the adolescent population in Greece. Furthermore, data were collected during 2018, making findings deriving from this analysis quite current.

In conclusion, we found evidence that specific diet-related behaviors such as skipping breakfast, eating meals/snacks in front of a screen, eating in fast-food restaurants and eating infrequently with the family were quite prevalent in a representative sample of school-aged adolescents living in Greece and that all these behaviors were associated with less favorable diet quality. Modifying or preventing the establishment of these behaviors during childhood and adolescence through the implementation of targeted, multifaceted health promotion and education initiatives may lead to healthier dietary choices and better diet quality.

Author Contributions: Conceptualization, V.B., A.F. and A.K. (Anna Kokkevi); formal analysis, A.K. (Afroditi Kanellopoulou), E.K. and P.O.; methodology, V.B., E.K., A.F., M.S., C.R. and A.K. (Anna Kokkevi); project administration, A.K. (Anna Kokkevi); writing—original draft, V.B., A.K. (Afroditi Kanellopoulou) and P.O.; writing—review and editing, V.B., A.K. (Afroditi Kanellopoulou), E.K., A.F., M.S., C.R., P.O. and A.K. (Anna Kokkevi). All authors have read and agreed to the published version of the manuscript.

Acknowledgments: The implementation of the 2018 HBSC survey in Greece was made possible by partial financial support from the Greek Organization Against Drugs (OKANA) and the non-profit organization "Advancement of knowledge on Mental Disorders". The data collection was carried out thanks to the cooperation of a nationwide network of university academic staff and students. The authors would like to thank all participating schools and students for their cooperation.

References

1. Sawyer, S.M.; Afifi, A.R.; Bearinger, L.H.; Blakemore, S.-J.; Dick, B.; Ezeh, A.C.; Patton, G.C. Adolescence: A foundation for future health. *Lancet* **2012**, *379*, 1630–1640. [CrossRef]
2. World Health Organization. *Guideline: Implementing Effective Actions for Improving Adolescent Nutrition*; WHO: Geneva, Switzerland, 2018; Available online: https://www.who.int/nutrition/publications/guidelines/effective-actions-improving-adolescent/en/ (accessed on 1 September 2020).
3. Spear, B.A. Adolescent growth and development. *J. Acad. Nutr. Diet.* **2002**, *102*, S23–S29. [CrossRef]
4. Prentice, A.M.; Ward, K.A.; Goldberg, G.R.; Jarjou, L.M.; Moore, S.E.; Fulford, A.J.; Prentice, A. Critical windows for nutritional interventions against stunting. *Am. J. Clin. Nutr.* **2013**, *97*, 911–918. [CrossRef] [PubMed]
5. Story, M.; Neumark-Sztainer, D.; French, S. Individual and Environmental Influences on Adolescent Eating Behaviors. *J. Am. Diet. Assoc.* **2002**, *102*, S40–S51. [CrossRef]
6. Rampersaud, G.C.; Pereira, M.A.; Girard, B.L.; Adams, J.; Metzl, J.D. Breakfast Habits, Nutritional Status, Body Weight, and Academic Performance in Children and Adolescents. *J. Am. Diet. Assoc.* **2005**, *105*, 743–760. [CrossRef]

7. Kenney, E.L.; Gortmaker, S.L. United States Adolescents' Television, Computer, Videogame, Smartphone, and Tablet Use: Associations with Sugary Drinks, Sleep, Physical Activity, and Obesity. *J. Pediatr.* **2017**, *182*, 144–149. [CrossRef]
8. Monzani, A.; Ricotti, R.; Caputo, M.; Caputo, M.; Archero, F.; Bellone, S.; Prodam, F. A Systematic Review of the Association of Skipping Breakfast with Weight and Cardiometabolic Risk Factors in Children and Adolescents. What Should We Better Investigate in the Future? *Nutrients* **2019**, *11*, 387. [CrossRef]
9. Blondin, S.A.; Anzman-Frasca, S.; Djang, H.C.; Economos, C.D. Breakfast consumption and adiposity among children and adolescents: An updated review of the literature. *Pediatr. Obes.* **2016**, *11*, 333–348. [CrossRef]
10. Adolphus, K.; Lawton, C.L.; Champ, C.L.; Dye, L. The Effects of Breakfast and Breakfast Composition on Cognition in Children and Adolescents: A Systematic Review. *Adv. Nutr.* **2016**, *7*, 590S–612S. [CrossRef]
11. Lachat, C.; Nago, H.E.S.; Verstraeten, R.; Roberfroid, D.; Van Camp, J.; Kolsteren, P. Eating out of home and its association with dietary intake: A systematic review of the evidence. *Obes. Rev.* **2012**, *13*, 329–346. [CrossRef]
12. Poti, J.M.; Duffey, K.J.; Popkin, B.M. The association of fast food consumption with poor dietary outcomes and obesity among children: Is it the fast food or the remainder of the diet? *Am. J. Clin. Nutr.* **2014**, *99*, 162–171. [CrossRef] [PubMed]
13. Taher, A.K.; Evans, N.; Evans, C.E.L. The cross-sectional relationships between consumption of takeaway food, eating meals outside the home and diet quality in British adolescents. *Public Health Nutr.* **2018**, *22*, 63–73. [CrossRef]
14. Larson, N.; MacLehose, R.F.; Fulkerson, J.A.; Berge, J.M.; Story, M.; Neumark-Sztainer, D. Eating Breakfast and Dinner Together as a Family: Associations with Sociodemographic Characteristics and Implications for Diet Quality and Weight Status. *J. Acad. Nutr. Diet.* **2013**, *113*, 1601–1609. [CrossRef] [PubMed]
15. Berge, J.M.; Truesdale, K.P.; Sherwood, N.E.; Mitchell, N.; Heerman, W.J.; Barkin, S.; Matheson, D.; Levers-Landis, C.E.; French, S.A.; Ievers-Landis, C.E. Beyond the dinner table: Who's having breakfast, lunch and dinner family meals and which meals are associated with better diet quality and BMI in pre-school children? *Public Health Nutr.* **2017**, *20*, 3275–3284. [CrossRef] [PubMed]
16. Neumark-Sztainer, D.; Hannan, P.J.; Story, M.; Croll, J.; Perry, C. Family meal patterns: Associations with sociodemographic characteristics and improved dietary intake among adolescents. *J. Am. Diet. Assoc.* **2003**, *103*, 317–322. [CrossRef] [PubMed]
17. Tambalis, K.D.; Panagiotakos, D.B.; Psarra, G.; Sidossis, L. Breakfast skipping in Greek schoolchildren connected to an unhealthy lifestyle profile. Results from the National Action for Children's Health program. *Nutr. Diet.* **2019**, *76*, 328–335. [CrossRef] [PubMed]
18. Hallström, L.; Vereecken, C.A.; Labayen, I.; Ruiz, J.R.; Le Donne, C.; Cuenca-Garcia, M.; Gilbert, C.C.; Martínez, S.G.; Grammatikaki, E.; Huybrechts, I.; et al. Breakfast habits among European adolescents and their association with sociodemographic factors: The HELENA (Healthy Lifestyle in Europe by Nutrition in Adolescence) study. *Public Health Nutr.* **2012**, *15*, 1879–1889. [CrossRef]
19. Tambalis, K.D.; Panagiotakos, D.B.; Psarra, G.; Sidossis, L. Association between fast-food consumption and lifestyle characteristics in Greek children and adolescents; results from the EYZHN (National Action for Children's Health) programme. *Public Health Nutr.* **2018**, *21*, 3386–3394. [CrossRef]
20. Tambalis, K.D.; Panagiotakos, D.B.; Moraiti, I.; Psarra, G.; Sidossis, L.S.; the EYZHN Study Group. Poor dietary habits in Greek schoolchildren are strongly associated with screen time: Results from the EYZHN (National Action for Children's Health) Program. *Eur. J. Clin. Nutr.* **2018**, *72*, 572–580. [CrossRef]
21. Yannakoulia, M.; Karayiannis, D.; Terzidou, M.; Kokkevi, A.; Sidossis, L.S. Nutrition-related habits of Greek adolescents. *Eur. J. Clin. Nutr.* **2004**, *58*, 580–586. [CrossRef]
22. Currie, C.; Gabhainn, N.S.; Godeau, E.; the International HBSC Network Coordinating Committee. The Health Behaviour in School-aged Children: WHO Collaborative Cross-National (HBSC) Study: Origins, concept, history and development 1982–2008. *Int. J. Public Health* **2009**, *54*, 131–139. [CrossRef] [PubMed]
23. Kastorini, C.-M.; Critselis, E.; Zota, D.; Coritsidis, A.L.; Nagarajan, M.K.; Papadimitriou, E.; Belogianni, K.; Benetou, V.; Linos, A.; on behalf of the Greek National Dietary Guidelines Scientific Team. National Dietary Guidelines of Greece for children and adolescents: A tool for promoting healthy eating habits. *Public Health Nutr.* **2019**, *22*, 2688–2699. [CrossRef] [PubMed]

24. Inchley, J.; Currie, D.; Budisavljevic, S.; Torsheim, T.; Jastad, A.; Cosma, A.; Kelly, C.; Arnarsson, Á.M.; Barnekow, V.; Weber, M.M. *Spotlight on Adolescent Health and Well-Being. Findings from the 2017/2018 Health Behaviour in School-Aged Children (HBSC) Survey in Europe and Canada*; International Report, Key Data; WHO Regional Office for Europe: Copenhagen, Denmark, 2020; Volume 2.
25. Matthys, C.; De Henauw, S.; Bellemans, M.; De Maeyer, M.; De Backer, G. Breakfast habits affect overall nutrient profiles in adolescents. *Public Health Nutr.* **2007**, *10*, 413–421. [CrossRef] [PubMed]
26. O'Neil, C.E.; Nicklas, T.A.; Fulgoni, V.L. Nutrient Intake, Diet Quality, and Weight Measures in Breakfast Patterns Consumed by Children Compared with Breakfast Skippers: NHANES 2001–2008. *AIMS Public Health* **2015**, *2*, 441–468. [CrossRef] [PubMed]
27. O'Neil, C.E.; Nicklas, T.A.; Fulgoni, V.L. Nutrient intake, diet quality, and weight/adiposity parameters in breakfast patterns compared with no breakfast in adults: National Health and Nutrition Examination Survey 2001–2008. *J. Acad. Nutr. Diet.* **2014**, *114*, S27–S43. [CrossRef]
28. Larson, N.; Miller, J.M.; Watts, A.W.; Story, M.T.; Neumark-Sztainer, D.R. Adolescent Snacking Behaviors Are Associated with Dietary Intake and Weight Status. *J. Nutr.* **2016**, *146*, 1348–1355. [CrossRef]
29. Ciccone, J.; Woodruff, S.J.; Fryer, K.; Campbell, T.; Cole, M. Associations among evening snacking, screen time, weight status, and overall diet quality in young adolescents. *Appl. Physiol. Nutr. Metab.* **2013**, *38*, 789–794. [CrossRef]
30. Hobbs, M.; Pearson, N.; Foster, P.J.; Biddle, S.J.H. Sedentary behaviour and diet across the lifespan: An updated systematic review. *Br. J. Sports Med.* **2014**, *49*, 1179–1188. [CrossRef]
31. Rosenheck, R. Fast food consumption and increased caloric intake: A systematic review of a trajectory towards weight gain and obesity risk. *Obes. Rev.* **2008**, *9*, 535–547. [CrossRef]
32. Rockett, H.R. Family Dinner: More than Just a Meal. *J. Am. Diet. Assoc.* **2007**, *107*, 1498–1501. [CrossRef]
33. McCarthy, R.; Kehoe, L.; Flynn, A.; Walton, J. The role of fruit and vegetables in the diets of children in Europe: Current state of knowledge on dietary recommendations, intakes and contribution to energy and nutrient intakes. *Proc. Nutr. Soc.* **2020**, 1–8. [CrossRef] [PubMed]

2

Association of Infant Feeding Patterns with Taste Preferences in European Children and Adolescents: A Retrospective Latent Profile Analysis

Elida Sina [1,†], Christoph Buck [1,†], Hannah Jilani [1,2], Michael Tornaritis [3], Toomas Veidebaum [4], Paola Russo [5], Luis A. Moreno [6], Denes Molnar [7], Gabriele Eiben [8], Staffan Marild [9], Valeria Pala [10], Wolfgang Ahrens [1,11] and Antje Hebestreit [1,*]

1 Leibniz Institute for Prevention Research and Epidemiology—BIPS, Achterstr. 30, 28359 Bremen, Germany; sina@leibniz-bips.de (E.S.); buck@leibniz-bips.de (C.B.); jilani@leibniz-bips.de (H.J.); ahrens@leibniz-bips.de (W.A.)
2 Institute for Public Health and Nursing Research—IPP, University of Bremen, 28359 Bremen, Germany
3 Research and Education Institute of Child Health, 2035 Lefcosia, Cyprus; tor.michael@cytanet.com.cy
4 Department of Chronic Diseases, National Institute for Health Development, 11619 Tallin, Estonia; toomas.veidebaum@tai.ee
5 Institute of Food Sciences, National Research Council, 83100 Avellino, Italy; prusso@isa.cnr.it
6 GENUD (Growth, Exercise, Nutrition and Development) Research Group, Instituto Agroalimentario de Aragón (IA2), Instituto de Investigación Sanitaria Aragón (IIS Aragón), Centro de Investigación Biomédica en Red Fisiopatología de la Obesidad y Nutrición (CIBERObn), University of Zaragoza, 50009 Zaragoza, Spain; lmoreno@unizar.es
7 Department of Pediatrics, Medical School, University of Pécs, 7623 Pécs, Hungary; denes.molnar@aok.pte.hu
8 Department of Biomedicine and Public Health, School of Health and Education, University of Skövde, 54128 Skövde, Sweden; gabriele.eiben@his.se
9 Department. of Pediatrics, Institute of Clinical Sciences, Sahlgrenska Academy at University of Gothenburg, 40530 Gothenburg, Sweden; staffan.marild@pediat.gu.se
10 Department of Preventive and Predictive Medicine, Fondazione IRCCS, Istituto Nazionale dei Tumori, 20133 Milan, Italy; Valeria.Pala@istitutotumori.mi.it
11 Faculty of Mathematics/Computer Science, University of Bremen, 28359 Bremen, Germany
* Correspondence: hebestr@leibniz-bips.de
† Shared first authorship.

Abstract: The aim was to investigate associations between the duration of infant feeding practices (FP) and taste preferences (TP) in European children and adolescents. A total of 5526 children (6–16 years old) of the I.Family study completed a Food and Beverage Preference Questionnaire to measure their preferences for sweet, fatty and bitter tastes. Mothers retrospectively reported the FPs duration in months: exclusive breastfeeding (EBF), exclusive formula milk feeding (EFMF), combined breastfeeding (BF&FMF) and the age at the introduction of complementary foods (CF). Using logistic regression analyses and latent class analysis (latent profiles of FP and CF were identified), we explored associations between profiles and TP, adjusting for various covariates, including the Healthy Diet Adherence Score (HDAS). A total of 48% of children had short durations of EBF (≤4 months) and BF&FMF (≤6 months) and were introduced to CF early (<6 months). No significant relationship was observed between the single FPs and TP, even when considering common profiles of FP. HDAS was inversely associated with sweet and fatty TP, but positively with bitter TP. Contrary to our hypotheses, we did not observe associations between FP and children's TP later in life. Further studies with higher FP variation and longitudinal design are needed to investigate the causal associations between infant FP and taste preferences later in life.

Keywords: breastfeeding; formula milk; taste preference; healthy diet adherence; children; IDEFICS study; I.Family

---

1. Introduction

Taste preference (TP) is one of the factors that affect the children's food intake and eating habits [1]. Humans can perceive 6 main basic tastes: (1) Sweet taste is caused by sugar and its derivatives such as fructose or lactose, but other substances such as amino acids and alcohol in fruit juices or alcoholic drinks can also activate the sensory cells that respond to sweetness; (2) Sour taste is mostly perceived via acidic solutions such as lemon juice or organic acids and is caused by hydrogen ions; (3) Salty taste is mainly perceived through foods containing table salt. Its chemical basis is the salt crystal, which consists of sodium and chloride. The sensation of saltiness can be caused by other mineral salts such as potassium or magnesium salts [2]; (4) Bitter taste is brought by a variety of components such as 6-*n*-propylthiouracil (PROP), sinigrin and goitrin, found in cruciferous vegetables (e.g., broccoli). There are 25 bitter taste receptors in humans but the most studied is *TAS2R38*. Genetic variations in this receptor cause different responses in taste sensitivity to bitter compounds from one human to another [3]; (5) Umami taste is caused by glutamic acid or aspartic acid and is similar to the taste of meat broth. It is also found in some plants, such as ripe tomatoes or asparagus [4]; (6) Fatty taste, called Oleogustus, has been described as the sixth basic taste. The stimuli devoted to the detection of dietary fat taste are the Non-Esterified Fatty Acids (NEFA). In particular, medium and long-chain fatty acids have a distinct taste sensation compared to other basic tastes (sweet, bitter, sour and salty) [5,6].

Evidence for the influencing role of genetic and environmental factors on the development of TP is well established [7]. Infants prefer the sweet taste and reject the sour and bitter tastes [7], while the preference for salt appears at about 4 months postnatally [8,9]. TP are learned during contact with food and the eating environment. An infant's experience with flavors begins in the mother's womb and during lactation, when flavors from the mother's diet are transmitted to her amniotic fluid, and later to her colostrum and milk. The infant-feeding method parents choose, whether it is breast or formula milk, will later influence their child-feeding practices [10,11] and the development of their children's food preferences and food acceptance patterns [12].

The fundamental role of breastfeeding on different physiological functions and on the infant's early immunity has been recognized through international nutritional policies, such as the World Health Organization guidelines on early life feeding, which recommends the exclusive breastfeeding of infants up to the age of 6 months and at least for the first 4 months of life [13]. Exclusive breastfeeding is crucial for the growth and development of infants [14], has a long term impact in shaping children's eating behaviors, and predicts the Body Mass Index (BMI) during childhood [15] and later in adult life [16]. Previous studies have pointed out the positive influence of breastfeeding duration on food variety and higher intake of fruits and vegetables in preschoolers [17,18], including in 4 European cohorts [19] and in school-aged children [20,21]. Vital compounds in the human milk provide a specific taste, such as lactose for the sweet taste, glutamate for the umami or savory taste, sodium for the salty taste, urea for the bitter taste and long-chain fatty acids for the fatty taste [22,23].

The introduction of formula milk and other complementary foods represents a crucial period for establishing infants' taste preferences and attitudes towards food, as well as for obesity prevention [24]. Children who were fed exclusively with formula milk do not benefit from the rich flavor profile of their mother's milk: their flavor experience is poorer as they don't experience the flavors from the variety of foods in the mother's diet. Various types and brands of formula milk products offer a diversity of flavors: milk-based formulas are described as having low levels of sweetness and 'sour and cereal-type'; soy-based formulas are described as tasting sweeter, more sour and bitter, and having a 'hay/beany' odor, whereas the hydrolysate formulas are extremely unpalatable to adults due to their sourness and bitterness [25]. Formula-fed infants learn to prefer the flavors associated with the formula milk they were fed and this has been found to influence taste preferences later in life [3,25]. Infant formulas might differ in protein, fat and carbohydrate composition and/or structure, and these differences may, in turn, affect growth, health outcomes and taste preferences [26].

Scott et al. demonstrated that breastfeeding duration is directly associated with the food variety at two years of age [18], independent of factors that are known to influence diet quality in children, such as maternal age and education [27,28]. Another study found that having been breastfed was positively associated with a healthier dietary pattern amongst older Australian children [20]. Burnier et al. [29] investigated longitudinal data from the Quebec Longitudinal Study of Child Development and observed that 3 or more months of exclusive breastfeeding appeared to be a predictive factor for the higher consumption of vegetables in preschool age children. Nicklaus and colleagues found that 2–8 year old children who were breastfed for at least three or more months were more likely to eat vegetables compared to those who were breastfed for a shorter time [30]. A number of animal studies [31,32] and experimental studies in humans [33,34] indicated that breastfeeding is associated with a greater acceptability of new food and flavors during the weaning period. Breastfeeding can contribute towards reducing infants' fears to try new foods and facilitate the transition from milk feeding to solid food eating with lower resistance. Consequently, this can lead to an intake of a higher food variety in breastfed children [3,21,35,36].

Although research has shown that breastfeeding influences infants' food acceptance [22,37–39], to our knowledge, no studies have examined whether it shapes taste preferences in later stages of life. This study seeks to fill this gap by examining how breastfeeding practices—in comparison to formula milk feeding—during infancy, affect food TP in later childhood and adolescence, in a population-based cohort of normal, healthy developing children aged 6 to 16 years old, in 7 European countries: Cyprus, Estonia, Germany, Hungary, Italy, Spain and Sweden.

To be exact, we examined the association between infant feeding practices duration (FP): (1) exclusive breastfeeding (EBF), (2) exclusive formula milk feeding (EFMF) and (3) combined strategy (BF&FMF), and taste preferences (TP) evaluated in our study: sweet, fatty and bitter. We further considered a latent class analysis to identify feeding patterns from a combination of feeding practices and food introduction, and their association with taste preferences.

2. Materials and Methods

2.1. Study Sample

I.Family builds on the IDEFICS (Identification and prevention of Dietary and lifestyle-induced health Effects in Children and InfantS) study, whereby it additionally engages the families of the children who were examined during the IDEFICS baseline (T0) and/or follow-up survey (T1) [40,41]. During the IDEFICS study in 2007/2008, 16,229 children aged 2–9 years from Belgium, Cyprus, Estonia, Germany, Hungary, Italy, Spain and Sweden participated in the baseline survey (T0). Two years later (T1), 13,596 children were examined, 11,041 of whom had previously participated in T0 (68%). In 2013/2014, I.Family (T3) collected further data on the lifestyle-related diseases of 7105 (52% of T1) children, who were then between 7 and 17 years old [42]. Data of 5526 children aged 6–16 years old who completed the Food and Beverage Preference Questionnaire (FBP) during I.Family were used. For the purpose of this investigation, Belgian participants were excluded as their data on food and beverage preference were not collected. Further, retrospective information from the Pregnancy and Early Childhood Questionnaire concerning breastfeeding and formula milk feeding practices and their respective durations during infancy and early childhood reported by mothers in both the IDEFICS study and I.Family were linked. Parents provided written informed consent for all examinations. Each child was informed orally about the measurements by field workers and asked for his/her consent immediately before the examination.

2.2. Core Questionnaire

Information on sex, age, country, migration and socio-economic status (SES) of I.Family participants were collected using a self-administered questionnaire. A validated [43,44] and reproducibility tested [45] food frequency questionnaire (FFQ) containing 59 food and beverage items was completed for each participant. The response categories were 'never/less than once a week', '1–3 times a week', '4–6 times a week', '1 time/day', '2 times a day', '3 times a day' and 'I have no idea'. Based on the FFQ data, a Healthy Diet Adherence Score (HDAS) was developed for all 7 countries [46,47], as a proxy-indicator of children's adherence to healthy dietary guidelines including a high consumption of fruits and vegetables, of whole meals, fish consumption of 2–3 times per week and a reduced intake of refined sugars and fat. The HDAS was used for the present analyses as a continuous variable and ranged from 0 to 50. A higher score represented a higher adherence to healthy dietary guidelines. The self-reported educational level of parents was assessed based on the International Standard Classification of Education (ISCED) [48] and used as a proxy indicator for SES. For the present analyses, it was classified into two main categories: "low-medium education", and "high education". Children's migration background was assessed based on whether the parents were born outside the respective country of residence and recorded as the migration status in the categories "both parents", "one parent", "none of the parents".

All questionnaires were developed in English and translated into the respective national languages. They were then back-translated into English to check for translation errors. Children aged 12 years and above self-completed the questionnaire, while parents proxy-reported the relevant questions for children below 12 years of age. The cut-off of 12 years was chosen because children have been shown to be reliable reporters of their food intake at this age [49].

2.3. Food and Beverage Preference Questionnaire

The questionnaire was constructed as part of the I.Family survey to assess the preferences for sweet, fatty, bitter and salty tasting foods and beverages and was administered to children and adolescents. It contained food photographs of 63 items, including single foods (e.g., broccoli, banana, lettuce), mixed foods (e.g., lasagna, donut), condiments (e.g., nougat spread, butter), and drinks (e.g., fruit juice, lemonade). Using a 1–5 point Likert (smiley) scale, children indicated how much they like the taste of the food given in the photograph, with 1 meaning "do not like at all" and 5 meaning "I like it very much". Participants were also given the chance to indicate if they had never tried (don't know) a specific food/drink item (Figure 1). A pre-test was conducted in every center to ensure the availability of all food items across countries. Furthermore, the FBP questionnaire has been shown to provide valid data that are useful for characterizing taste phenotypes in epidemiological studies [50]. For the present analyses, the preferences for sweet and fatty taste were used as proxy-indicators for unhealthy foods [51,52], while bitter taste was used as a proxy-indicator for healthy foods [3]. Our study only focused on taste preferences that are linked to current obesogenic dietary intake in children, characterized by nutrient-dense foods high in fat and sugar and low in fiber [53,54], hence, salty and sour taste were not assessed. Umami taste is under discussion for healthy (e.g., tomatoes) and unhealthy food preferences (e.g., crisps); thus we also did not consider the preference for umami taste. For the sake of clarity, the term "taste preference" will be used instead of preferences for sweet, fatty and bitter tasting foods and beverages, hereafter.

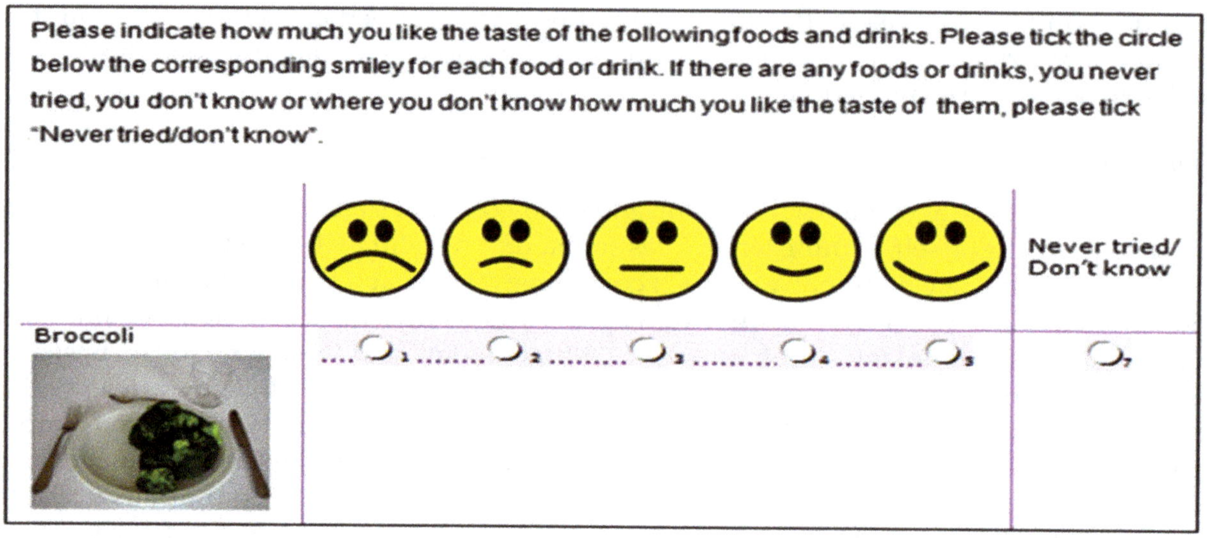

Figure 1. A screenshot of a food item from the Food and Beverage Preference Questionnaire [55].

2.4. *Taste Preference Scores*

The food and beverages included in our analyses were chosen based on factor analyses conducted by Jilani and colleagues [55] that assigned foods to respective taste modalities. In accordance with the factor analyses, we computed scores for the liking of three specific taste modalities: sweet, fatty and bitter, by calculating the mean liking of the foods and drinks included in each of the 3 categories. To control for differences of age and sex in the liking of each taste, the scores were first calculated separately for boys under 12 years old, girls under 12 years, boys aged 12 years and above and girls aged 12 years and above. The cut off of 12 years was chosen as the median age where children enter the age of puberty and further physiological and anatomical developments occur [56]. The scores were then merged into one unique score for each taste modality, in order to assess the association between taste preference scores and infant FP, independent of the age and sex of subjects. The sum of the ratings for the foods and drinks was then calculated and divided by the total number of foods and drinks that were included in the specific taste modality group. The taste preference scores were then categorized as "high" vs. "low", depending on the children's answers. Based on the median value, those who reported 4 or 5 on the smiley scale were included in the "high" preference category, while children who reported 3 or below on the Likert scale were categorized in the "low" preference category. Due to missing values in the taste preference scores, the sample size varied. For instance, when analyzing the sweet score, the sample size was higher than for the bitter score, because children recognized the sweet tasting foods more than the bitter tasting ones.

2.5. *Pregnancy and Early Childhood Questionnaire*

During the IDEFICS surveys (2007/2008 and 2009/2010) and the I.Family survey (2013/2014), mothers were asked to retrospectively report on the feeding strategies they had chosen during infancy and the early life stage of their children. The FP included the duration of

1. Exclusive breastfeeding (EBF): calculated as the difference in months between age at start of other forms of feeding (formula or other complementary foods) and the age at the start of EBF (at birth); EBF was then classified in categories "None", "Up to 4 months" and "More than 4 months",
2. Combined breastfeeding (BF&FMF): calculated as the total duration of breastfeeding after birth (breastfeeding combined with any other type of feeding, formula or complementary foods) and classified as "None", "Up to 6 months" and "More than 6 months".
3. Exclusive formula milk feeding (EFMF): calculated as the difference of total duration of formula milk feeding in combination with other types of feeding and the duration of either EBF or BF&FMF. It was then categorized as "None", "Up to 6 months", "More than 6 months".

The categories for the infant feeding variables were chosen to try and accommodate the restricted sample size for smaller categories and to facilitate the interpretability of the results. The cut off of 4 months for EBF was chosen based on the WHO recommendations to breastfeed infants exclusively with breastmilk for at least the first 4 months of life [13]., As the introduction of complementary foods and the duration of FP in many countries varies, the cut off of 6 months was chosen for the BF&FMF and EFMF. This is in accordance with WHO observations and findings of other studies [13,22]. Mothers also provided information on the age at first introduction of any of the five food categories: cereals (or foods containing rye, wheat or barley), vegetables, fruits, meat and cow milk. These categories were then merged into one unique variable—the minimum age at the first introduction of any food category—which was then categorized as "up to 6 months", "later than 6 months" and "missing". This was again based on WHO observations of the introduction of complementary feeding [13]. From here on, we will refer to these categories as complementary food introduction (CF).

2.6. Statistical Analyses

Descriptive analyses of FP during infancy were conducted by calculating the mean, median and range of the duration of EBF, BF&FMF and EFMF. Furthermore, the following study characteristics were described, i.e., N and proportions, based on categories of BF&FMF for categorical covariates included in the analyses, such as age groups, sex, SES, migration status, the age of the first introduction of complementary food categories, preference scores for each taste modality and country. In order to evaluate the association between each of the three different FP (independent variables) and taste preferences (dependent variables), i.e., sweet, fatty and bitter, logistic regression analyses to calculate Odds Ratios (OR) and 95% confidence limits adjusted for covariates (country, age, sex, HDAS, CF introduction, parents' migration status and SES) were conducted. As a combined analysis showed a high multicollinearity of feeding practices and did not yield interpretable results, a latent class analysis (LCA) was conducted in order to identify latent profiles considering categories of FP and age of complementary food introduction [57]. LCA was conducted considering three, four or five latent profiles of seven variables (three FP variables and four separate variables for the introduction of food items). The different LCA were compared by considering the Bayesian Information Criterium (BIC) and a clear distinction of latent profiles in terms of conditional probabilities. The chosen profiles were then used in logistic regression models as independent variables for each of the TP to again calculate Odds Ratios and 95% confidence limits adjusted for the remaining covariates. All statistical analyses were performed using the statistical software SAS, version 9.3 (Statistical Analyses System, SAS Institute Inc., Cary, NC, USA). The latent class analysis was conducted using the PROC LCA Macro (version 1.3.2, University Park: The Methodology Center, Penn State, PA, USA) [58] in SAS 9.3. Level of significance was set to $\alpha = 0.05$.

3. Results

3.1. Study Characteristics

The descriptive analyses of the three main feeding practices, as shown in Table 1, indicated that the median for EBF was 4 months, ranging from not breastfed at all to 36 months of EBF. The BF&FMF had a median of 6 months, varying from 0 to 36 months of total breastfeeding (BF combined with other types of feeding). The EFMF had a maximum of 48 months, with a median of 0 months of formula milk feeding.

Half of the study population was female (Table 2) and the mean age was 11.6 years (SD = 1.9), whereby 53.3 % of the participants were less than 12 years old. Both parents of a small proportion of the children were migrants (5.4%), while 9.8 % had one parent who was a migrant. Half of the children (50.5%) came from highly educated families and 78.1% of them were introduced to complementary foods early (≤6 months). The HDAS ranged from 0 to 44, with a median of 18.

Table 1. The duration of feeding practices during infancy.

Types of Feeding Practices (N = 5526) Duration in Months	Mean/SD	Median	Min/Max
Exclusive Breastfeeding (EBF)	3.3/2.7	4.0	0.0/36.0
Combined Breastfeeding (BF&FMF)	7.2/6.3	6.0	0.0/36.0
Exclusive Formula Milk Feeding (EFMF)	4.1/8.1	0	0.0/48.0

Table 2. The study characteristics of participants according to the duration of combined breastfeeding (BF&FMF).

	Combined Breastfeeding (BF&FMF)						All	
Variables	None		Up to 6 Months		More Than 6 Months			
	N	%	*N*	%	*N*	%	*N*	%
All	798	100.0	2318	100.0	2410	100.0	5526	100.0
Age Groups								
<12 years	404	50.6	1184	51.1	1359	56.4	2947	53.3
≥12 years	394	49.4	1134	48.9	1051	43.6	2579	46.7
Sex								
Boys	410	51.4	1147	49.5	1203	49.9	2760	49.9
Girls	388	48.6	1171	50.5	1207	50.1	2766	50.1
SES								
Low –Medium	511	64.0	1306	56.3	921	38.2	2738	49.5
High	287	36.0	1012	43.7	1489	61.8	2788	50.5
Migrant Status								
Both Parents	69	8.6	107	4.6	122	5.1	298	5.4
One parent	94	11.8	276	11.9	170	7.1	540	9.8
Neitherparent	635	79.6	1935	83.5	2118	87.9	4688	84.8
Complementary Food Introduction								
Missing	76	9.5	153	6.6	86	3.6	315	5.7
≤6 months	592	74.2	1892	81.6	1833	76.1	4317	78.1
>6 months	130	16.3	273	11.8	491	20.4	894	16.2
Sweet Taste Preference								
Low	350	43.9	950	41.0	918	38.1	2218	40.1
High	448	56.1	1368	59.0	1485	61.6	3301	59.7
Missing [1]	0	0	0	0	7	0.3	7	0.1
Fatty Taste Preference								
Low	317	39.7	855	36.9	948	39.3	2120	38.4
High	481	60.3	1463	63.1	1460	60.6	3404	61.6
Missing [1]	0	0	0	0	2	0.1	2	0.0
Bitter Taste Preference								
Low	546	68.4	1583	68.3	1624	67.4	3753	67.9
High	223	27.9	666	28.7	707	29.3	1596	28.9
Missing [1]	29	3.6	69	3.0	79	3.3	177	3.2
Country								
Italy	170	21.3	652	28.1	224	9.3	1046	18.9
Estonia	57	7.1	265	11.4	554	23.0	876	15.9
Cyprus	228	28.6	508	21.9	169	7.0	905	16.4
Sweden	41	5.1	208	9.0	433	18.0	682	12.3
Germany	181	22.7	310	13.4	315	13.1	806	14.6
Hungary	60	7.5	242	10.4	509	21.1	811	14.7
Spain	61	7.6	133	5.7	206	8.5	400	7.2

[1] Missing values were generated when calculating the taste preference scores for each taste group. N is the number of participants in the BF&FMF categories.

Almost 42% of the study population was breastfed for up to 6 months, while 43.6% had a longer duration of more than 6 months and 14.4% were never breastfed. Looking at the proportions of taste preference categories (low vs. high) according to BF&FMF, the children reported high sweet and fatty taste preferences, independent of the duration of BF&FMF during infancy. The contrary was however shown for bitter taste preferences.

3.2. *Association between Exclusive Breastfeeding and Taste Preference*

The results of the logistic regression analyses showed no associations between EBF and preferences for sweet, fatty and bitter tastes (Table 3). An increase in the HDAS was observed to significantly decrease the chance for high sweet taste preferences (OR = 0.88, 95% CI [0.82; 0.96]) and high-fat taste preferences (OR = 0.88, 95% CI [0.81; 0.95]), while on the other hand significantly increasing the chance for a high bitter taste preference (OR = 1.31, 95% CI [1.20; 1.43]). A late introduction to complementary foods (≤6 months) was found to significantly decrease the odds for a high-fat taste preference (OR = 0.81, 95% CI [0.68; 0.95]). Compared to having parents with a high SES, having parents with a low/medium SES significantly increased the odds for a high-fat taste preference (OR = 1.14, 95% CI [1.009; 1.30]).

Table 3. The association between exclusive breastfeeding (EBF) duration and taste preferences in 6–16 year old children and adolescents who participated in the IDEFICS/I.Family studies.

	Sweet Taste (*N* = 5191)			**Fatty Taste (*N* = 5196)**			**Bitter Taste (*N* = 5029)**		
	OR	**95% CI**		**OR**	**95% CI**		**OR**	**95% CI**	
EBF									
(ref: None)	1.00			1.00			1.00		
≤4 months	1.12	0.97	1.29	1.04	0.90	1.21	0.98	0.84	1.15
>4 months	1.10	0.95	1.29	1.02	0.87	1.19	0.95	0.80	1.12
Healthy Diet Adherence Score (HDAS) $	0.88	0.82	0.96	0.88	0.81	0.95	1.31	1.20	1.43
Complementary Food Introduction									
(ref. ≤6 months)									
>6 months	0.91	0.77	1.07	0.81	0.68	0.95	1.02	0.86	1.22
Missing	0.88	0.67	1.14	0.82	0.62	1.07	1.02	0.75	1.38
SES									
(ref. high)									
Low- medium	1.11	0.98	1.26	1.14	1.009	1.30	0.88	0.77	1.017

$ OR is calculated for difference in one unit from the mean. (Logistic regression models were adjusted also for age, sex, migrant background and country—OR not reported).

3.3. *Association between Combined Breastfeeding and Taste Preference*

The logistic regression analyses did not show an association between the duration of BF&FMF and taste preferences (sweet, fatty and bitter) (Table 4). As observed for EBF, significant associations were observed between HDAS and taste preferences, with having a higher HDAS significantly decreasing the odds for high sweet and fatty taste preference but significantly increasing the odds for high bitter taste preference (Table 4). A late introduction of complementary foods significantly decreased the odds for a high-fat taste preference (OR = 0.82, 95% CI [0.70; 0.97]) compared to an introduction of complementary foods before the age of 6 months. Having parents with a low/medium SES again significantly increased the odds for a high-fat taste preference (OR = 1.14, 95% CI [1.004; −1.29]).

Table 4. The association between combined breastfeeding (BF&FMF) duration and taste preference in 6–16 year old children and adolescents who participated in the IDEFICS/I.Family studies.

	Sweet Taste (N = 5191)			Fatty Taste (N = 5196)			Bitter Taste (N = 5029)		
	OR	95% CI		OR	95% CI		OR	95% CI	
BF&FMF									
(ref. None)	1.00			1.00			1.00		
≤6 months	1.11	0.93	1.32	1.15	0.96	1.37	0.98	0.81	1.19
>6 months	1.10	0.92	1.32	1.03	0.85	1.24	1.09	0.89	1.33
HDAS $	0.88	0.81	0.96	0.88	0.81	0.95	1.31	1.20	1.43
Complementary Food Introduction									
(ref. ≤6 months)									
>6 months	0.91	0.78	1.07	0.82	0.70	0.97	0.99	0.83	1.18
Missing	0.88	0.67	1.15	0.82	0.63	1.08	1.01	0.74	1.37
SES									
(ref. High)									
Low- medium	1.11	0.98	1.26	1.14	1.004	1.29	0.90	0.78	1.03

$ OR is calculated for difference in one unit from the mean. (Logistic regression models were adjusted also for age, sex, migration status and country—OR not reported.

3.4. Association between Exclusive Formula Feeding and Taste Preference

No significant association was observed between the EFMF duration and preferences for sweet, fatty and bitter taste (Table 5). HDAS was again significantly associated with sweet and fatty taste preferences, (OR = 0.88, 95% CI [0.81; 0.96]) and OR = 0.88, 95% CI [0.81; 0.95]) respectively, as well as with a high bitter taste preference (OR = 1.31, 95% CI [1.20; 1.42]). Furthermore, a late introduction of complementary foods decreased the chance for a high preference of fatty taste (OR = 0.82, 95% CI [0,70; 0.97]) at a later age, compared to an early introduction. Compared to having a high SES background, having a low/medium SES background increased the odds to prefer a high-fat taste (OR = 1.14, 95% CI [1.00; 1.29]).

Table 5. The association between exclusive formula milk feeding (EFMF) duration and taste preference in 6–16 years old children and adolescents who participated in the IDEFICS/I.Family studies.

	Sweet Taste (N = 5191)			Fatty Taste (N = 5196)			Bitter Taste (N = 5029)		
	OR	95% CI		OR	95% CI		OR	95% CI	
EFMF									
(ref. None)									
≤6 months	1.001	0.84	1.18	1.09	0.92	1.29	0.85	0.71	1.02
>6 months	1.009	0.85	1.18	1.008	0.85	1.18	0.95	0.80	1.13
HDAS $	0.88	0.82	0.96	0.88	0.81	0.96	1.31	1.20	1.43
Complementary Food Introduction									
(ref. ≤6 months)									
>6 months	0.91	0.78	1.07	0.81	0.69	0.95	1.004	0.84	1.19
Missing	0.87	0.67	1.14	0.82	0.62	1.07	1.01	0.75	1.37
SES									
(ref. High)									
Low- medium	1.10	0.97	1.25	1.14	1.004	1.29	0.90	0.78	1.03

$ OR is calculated for difference in one unit from the mean. (Logistic regression models were adjusted also for age, sex, migration status and country—OR not reported).

3.5. Association between Latent Profiles of Feeding Practices and Taste Preferences

With regard to the four latent profiles, the LCA showed the lowest BIC and a clear interpretable distinction of conditional probabilities for the respective variables. Results of the latent class profiles are presented in Table 6, where names of the profiles were chosen according to the highest conditional probabilities. Almost half of the children and adolescents (48%) had a short duration of EBF (up to

4 months), then were breastfed in combination with formula milk and introduced to complementary foods early (before 6 months). About a quarter (24%) were exclusively breastfed for a long period, were never exclusively fed formula milk and had a late introduction to complementary foods (later than 6 months). A total of 14% were fed formula milk as the main alternative to breastmilk and were as well introduced to complementary foods at a later age. Only 13% were exclusively fed formula milk and were introduced to complementary foods early.

Table 6. The latent class profiles and highest conditional probabilities (ϱ-estimate) of categories within each profile.

Latent Profiles of Feeding Practices			**Frequency**	**%**
1. Long period of EBF and mixed breastfeeding, no exclusive use of formula milk, late introduction of complementary foods			1334	24.14
Variable	Category	ϱ-estimate		
Mixed feeding	more than 6 months	0.869		
Exclusive breastfeeding	more than 4 months	0.853		
Exclusive formula milk feeding	None	0.952		
Introduction of vegetables	after month 6	0.674		
Introduction of fruit	after month 6	0.562		
Introduction of meat	after month 6	0.981		
Introduction of cow milk	after month 6	0.988		
2. Predominantly formula milk feeding (mixed and exclusive) and late introduction of complementary foods			774	14.01
Variable	Category	ϱ-estimate		
Mixed feeding	0–6 months	0.702		
Exclusive breastfeeding	0–4 months	0.464		
Exclusive formula milk feeding	more than 6 months	0.619		
Introduction of vegetables	after month 6	0.832		
Introduction of fruit	after month 6	0.657		
Introduction of meat	after month 6	0.997		
Introduction of cow milk	after month 6	0.973		
3. Short duration of EBF and mixed BF without exclusive formula milk use, early introduction of main complementary foods			2700	48.86
Variable	Category	ϱ-estimate		
Mixed feeding	0–6 months	0.541		
Exclusive breastfeeding	0–4 months	0.627		
Exclusive formula milk feeding	None	0.764		
Introduction of vegetables	before month 6	0.964		
Introduction of fruit	before month 6	0.988		
Introduction of meat	before month 6	0.681		
Introduction of cow milk	after month 6	0.824		
4. No breastfeeding, but exclusive formula milk use, early introduction of main complementary foods.			718	12.99
Variable	Category	ϱ-estimate		
Mixed feeding	None	0.841		
Exclusive breastfeeding	None	0.994		
Exclusive formula milk feeding	more than 6 months	0.583		
Introduction of vegetables	before month 6	0.911		
Introduction of fruit	before month 6	0.983		
Introduction of meat	before month 6	0.645		
Introduction of cow milk	after month 6	0.806		

Profile number 4 was considered to reflect the least advisable feeding strategy (no breastfeeding, only formula milk, early introduction) and served as a reference for the logistic regression analyses presented in Table 7. No significant associations of profiles of feeding practices with taste preferences for sweet, fatty and bitter tastes were observed. Again, the HDAS was significantly negatively associated with sweet (OR = 0.88, 95% CI [0.82; 0.96]) and fatty taste preferences (OR = 0.88, 95% CI [0.81; 0.95]) and significantly positively associated with a bitter taste preference (OR = 1.31, 95% CI [1.20; 1.43]).

In addition, children from low/medium SES families were observed to have a higher chance of having a high-fat taste preference (OR = 1.14, 95% CI [1.00; 1.29]).

Table 7. The results of logistic regression models investigating the association between latent profiles of feeding practices (FP) and taste preferences of 6–16 year old children and adolescents who participated in the IDEFICS/I.Family studies.

	Sweet Taste (N = 5191)			**Fatty Taste (N = 5196)**			**Bitter Taste (N = 5029)**		
Variables	**OR**	**95% CI**		**OR**	**95% CI**		**OR**	**95% CI**	
Profile of FP									
(ref: profile 4)	1.00			1.00			1.00		
Profile 1	0.99	0.81	1.20	0.97	0.79	1.19	1.09	0.88	1.36
Profile 2	0.90	0.72	1.13	1.13	0.90	1.43	1.05	0.82	1.35
Profile 3	1.09	0.91	1.30	1.11	0.92	1.33	1.06	0.87	1.29
HDAS $	0.88	0.82	0.96	0.88	0.81	0.95	1.31	1.20	1.43
SES (ref: high)									
Low/medium	1.11	0.97	1.25	1.14	1.004	1.29	0.89	0.78	1.02

$ OR is calculated for difference in one unit from the mean. (Logistic regression models were adjusted also for age, sex, migration status and country—OR not reported).

4. Discussion

To our knowledge, this is the first study assessing the association between different infant FPs and children's taste preferences in later stages in life which included retrospective and current data from 7 European countries. Our results indicate that European children were predominantly breastfed exclusively for at least 4 months, which is in line with the WHO guidelines [13]. In addition, almost half of the subjects had a long duration of BF&FMF and only a minority (13%) was exclusively fed FM. The feeding strategy parents used seemed not to play a role in the development of taste preferences later in life, irrespective of whether it was EBF, EFMF or a combination. Using both single logistic regression analyses and LCA methods, in which latent profiles of all FP and introduction of complementary food categories were identified, a higher quality diet (HDAS) was observed to be associated with lower chances for a high sweet and high-fat taste preference and increased chances for high bitter taste preference. This suggests that current food choices can actually mold children's preferences for sweet, fat and bitter tastes, independent of their infant feeding patterns. SES also seemed to play a role, as children who came from a lower SES background were more likely to prefer the fatty taste compared to those from a higher SES background. Our results indicate that a variation in food choice and parental education can affect children's behaviors towards healthy food choices and preferences.

Our findings are supported by the current evidence, which suggests that children have innate preferences for sweet taste as signalers of high energy foods [3,8]. Further, Schwartz et al. reported that infants' sweet acceptance was not related to longer durations of EBF [22]. In a longitudinal study, Desor and colleagues measured the sweet preference in children at the age of 11–15 years and again when they were 19–25 years of age, and found that the preferred levels of sucrose decreased over time [59]. Other studies have suggested that children learn to prefer flavors associated with a high dietary fat content [60,61]. Previous findings from the IDEFICS study indicated that children from low educational backgrounds tended to eat more high energy-dense foods, such as sugar-rich and fat-rich foods, compared to those whose parents had a high education [62]. In contrast, children of parents with a higher education tended to eat more fruits and vegetables, generally eating less unhealthy foods. They were also more likely to eat breakfast on a daily basis, emphasizing the influence of parental education on children's eating habits [47,63–67]. Furthermore, a higher number of fruits and vegetables at 14 months has been shown to increase the preference for these foods and improve the quality of the diet at 3.7 years of age [68]. Our results, which are supported by the current evidence, suggest that taste preferences in children are learned via food experience and are significantly influenced by the food choice and diet literacy of parents. Thus, public health education programs should emphasize the role of food variety in shaping children's preferences for bitter tasting foods in the long term. Particular attention needs to be paid to parents and other caretakers of low to medium socio-economic status families in order to help them reduce their children's preferences for high energy-dense foods.

5. Strengths and Limitations

One of the main strengths of our study is the large sample size of 5526 children and adolescents from 7 European countries, which allowed us to have a detailed picture of FP and its potential association with taste preferences in later stages of life. The standardized protocol and the pre-test conducted in a subsample of children showed that the Food and Beverage Preference Questionnaire is a feasible instrument for assessing preferences of food and beverages in children and adolescents.

Furthermore, having information on covariates such as country of residence, age, sex, HDAS, the timing of the first introduction of complementary feeding, parental education level and migration status allowed us to make adjustments and to control for confounding.

Nevertheless, there are important methodological limits concerning our research. The scale of the taste preference was slightly limited as it was calculated based on measuring the food preference with only 5 points. This limited our ability to clearly distinguish between extreme taste preferences. Further, in the BF&FMF category, information on the proportion of actual formula milk and breastmilk feeding was not provided. Thus, we have to acknowledge this as a limitation as it hampers a critical discussion on the potential effects of a mixed strategy of feeding on taste preference.

Since mothers self-reported the details of their infants' FP (age at starting and termination of infant feeding, the timing of the first introduction of complementary foods) and as adolescents tend to self-report a lower preference for energy-dense (fatty and sweet) foods and beverages [69,70], we cannot entirely exclude social desirability bias. As we used retrospective information on feeding practices, recall bias also potentially affected our data. The reproducibility testing of the early infant parameters showed a weak reproducibility of maternal reports on early infant nutrition, a further potential limitation [71]. Nevertheless, research has shown that mothers recall breastfeeding duration accurately [72,73], while the recall of age at introduction of complementary food is less satisfactory [73]. Moreover, the parents of half of our sample had a high educational status, a fact which might also bias the results with regard to socio-economic status. In addition, we did not have information on other confounding factors such as the role of the maternal diet during breastfeeding and the family diet, factors that have been found to influence taste preference and food intake in children [3,55,74]. Lastly, our research was conducted using only cross-sectional data enriched with retrospective information. We strongly recommend further longitudinal research, e.g., through birth cohorts, that can evaluate the effects of FP during infancy and changes of taste preferences during different stages of life, particularly accounting for the interplay between food choice and socio-economic background.

6. Conclusions

In contrast to our hypotheses, we did not observe an association between infant feeding practices and taste preferences in school children and adolescents, neither regarding the single FPs or as a mixed strategy, nor considering common profiles of FP. Instead, the current diet quality through food choice and educational status of parents consistently showed an association with the current taste preference for sweet, fatty or bitter tastes. Hence, further studies with higher FP variations and using longitudinal data are necessary in order to investigate causal associations between infant feeding practices and taste preferences in later stages of life.

Author Contributions: The authors' responsibilities were as follows: E.S. wrote the paper; E.S., C.B. and A.H. had primary responsibility for the final content; E.S. and C.B. performed the data analysis. H.J., M.T., T.V., P.R., L.A.M., D.M., G.E., S.M., V.P. and W.A. participated in the coordination of the data collection and the project administration. All authors were responsible for critical revisions and final approval of the manuscript. This manuscript represents original work that has not been published previously and is not currently being considered by another journal. If accepted, it will not be published elsewhere, including electronically in the same form, in English or in any other language, without the written consent of the copyright holder.

Acknowledgments: This work was done as part of the IDEFICS (http://www.idefics.eu) and I. Family studies (http://www.ifamilystudy.eu/).We thank the IDEFICS and I.Family children and their parents for participating in this extensive examination. We are grateful for the support from school boards, headmasters, and communities.

References

1. Drewnowski, A. Taste preferences and food intake. *Annu. Rev. Nutr.* **1997**, *17*, 237–253. [CrossRef] [PubMed]
2. IQWiG (Institute for Quality and Efficiency in Health Care). *How Does Our Sense of Taste Work?* IQWiG (Institute for Quality and Efficiency in Health Care): Cologne, Germany, 2011.
3. Mennella, J.A. Ontogeny of taste preferences: Basic biology and implications for health. *Am. J. Clin. Nutr.* **2014**, *99*, 704s–711s. [CrossRef]
4. Ikeda, K. New seasonings. *Chem. Senses* **2002**, *27*, 847–849. [CrossRef] [PubMed]
5. Running, C.A.; Craig, B.A.; Mattes, R.D. Oleogustus: The unique taste of fat. *Chem. Senses* **2015**, *40*, 507–516. [CrossRef]
6. Besnard, P.; Passilly-Degrace, P.; Khan, N.A. Taste of fat: A sixth taste modality? *Physiol. Rev.* **2016**, *96*, 151–176. [CrossRef] [PubMed]
7. Birch, L.L. Development of food preferences. *Annu. Rev. Nutr.* **1999**, *19*, 41–62. [CrossRef]
8. Beauchamp, G.K.; Cowart, B.J.; Mennella, J.A.; Marsh, R.R. Infant salt taste: Developmental, methodological, and contextual factors. *Dev. Psychobiol.* **1994**, *27*, 353–365. [CrossRef]
9. Beauchamp, G.K.; Cowart, B.J.; Moran, M. Developmental changes in salt acceptability in human infants. *Dev. Psychobiol.* **1986**, *19*, 17–25. [CrossRef]
10. Fisher, J.O.; Birch, L.L.; Smiciklas-Wright, H.; Picciano, M.F. Breast-feeding through the first year predicts maternal control in feeding and subsequent toddler energy intakes. *J. Am. Diet. Assoc.* **2000**, *100*, 641–646. [CrossRef]
11. Li, R.; Scanlon, K.S.; May, A.; Rose, C.; Birch, L. Bottle-feeding practices during early infancy and eating behaviors at 6 years of age. *Pediatrics* **2014**, *134* (Suppl. 1), S70–S77. [CrossRef]
12. Sullivan, S.A.; Birch, L.L. Infant dietary experience and acceptance of solid foods. *Pediatrics* **1994**, *93*, 271–277.
13. Michaelsen, K.F.; Europe, W.R.O.f.; Europe, W.H.O.R.O.f. *Feeding and Nutrition of Infants and Young Children: Guidelines for the Who European Region, with Emphasis on the Former Soviet Countries*; WHO Regional Office for Europe: Copenhagen, Denmark, 2000.
14. Carling, S.J.; Demment, M.M.; Kjolhede, C.L.; Olson, C.M. Breastfeeding duration and weight gain trajectory in infancy. *Pediatrics* **2015**, *135*, 111–119. [CrossRef] [PubMed]
15. Imai, C.M.; Gunnarsdottir, I.; Thorisdottir, B.; Halldorsson, T.I.; Thorsdottir, I. Associations between infant feeding practice prior to six months and body mass index at six years of age. *Nutrients* **2014**, *6*, 1608–1617. [CrossRef]
16. De Kroon, M.L.; Renders, C.M.; Buskermolen, M.P.; Van Wouwe, J.P.; van Buuren, S.; Hirasing, R.A. The terneuzen birth cohort. Longer exclusive breastfeeding duration is associated with leaner body mass and a healthier diet in young adulthood. *BMC Pediatr.* **2011**, *11*, 33. [CrossRef] [PubMed]
17. Okubo, H.; Miyake, Y.; Sasaki, S.; Tanaka, K.; Hirota, Y. Feeding practices in early life and later intake of fruit and vegetables among Japanese toddlers: The Osaka maternal and child health study. *Public Health Nutr.* **2016**, *19*, 650–657. [CrossRef] [PubMed]
18. Scott, J.; Chih, T.; Oddy, W. Food variety at 2 years of age is related to duration of breastfeeding. *Nutrients* **2012**, *4*, 1464–1474. [CrossRef] [PubMed]
19. De Lauzon-Guillain, B.; Jones, L.; Oliveira, A.; Moschonis, G.; Betoko, A.; Lopes, C.; Moreira, P.; Manios, Y.; Papadopoulos, N.G.; Emmett, P.; et al. The influence of early feeding practices on fruit and vegetable intake among preschool children in 4 European birth cohorts. *Am. J. Clin. Nutr.* **2013**, *98*, 804–812. [CrossRef]
20. Grieger, J.A.; Scott, J.; Cobiac, L. Dietary patterns and breast-feeding in Australian children. *Public Health Nutr.* **2011**, *14*, 1939–1947. [CrossRef]
21. Skinner, J.D.; Carruth, B.R.; Bounds, W.; Ziegler, P.; Reidy, K. Do food-related experiences in the first 2 years of life predict dietary variety in school-aged children? *J. Nutr. Educ. Behav.* **2002**, *34*, 310–315. [CrossRef]

22. Schwartz, C.; Chabanet, C.; Laval, C.; Issanchou, S.; Nicklaus, S. Breast-feeding duration: Influence on taste acceptance over the first year of life. *Br. J. Nutr.* **2013**, *109*, 1154–1161. [CrossRef]
23. Andreas, N.J.; Kampmann, B.; Le-Doare, K.M. Human breast milk: A review on its composition and bioactivity. *Early Hum. Dev.* **2015**, *91*, 629–635. [CrossRef]
24. De Cosmi, V.; Scaglioni, S.; Agostoni, C. Early taste experiences and later food choices. *Nutrients* **2017**, *9*, 107. [CrossRef]
25. Mennella, J.A.; Beauchamp, G.K. Flavor experiences during formula feeding are related to preferences during childhood. *Early Hum. Dev.* **2002**, *68*, 71–82. [CrossRef]
26. Trabulsi, J.C.; Mennella, J.A. Diet, sensitive periods in flavour learning, and growth. *Int. Rev. Psychiatry (Abingdon Engl.)* **2012**, *24*, 219–230. [CrossRef]
27. North, K.; Emmett, P. Multivariate analysis of diet among three-year-old children and associations with socio-demographic characteristics. The Avon longitudinal study of pregnancy and childhood (alspac) study team. *Eur. J. Clin. Nutr.* **2000**, *54*, 73–80. [CrossRef]
28. Robinson, S.; Marriott, L.; Poole, J.; Crozier, S.; Borland, S.; Lawrence, W.; Law, C.; Godfrey, K.; Cooper, C.; Inskip, H. Dietary patterns in infancy: The importance of maternal and family influences on feeding practice. *Br. J. Nutr.* **2007**, *98*, 1029–1037. [CrossRef]
29. Burnier, D.; Dubois, L.; Girard, M. Exclusive breastfeeding duration and later intake of vegetables in preschool children. *Eur. J. Clin. Nutr.* **2011**, *65*, 196–202. [CrossRef] [PubMed]
30. Nicklaus, S. The role of food experiences during early childhood in food pleasure learning. *Appetite* **2016**, *104*, 3–9. [CrossRef]
31. Galef, B.G.; Henderson, P.W. Mother's milk: A determinant of the feeding preferences of weaning rat pups. *J. Comp. Physiol. Psychol.* **1972**, *78*, 213–219. [CrossRef]
32. Galef, B.G.; Sherry, D.F. Mother's milk: A medium for transmission of cues reflecting the flavor of mother's diet. *J. Comp. Physiol. Psychol.* **1973**, *83*, 374–378. [CrossRef]
33. Mennella, J.A.; Forestell, C.A.; Morgan, L.K.; Beauchamp, G.K. Early milk feeding influences taste acceptance and liking during infancy. *Am. J. Clin. Nutr.* **2009**, *90*, 780s–788s. [CrossRef] [PubMed]
34. Mennella, J.A.; Beauchamp, G.K. Mothers' milk enhances the acceptance of cereal during weaning. *Pediatr. Res.* **1997**, *41*, 188–192. [CrossRef]
35. Galloway, A.T.; Lee, Y.; Birch, L.L. Predictors and consequences of food neophobia and pickiness in young girls. *J. Am. Diet. Assoc.* **2003**, *103*, 692–698. [CrossRef]
36. Cooke, L.J.; Wardle, J.; Gibson, E.L.; Sapochnik, M.; Sheiham, A.; Lawson, M. Demographic, familial and trait predictors of fruit and vegetable consumption by pre-school children. *Public Health Nutr.* **2004**, *7*, 295–302. [CrossRef] [PubMed]
37. Mennella, J.A.; Daniels, L.M.; Reiter, A.R. Learning to like vegetables during breastfeeding: A randomized clinical trial of lactating mothers and infants. *Am. J. Clin. Nutr.* **2017**, *106*, 67–76. [CrossRef] [PubMed]
38. Hausner, H.; Nicklaus, S.; Issanchou, S.; Molgaard, C.; Moller, P. Breastfeeding facilitates acceptance of a novel dietary flavour compound. *Clin. Nutr. (Edinb. Scotl.)* **2010**, *29*, 141–148. [CrossRef] [PubMed]
39. Forestell, C.A.; Mennella, J.A. Early determinants of fruit and vegetable acceptance. *Pediatrics* **2007**, *120*, 1247–1254. [CrossRef] [PubMed]
40. Ahrens, W.; Bammann, K.; Siani, A.; Buchecker, K.; De Henauw, S.; Iacoviello, L.; Hebestreit, A.; Krogh, V.; Lissner, L.; Mårild, S.; et al. The idefics cohort: Design, characteristics and participation in the baseline survey. *Int. J. Obes.* **2011**, *35* (Suppl. 1), S3–S15. [CrossRef]
41. Hebestreit, A.; Intemann, T.; Siani, A.; De Henauw, S.; Eiben, G.; Kourides, Y.A.; Kovacs, E.; Moreno, L.A.; Veidebaum, T.; Krogh, V.; et al. Dietary patterns of european children and their parents in association with family food environment: Results from the i.Family study. *Nutrients* **2017**, *9*, 126. [CrossRef]
42. Ahrens, W.; Siani, A.; Adan, R.; De Henauw, S.; Eiben, G.; Gwozdz, W.; Hebestreit, A.; Hunsberger, M.; Kaprio, J.; Krogh, V.; et al. Cohort profile: The transition from childhood to adolescence in European children-how i.Family extends the idefics cohort. *Int. J. Epidemiol.* **2017**, *46*, 1394–1395j. [CrossRef]
43. Bel-Serrat, S.; Mouratidou, T.; Pala, V.; Huybrechts, I.; Börnhorst, C.; Fernández-Alvira, J.; Moreno, L. Relative validity of the children's eating habits questionnaire–food frequency section among young european children: The idefics study. *Public Health Nutr.* **2014**, *17*, 266–276. [CrossRef]

44. Huybrechts, I.; Börnhorst, C.; Pala, V.; Moreno, L.A.; Barba, G.; Lissner, L.; Fraterman, A.; Veidebaum, T.; Hebestreit, A.; Sieri, S.; et al. Evaluation of the children's eating habits questionnaire used in the idefics study by relating urinary calcium and potassium to milk consumption frequencies among european children. *Int. J. Obes.* **2011**, *35* (Suppl. 1), S69–S78. [CrossRef]
45. Lanfer, A.; Hebestreit, A.; Ahrens, W.; Krogh, V.; Sieri, S.; Lissner, L.; Eiben, G.; Siani, A.; Huybrechts, I.; Loit, H.M.; et al. Reproducibility of food consumption frequencies derived from the children's eating habits questionnaire used in the idefics study. *Int. J. Obes.* **2011**, *35* (Suppl. 1), S61–S68. [CrossRef]
46. Arvidsson, L.; Eiben, G.; Hunsberger, M.; De Bourdeaudhuij, I.; Molnar, D.; Jilani, H.; Thumann, B.; Veidebaum, T.; Russo, P.; Tornatitis, M.; et al. Bidirectional associations between psychosocial well-being and adherence to healthy dietary guidelines in european children: Prospective findings from the idefics study. *BMC Public Health* **2017**, *17*, 926. [CrossRef]
47. Jilani, H.S.; Pohlabeln, H.; Buchecker, K.; Gwozdz, W.; De Henauw, S.; Eiben, G.; Molnar, D.; Moreno, L.A.; Pala, V.; Reisch, L.; et al. Association between parental consumer attitudes with their children's sensory taste preferences as well as their food choice. *PLoS ONE* **2018**, *13*, e0200413. [CrossRef]
48. UNESCO. International Standard Classification of Education 2012. Available online: http://uis.Unesco.Org/sites/default/files/documents/international-standard-classification-of-education-isced-2011-en.Pdf (accessed on 27 October 2016).
49. Livingstone, M.B.; Robson, P.J. Measurement of dietary intake in children. *Proc. Nutr. Soc.* **2000**, *59*, 279–293. [CrossRef] [PubMed]
50. Jilani, H.P.H.; De Henauw, S.; Eiben, G.; Hunsberger, M.; Molnar, D.; Moreno, L.; Pala, V.; Russo, P.; Solea, A.; Veidebaum, T.; et al. Relative validity of a food and beverage preference questionnaire to characterise taste phenotypes in children, adolescents and adult. *Nutrient* **2019**. under revision.
51. Ricketts, C.D. Fat preferences, dietary fat intake and body composition in children. *Eur. J. Clin. Nutr.* **1997**, *51*, 778–781. [CrossRef] [PubMed]
52. Ventura, A.K.; Mennella, J.A. Innate and learned preferences for sweet taste during childhood. *Curr. Opin. Clin. Nutr. Metab. Care* **2011**, *14*, 379–384. [CrossRef]
53. Paes, V.M.; Ong, K.K.; Lakshman, R. Factors influencing obesogenic dietary intake in young children (0–6 years): Systematic review of qualitative evidence. *BMJ Open* **2015**, *5*, e007396. [CrossRef] [PubMed]
54. Johnson, L.; Mander, A.P.; Jones, L.R.; Emmett, P.M.; Jebb, S.A. Energy-dense, low-fiber, high-fat dietary pattern is associated with increased fatness in childhood. *Am. J. Clin. Nutr.* **2008**, *87*, 846–854. [CrossRef]
55. Jilani, H.S.; Intemann, T.; Bogl, L.H.; Eiben, G.; Molnar, D.; Moreno, L.A.; Pala, V.; Russo, P.; Siani, A.; Solea, A.; et al. Familial aggregation and socio-demographic correlates of taste preferences in european children. *BMC Nutr.* **2017**, *3*, 87. [CrossRef]
56. Parent, A.-S.; Teilmann, G.; Juul, A.; Skakkebaek, N.E.; Toppari, J.; Bourguignon, J.-P. The timing of normal puberty and the age limits of sexual precocity: Variations around the world, secular trends, and changes after migration. *Endocr. Rev.* **2003**, *24*, 668–693. [CrossRef] [PubMed]
57. Lanza, S.T.; Flaherty, B.P.; Collins, L.M. Latent class and latent transition analysis. In *Handbook of Psychology*; Weiner, I.B., Ed.; John Wiley & Sons, Inc.: New York, NY, USA, 2003.
58. Lanza, S.T.; Dziak, J.J.; Huang, L.; Xu, S.; Collins, L.M. *PROC LCA & PROC LTA Users' Guide (Version 1.3.2)*; The Methodology Center; Penn State: University Park, PA, USA, 2011.
59. Desor, J.A.; Beauchamp, G.K. Longitudinal changes in sweet preferences in humans. *Physiol. Behav.* **1987**, *39*, 639–641. [CrossRef]
60. Johnson, S.L.; McPhee, L.; Birch, L.L. Conditioned preferences: Young children prefer flavors associated with high dietary fat. *Physiol. Behav.* **1991**, *50*, 1245–1251. [CrossRef]
61. Kern, D.L.; McPhee, L.; Fisher, J.; Johnson, S.; Birch, L.L. The postingestive consequences of fat condition preferences for flavors associated with high dietary fat. *Physiol. Behav.* **1993**, *54*, 71–76. [CrossRef]
62. Fernandez-Alvira, J.M. Parental education and frequency of food consumption in European children: The idefics study. *Public Health Nutr.* **2013**, *16*, 487–498. [CrossRef] [PubMed]
63. Van Ansem, W.J.; Schrijvers, C.T.; Rodenburg, G.; van de Mheen, D. Maternal educational level and children's healthy eating behaviour: Role of the home food environment (cross-sectional results from the inpact study). *Int. J. Behav. Nutr. Phys. Act.* **2014**, *11*, 113. [CrossRef] [PubMed]
64. Cribb, V.L.; Jones, L.R.; Rogers, I.S.; Ness, A.R.; Emmett, P.M. Is maternal education level associated with diet in 10-year-old children? *Public Health Nutr.* **2011**, *14*, 2037–2048. [CrossRef] [PubMed]

65. Sausenthaler, S.; Standl, M.; Buyken, A.; Rzehak, P.; Koletzko, S.; Bauer, C.P.; Schaaf, B.; von Berg, A.; Berdel, D.; Borte, M.; et al. Regional and socio-economic differences in food, nutrient and supplement intake in school-age children in germany: Results from the giniplus and the lisaplus studies. *Public Health Nutr.* **2011**, *14*, 1724–1735. [CrossRef]
66. Sausenthaler, S.; Kompauer, I.; Mielck, A.; Borte, M.; Herbarth, O.; Schaaf, B.; von Berg, A.; Heinrich, J. Impact of parental education and income inequality on children's food intake. *Public Health Nutr.* **2007**, *10*, 24–33. [CrossRef]
67. Lehto, E.; Ray, C.; Te Velde, S.; Petrova, S.; Duleva, V.; Krawinkel, M.; Behrendt, I.; Papadaki, A.; Kristjansdottir, A.; Thorsdottir, I.; et al. Mediation of parental educational level on fruit and vegetable intake among schoolchildren in ten european countries. *Public Health Nutr.* **2015**, *18*, 89–99. [CrossRef]
68. Mallan, K.M.; Fildes, A.; Magarey, A.M.; Daniels, L.A. The relationship between number of fruits, vegetables, and noncore foods tried at age 14 months and food preferences, dietary intake patterns, fussy eating behavior, and weight status at age 3.7 years. *J. Acad. Nutr. Diet.* **2016**, *116*, 630–637. [CrossRef]
69. Perl, M.A.; Mandic, M.L.; Primorac, L.; Klapec, T.; Perl, A. Adolescent acceptance of different foods by obesity status and by sex. *Physiol. Behav.* **1998**, *65*, 241–245. [CrossRef]
70. Tilgner, L.; Wertheim, E.H.; Paxton, S.J. Effect of social desirability on adolescent girls' responses to an eating disorders prevention program. *Int. J. Eat. Disord.* **2004**, *35*, 211–216. [CrossRef]
71. Herrmann, D.; Suling, M.; Reisch, L.; Siani, A.; De Bourdeaudhuij, I.; Maes, L.; Santaliestra-Pasias, A.M.; Veidebaum, T.; Molnar, D.; Pala, V.; et al. Repeatability of maternal report on prenatal, perinatal and early postnatal factors: Findings from the idefics parental questionnaire. *Int. J. Obes. (Lond.)* **2011**, *35* (Suppl. 1), S52–S60. [CrossRef]
72. Natland, S.T.; Andersen, L.F.; Nilsen, T.I.L.; Forsmo, S.; Jacobsen, G.W. Maternal recall of breastfeeding duration twenty years after delivery. *BMC Med. Res. Methodol.* **2012**, *12*, 179. [CrossRef] [PubMed]
73. Li, R.; Scanlon, K.S.; Serdula, M.K. The validity and reliability of maternal recall of breastfeeding practice. *Nutr. Rev.* **2005**, *63*, 103–110. [CrossRef] [PubMed]
74. Birch, L.L. The relationship between children's food preferences and those of their parents. *J. Nutr. Educ.* **1980**, *12*, 14–18. [CrossRef]

3

Development of a Quality Score for the Home Food Environment Using the Home-IDEA2 and the Healthy Eating Index-2010

Sarah K. Hibbs-Shipp [1], Richard E. Boles [2], Susan L. Johnson [2], Morgan L. McCloskey [1], Savannah Hobbs [1] and Laura L. Bellows [1,*]

1 Department of Food Science and Human Nutrition, Colorado State University, Fort Collins, CO 80523, USA; sarah.hibbs-shipp@colostate.edu (S.K.H.-S.); morgan.mccloskey@colostate.edu (M.L.M.); savannah.hobbs@colostate.edu (S.H.)

2 Department of Pediatrics, University of Colorado Anschutz Medical Campus, Aurora, CO 80045, USA; Richard.boles@ucdenver.edu (R.E.B.); Susan.Johnson@ucdenver.edu (S.L.J.)

* Correspondence: laura.bellows@colostate.edu

Abstract: The home food environment (HFE) is an important factor in the development of food preferences and habits in young children, and the availability of foods within the home reflects dietary intake in both adults and children. Therefore, it is important to consider the holistic quality of the HFE. The purpose of this study was to apply the Healthy Eating Index (HEI; a measure of diet quality in conformance to the Dietary Guidelines for Americans) algorithm to the Home-IDEA2, a valid and reliable food inventory checklist, to develop a Home-IDEA2 HEI Score. After an initial score was developed, it was psychometrically tested for content, criterion, and construct validity. Content validity testing resulted in 104 foods being retained. Internal criterion testing demonstrated that 42 foods (40%) changed component scores by >5%; however, no single food changed a total Home-IDEA2 HEI score by >5%. Testing of hypothetical HFEs resulted in a range of scores in the expected directions, establishing sensitivity to varied HFEs. This study resulted in a validated methodology to assess the overall quality of the HFE, thus contributing a novel approach for examining home food environments. Future research can test interventions modifying the HFE quality to improve individual dietary intake.

Keywords: home food environment; Healthy Eating Index; dietary quality; validation; psychometric

---

1. Introduction

In recent years, dietary research has expanded to assess not only the foods eaten, but also the context in which the food is eaten (e.g., at home versus away from home) [1–3] and where the food was obtained (e.g., fast-food [4], sit down restaurant [5], convenience store [6,7], grocery store [8,9], school/cafeteria [10], or vending machine [9]) [11,12]. One of these areas of expanding research is the home food environment (HFE), which provides context for individual and family dietary intake [13]. The HFE has received increasing attention as an important factor in the development of food preferences and habits in children, as a contributor to obesogenic environments, and as a modifiable factor for nutritional interventions, especially those targeting childhood obesity [13–15].

The HFE is influenced by factors that include food purchasing and preparation decisions, food availability, and food accessibility [16,17]. The HFE impacts children's diet not only through examples of eating habits, but also through the actual foods that are readily available and accessible in the home [18,19]. The availability of foods within the home has been shown to reflect intake in both adults and children, and as such, provides a potential dietary intervention point [3]. Intervention targets for improving children's dietary behaviors should focus on the availability and accessibility of a spectrum of foods, including increasing healthful foods as well as reducing foods and beverages that are energy-dense and nutrient poor [20].

This increasing recognition of the environmental context of dietary intake has led to a large increase in the number of tools available for assessing a given environment with regard to availability of foods. Often HFE tools were designed to fit the researchers' immediate questions and were brief, focused on only one aspect of food availability—such as high-fat foods, sugar-sweetened beverages, or fruits & vegetables—and had limited psychometric testing performed [21]. Small food sets and a lack of a complete listing of foods in most HFE assessments has limited researchers' abilities to examine the totality of the HFE and its contributions to dietary quality.

The Home Inventory to Describe Eating and Activity (Home-IDEA2) is one such assessment that has been found to be valid and reliable in assessing food, activity, and electronic home environments among low-income minority parents of preschoolers [22]. The Home-IDEA2 is a semi-comprehensive checklist designed to assess the foods present in the home at a single point in time. It includes foods sourced from the Allowable Foods List from the US Special Supplemental Nutrition Program for Women, Infants, and Children (WIC Program), the Block Food Frequency Questionnaire, and the modified Harvard Food Frequency Questionnaire (FFQ), allowing for application to diverse households.

Given the relationship between the HFE and dietary intake, it is important to consider the HFE beyond the presence and absence of individual foods, and examine the holistic quality of the entire HFE. The Healthy Eating Index (HEI), developed by the National Cancer Institute, is the method of choice in the US for assessing dietary quality [23]. The HEI is a formalized approach that includes rules and analysis algorithms allowing for effective comparisons in the overall quality of foods across different levels of the food supply [23,24]. HEI algorithms have been applied to the US food supply level [25], the community food environment (e.g., food assistance program offerings [26], supermarket sales circulars [27], menu offerings [4], corner stores [28], grocery purchases [29], by multiple food purchase locations [30]), and at the individual food intake level (e.g., comparing diet cost to diet quality [31], comparing different dietary patterns [32–35], and evaluating differences in mortality outcomes by diet quality [36]). To date, the HEI algorithm has been applied to the HFE in one recent study [37], which demonstrates a need for more rigorous validation and psychometric testing. Application of the HEI to the HFE provides a unique way of assessing overall quality of the HFE, and allows for direct comparison to dietary intake quality, thus providing the potential for further insights into the relationship between the HFE, dietary intake, and health outcomes.

For this study, the Home-IDEA2 was used as an instrument to apply the HEI algorithm to assess the quality of the HFE. Specific objectives were to (1) develop an initial Home-IDEA2 HEI Score, and (2) psychometrically test the Home-IDEA2 HEI Score for content, criterion, and construct validity.

2. Materials and Methods

2.1. Development of an Initial Home-IDEA2 Healthy Eating Index Score

2.1.1. Application of the HEI Algorithm to the Home-IDEA2

The Healthy Eating Index (HEI) is updated to conform to each edition of the Dietary Guidelines for Americans (DGA), with the HEI-2010 [23] reflecting diet patterning in conformance with the 2010-DGAs [38]. The HEI-2010 was used, as the HEI-2015 was not yet available during the development of the Home-IDEA2 HEI Score. Briefly, the HEI-2010 scores 12 dietary components for a total score ranging from 0–100 (Table 1), with total scores less than 51 categorized as 'poor,' 51–80 as 'needs improvement,' and greater than 80 as 'good' [39]. The HEI has been applied to other food supply levels using three steps: (1) identification of a set of foods, (2) determination of the amount of each dietary constituent associated with each food in the set, and (3) deriving ratios to score each HEI component using developed algorithms [40].

Table 1. Healthy Eating Index-2010 components and scoring standards.

HEI-2010 Components	Maximum Points	Standard for Maximum Score (per 1000 kcal) [a]	Standard for Minimum Score of Zero (per 1000 kcal) [a]
Adequacy			
Total Fruit [b]	5	≥0.8 cup equiv. (102 g)	No Fruit
Whole Fruit [c]	5	≥0.4 cup equiv. (51 g)	No Whole Fruit
Total Vegetables [d]	5	≥1.1 cup equiv. (141 g)	No Vegetables
Greens & Beans [d]	5	≥0.2 cup equiv. (26 g)	No Dark Green Vegetables or Beans/Peas
Whole Grains	10	≥1.5 oz equiv. (42 g)	No Whole Grains
Dairy [e]	10	≥1.3 cup equiv. (166 g)	No Dairy
Total Protein Foods [f]	5	≥2.5 oz equiv. (71 g)	No Protein Foods
Seafood & Plant Proteins [f,g]	5	≥0.8 oz equiv. (23 g)	No Seafood or Plant Proteins
Fatty Acid Ratio [h]	10	(PUFAs + MUFAs)/SFA ≥2.5	(PUFAs + MUFAs)/SFA ≤1.2
Moderation			
Refined Grains	10	≤1.8 oz equiv. (~51.0 g)	≥4.3 oz equiv. (122 g)
Sodium	10	≤1.1 g	≥2.0 g
Empty Calories [i]	20	≤19% of energy	≥50% of energy
Total Score [j]	100		

Adapted from the National Cancer Institute's HEI-2010 Components & Scoring Standards Table [41]. (Development of the scoring rubric has been previously described in detail [42]. [a] Amounts between the minimum and maximum scores are scored proportionately. [b] Includes 100% fruit juice. [c] Includes all forms except juice. [d] Includes any beans and peas not counted as total protein foods. [e] Includes all milk products, such as fluid milk, yogurt, and cheese, and fortified soy beverages. [f] Beans and peas are included here (and not with vegetables) when the total protein foods standard is otherwise not met. [g] Includes seafood, nuts, seeds, and soy products (other than beverages), as well as beans and peas counted as total protein foods. [h] Ratio of poly- and monounsaturated fatty acids (PUFAS and MUFAS) to saturated fatty acids (SFAs): (PUFAs + MUFAs)/SFA. [i] Calories from solid fats, alcohol, and added sugars; threshold for counting alcohol is >13 g/1000 kcal. [j] The Center for Nutrition Policy and Promotion categorizes total scores as poor (less than 51), needs improvement (51–80), and good (greater than 80) [39]. Abbreviations: HEI: Healthy Eating Index; equiv., equivalents; oz., ounces; g., grams.

The Home-IDEA2 (the self-report checklist that participants complete regarding availability of select food items in the home) includes 108 food items that represent a wide variety of potential types of foods in the home. For example, there are single-items, such as "apple," that represent all types of raw apples (Granny Smith, Macintosh, Red Delicious). There are also composite items that represent a "category" of similar items, such as "citrus fruits" representing oranges, tangerines, mandarins, grapefruit, lemons, limes, etc. All items, whether single or composite, are completed in terms of "Yes/No" availability in the home. No information is obtained as to how much of these items are in the home, rather, the presence or absence of the listed foods is assessed.

The Home-IDEA2 was chosen as the basis for developing a HFE quality score using the HEI for four reasons: (1) the high feasibility for individuals to complete the survey [22], (2) the included foods are relevant to socioeconomically, racially/ethnically, and geographically diverse families with young children [43,44], (3) it has been psychometrically validated [22,44], and (4) it has demonstrated positive associations with dietary intake for a broad range of foods ranging from healthy and less healthy foods in families with young children [43]. In order to apply the HEI to the Home-IDEA2, USDA's Center for Nutrition Policy and Promotion's recommended processes were modified to include the HFE, and a 3 step process was followed (Figure 1) [40]. Because all foods in the Home-IDEA2 are listed generically and without amounts, a 'representative' food identifying a specific food code that links to the Food and Nutrition Database for Dietary Studies (FNDDS) and a representative food amount for each Home-IDEA2 item needed to be assigned to apply nutrient values before ratios and HEI score components could be derived.

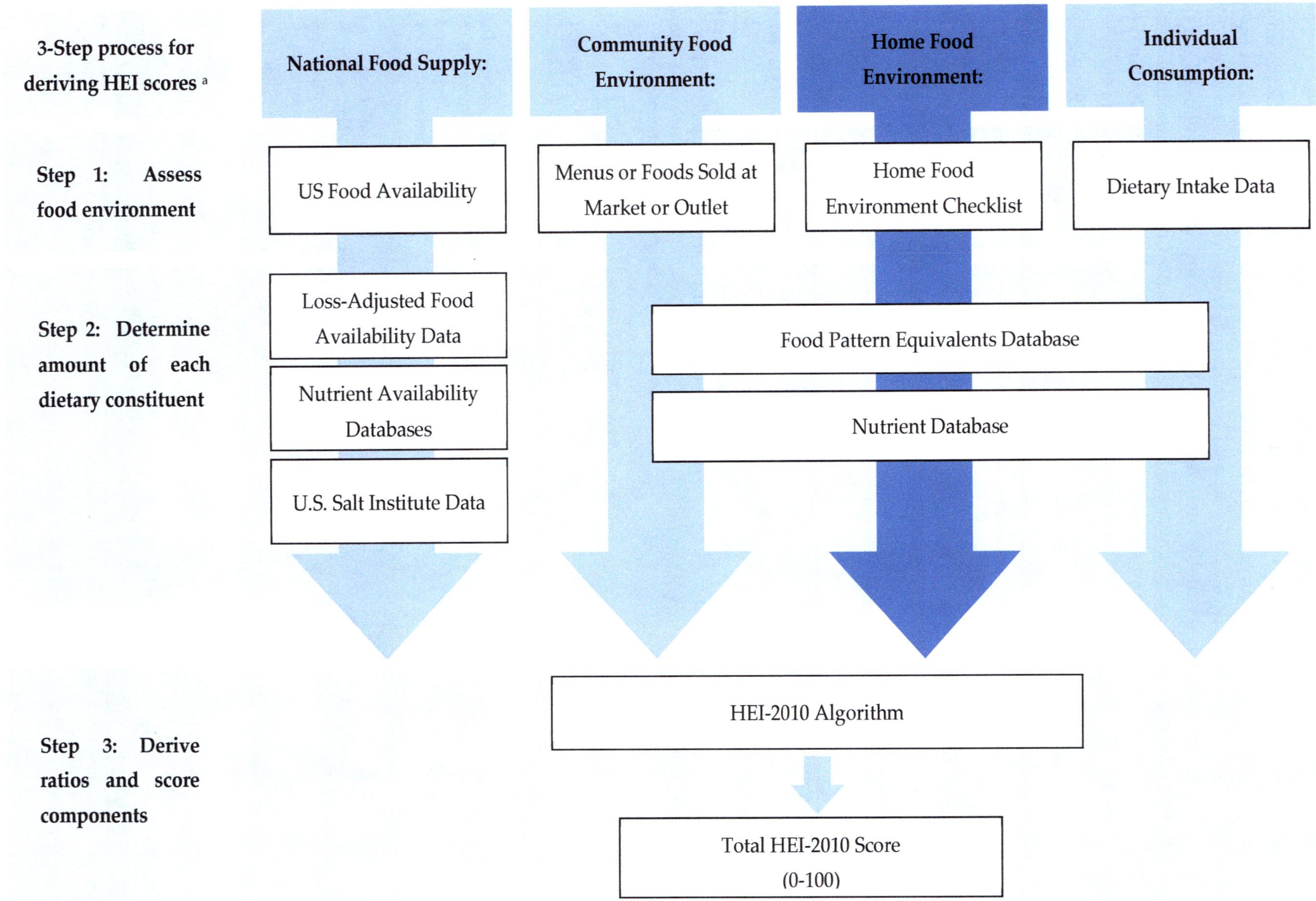

Figure 1. Three step process for deriving Healthy Eating Index (HEI) scores across different levels of the food system. [a] Figure adapted from Calculating HEI Scores at Different Levels, the HEI scoring illustration [45].

2.1.2. Representative Foods

The representative foods and food amounts for the Home-IDEA2 items were sourced from the FoodAPS, a national survey of 4826 ethnically and income-diverse U.S. households conducted by the USDA Economic Research Service (ERS) and Food and Nutrition Service (FNS) between April 2012 and January 2013 [46]. The publicly available, de-identified, food-at-home dataset was used for this study (faps_fahnutrients, downloaded 26 January 2017) [46]. A multi-part process was employed to identify a representative food for each Home-IDEA2 item. First, a keyword search within the FoodAPS file was conducted for foods that matched each Home-IDEA2 item. Next, four investigators with expertise in nutrition and psychometric testing evaluated the identified foods for face validity with Home-IDEA2 items and reasonableness for low-income, multi-ethnic households. These foods were discussed by the research team until consensus was achieved. Last, remaining options were evaluated for key nutrients/nutrient categories (e.g., sodium, whole fruit, whole grains) theorized to load into the HEI-2010 algorithm, with the food closest to the mean or median of the key nutrients/nutrient categories selected as the 'representative' food for each Home-IDEA2 item. Table 2 outlines key considerations for the selection of the representative food for citrus fruits.

Table 2. Sample considerations for the selection of the representative food for Home-IDEA2 Category of citrus fruits.

Potential Representative Food Item	HEI Component Score	Presence in Households [a]	Availability, Consumption and Other Considerations	Selection Decision
Oranges	Whole fruit; Total fruit	Common	*Availability:* Year-round; *Consumed:* As whole fruit	Selected (food code 61119010)
Clementines (Cuties®)	Whole fruit; Total fruit	Common	*Availability:* Seasonal; *Consumed:* As whole fruit	Not selected due to seasonality
Mandarins	Whole fruit; Total fruit; SOFAAS (added sugars)	Common	*Availability:* Seasonal (fresh); Year Round (packaged); *Consumed:* As whole fruit; *Other:* Packed in juice and syrup; contains added sugars	Not selected due to contribution of added sugars
Grapefruit	Whole fruit; Total fruit; SOFAAS (added sugars)	Less common	*Availability:* Seasonal (fresh); Year Round (packaged); *Consumed:* As whole fruit; *Other:* Packed in juice and syrup; contains added sugars	Not selected due low presence in households and contribution of added sugars
Tangerine	Whole fruit; Total fruit	Less common	*Availability:* Seasonal; *Consumed:* As whole fruit	Not selected due to low presence in households and seasonality
Lemons	Whole fruit; Total fruit	Common	*Availability:* Year-round; *Consumed:* Not typically eaten in whole as fruit	Not selected because not typically consumed as whole fruit
Limes	Whole fruit; Total fruit	Common	*Availability:* Year-round; *Consumed:* Not typically eaten in whole as fruit	Not selected because not typically consumed as whole fruit

[a] Presence in households was determined based on frequencies from Home-IDEA2 administered with a low-income, minority population (unpublished data). Abbreviations: HEI: Healthy Eating Index; Home-IDEA: Home Inventory Describing Eating and Activity; SoFAAS: Solid Fats, Alcohol, Added Sugars.

2.1.3. Food Amounts

For each representative food, food amounts were then selected. Within the FoodAPS dataset, the mean, median, and mode of available total edible gram weights were calculated for each representative food. Next, an internet search for standard consumer package sizes was performed. Calculated weights were adjusted to reflect reasonable package sizes for consistency across foods (e.g., milk varieties (whole, 2%, 1% skim, chocolate) were normalized to 1 gallon (3.8 L), cheese varieties (regular, low-fat) were normalized to 1 pound (454 g), meat varieties (chicken, beef) were normalized to 2 pounds (908 g), and for realistic purchase quantities (e.g., vegetable oil was reduced from 1 gallon (3.8 L) to 32 ounces (1 L)).

2.1.4. Ratios and HEI Score Components

The nutritional content for the representative foods and selected food amounts were merged with the Home-IDEA2 to create the Home-IDEA2 HEI Score database. The Home-IDEA2 captures a snapshot of the home at a single point in time, similar to a single dietary recall for one person; therefore, the HEI algorithm selected was "Calculating an individual's HEI-2010 score, using FPED, and one day of 24HR recall" [47]. Two nutrient files were created, mirroring the layout of individual dietary intake nutrient analysis files obtained from the Automated Self-Administered 24-h Recall System (ASA24), the INFMYPHEI (Items/Individuals Foods and Pyramid Equivalents Data), and TNMYPHEI (Total/Daily Total Nutrient and Pyramid Equivalents Data) files [48]. The algorithm was then applied to the Home-IDEA2 HEI Score database to generate HEI component and total scores.

2.2. Psychometric Testing on the Home-IDEA2 HEI Score

Extensive validation and psychometric testing was performed to test the functionality of the Home-IDEA2 HEI Score. Face validity was assessed throughout the selection of the representative foods and food amounts. Decisions were made to match the intention of Home-IDEA2 items and to control for foods that might reasonably be found in participants' homes. Content, internal criterion, and construct validity were also tested (Table 3).

Table 3. Development and initial validation of Home-IDEA2 HEI Score.

	Validity Measure	Research Question	Analysis Strategy
Objective 1: Develop an initial Home-IDEA2 HEI Score	Face	Do the representative food items and amounts selected represent the intent of each Home-IDEA2 item? Would the representative foods be reasonably found in the target population homes?	Expert review of representative foods and food amounts, including comparison to standard consumer packaging sizes
Objective 2: Psychometric Testing of Home-IDEA2 HEI Score	Content	Do the representative foods feed into the HEI component and total scores as theorized?	Iterative runs of the HEI-2010 algorithm on the Home-IDEA2 HEI Score Database; each food was removed individually and changes in scores were visually examined
	Criterion	Are there any individual representative foods that impact HEI component or total scores more substantially than other foods?	Iterative runs of the HEI-2010 algorithm on the Home-IDEA2 HEI Score Database; each food was removed individually and changes in scores were visually examined
	Construct	Does the Home-IDEA2 HEI Score identify different home food environments?	Test the Home-IDEA2 HEI Score on five sample Home-IDEA2 checklists representing varying diet patterns (CACFP, DASH, vegetarian, moderately processed, highly processed)

2.2.1. Content and Criterion Validity

Content and internal criterion validity were examined through over 300 rounds of iterative testing in the application of the HEI algorithm to the Home-IDEA2 HEI Score database. Iterative testing involved the removal of each food from the Home-IDEA2 HEI Score database to determine if the representative food was loading into the component scores as theorized (content validity), and to test the individual and cumulative group contributions of each food to component and total scores (internal criterion validity). The effect size was calculated by the percent change in both the component and total score after the removal of each individual food item from the total pattern. Due to the patterning nature of the HEI algorithm, it was necessary to test for inappropriately high effects of individual representative food loadings on component and total scores.

2.2.2. Construct Validity

Construct validity was assessed with five sample Home-IDEA2 checklists that were created to represent various diet patterns ranging from minimally healthful (theorized low HEI score) to very healthful (theorized high HEI score). These patterns included a highly processed pattern, a moderately processed pattern, a vegetarian pattern with minimal processed foods, and two dietary patterns that were used as evidence-based referent groups: the DASH diet [49], and a pattern based on the Dietary Guidelines for Americans (DGA) [50]. To test adherence to the DGA, a Child and Adult Care Food Program (CACFP) weekly menu was used to create the sample checklist. These food patterns were selected to examine sensitivity, and to evaluate if our tool and the resulting quality score would produce different scores for different home food environments. All analyses were conducted using SAS (version 9.4; SAS Institute Inc., Cary, NC, USA). The HEI-2010 algorithm was provided by the National Cancer Institute [40].

3. Results

3.1. Development of an Initial Home-IDEA2 HEI Score

In the process of determining representative foods from the FoodAPS, two Home-IDEA2 items were eliminated. "Unprepared mixes" was eliminated due to the complexity of options available, which did not allow for an accurate selection of a single representative food, and there were no options for "tortilla, other" outside of corn or flour, which were already captured as individual food items. In the process of determining food amounts, two additional Home-IDEA2 items were removed due to a lack of total edible gram (TEG) weights (rice cakes), and a TEG weight that had no comparable consumer purchase size (deer—the TEG from the FoodAPS database represented an entire deer carcass), leaving 104 foods in the Home-IDEA2 HEI Score database.

3.2. Psychometric Testing on the Home-IDEA2 HEI Score

3.2.1. Content and Criterion Validity

In testing content validity, results from iterative testing showed that two foods (those representing chocolate/candy and unsweetened cereal) did not load into component scores as initially hypothesized. Therefore, changes were made to the representative foods initially selected for chocolate/candy and unsweetened cereal to correct component score loading and maintain the original intent of the food within the Home-IDEA2. Inconsistent effects in component outcomes were also observed for processed food items and cooking oils/fats. Food amounts were adjusted to create similar effect sizes on component scores within each food category (e.g., fruits, processed foods, grains, cooking oils).

Iterative testing was then repeated to confirm changes in effect sizes for component and total scores. Internal criterion validity was demonstrated, as each representative food had larger percentage effect sizes in the relevant component score(s) than in the total score (Table 4). Five foods—ramen, brown rice, broccoli, grapes, and vegetable oil—were highlighted, as they were the foods in the

Home-IDEA2 HEI Score database that had the largest impact in a given component score: e.g., Sodium, Whole Grain, Whole Fruit, and Fatty Acid Ratios, respectively. Despite larger changes to component scores, there was no single food that resulted in a change of greater than 5% to the total score. For example, the absence of broccoli from a household yielded a 21.1% negative change to the Greens and Beans component score, but only a negative 1.2% change to the total score. Of the 104 foods in the Home-IDEA2 HEI Score database, 42 affected a change of at least 5% in one or more component scores when removed from analysis. Of those 42 foods, 13 affected a 10–20% change, with 2 affecting over a 20% change (broccoli: −21.1% change in Greens and Beans; vegetable oil: −31.1% change in Fatty Acid Ratio). This demonstrated internal criterion validity with regard to the intent of the algorithm (i.e., component scores represent individual food contribution, whereas the total score represents the overall patterning) [24].

Table 4. Criterion validity testing: percent (%) change values for HEI-2010 components and total score when specified food was removed from the Home-IDEA2 HEI Score database for 5 example foods.

	Percent (%) Change [a]				
HEI-2010 Component	**Ramen**	**Brown Rice**	**Broccoli**	**Grapes**	**Vegetable Oil**
Adequacy					
Total Fruit	2.0	0.7	0.1	−5.3	5.5
Whole Fruit	3.3	1.2	0.1	−10.7	5.1
Total Vegetables	2.0	0.7	−3.8	0.3	5.4
Greens and Beans	0.7	0.3	−21.1	0.1	2.0
Whole Grains	2.2	−7.3	0.1	0.3	5.9
Dairy	2.6	0.9	0.1	0.3	7.0
Total Protein Foods	3.0	1.1	0.1	0.4	8.2
Seafood and Plant Proteins	0.0	0.0	0.0	0.0	0.0
Fatty Acid Ratio	4.2	-0.1	0.0	0.0	−31.1
Moderation					
Refined Grains	5.4	−1.4	−0.1	−0.5	−10.5
Sodium	11.4	−1.7	0.0	−0.6	−12.7
SoFAAS Calories	1.5	−0.9	-0.1	−0.3	−7.0
Total Score	3.4	−0.9	−1.2	−0.9	−4.2

[a] Percent change was calculated relative to the maximum score for each component category, so the values presented are normalized to accurately reflect the correct weighting across categories. For example, if there was a change of 0.05 in a component with a maximum score of 5, the relative percent change is 1.0%, whereas a maximum score of 10 yields a percent change of 0.5%. Positive percent change values indicate that the component or total score has increased (become more aligned with the 2010 DGAs). Negative percent change values indicate that the component or total score has decreased (become less aligned with the 2010 DGAs). Abbreviations: HEI: Healthy Eating Index; Home-IDEA: Home Inventory Describing Eating and Activity; DGA: Dietary Guidelines for Americans; SoFAAS: Solid Fats, Alcohol, Added Sugars.

3.2.2. Construct Validity

The analyses of the five sample HFEs resulted in a range of scores in the expected directions for both component and total scores (Table 5). The highest total scores (out of 100) resulted from the minimally processed/vegetarian (93.8) and DASH (88.9) HFEs and are classified as 'good' (total score >80) according to the Center for Nutrition Policy and Promotion's standardized guidelines for HEI scores [39]. The CACFP HFE resulted in a nearly 'good' score, 78.9, with low scores for the seafood and plant proteins and fatty acid ratio components, as CACFP menus used to create the sample HFE did not include any food items that would contribute to the seafood and plant protein component. Moreover, while the CACFP menus contained substantial dairy (contributing saturated fatty acids to the denominator), they did not include foods that contained MUFAs and PUFAs (the numerator) for the fatty acid ratio component. All other component scores, excluding sodium, were maximized by the CACFP environment, thus indicating a high ability to detect adherence to the DGAs within the bounds of using the Home-IDEA2. The moderately and highly processed HFEs scored lower for most component scores and generated lower total scores (in the 'needs improvement' category and close to 'poor') than the more healthful HFEs, suggesting measurement sensitivity to different patterns in the anticipated directions.

Table 5. Construct validity: five sample home food environments and resulting HEI-2010 component and total scores.

HEI-2010 Components	Maximum Points	Home-IDEA2 (All Foods Present)	Sample Home Food Environments				
			Highly Processed	Moderately Processed	Minimally Processed, Vegetarian	DASH	CACFP
Adequacy							
Total Fruit	5	2.9	2.0	3.0	4.4	3.3	5.0
Whole Fruit	5	4.7	3.7	4.1	5.0	3.6	5.0
Total Vegetables	5	2.8	2.0	3.4	5.0	5.0	5.0
Greens & Beans	5	1.1	2.1	0.0	5.0	5.0	5.0
Whole Grains	10	6.2	0.5	0.5	10.0	8.0	10.0
Dairy	10	7.4	6.1	4.4	4.4	4.0	9.1
Total Protein Foods	5	4.3	4.7	4.3	5.0	5.0	5.0
Seafood & Plant Proteins	5	5.0	5.0	2.6	5.0	5.0	0.0
Fatty Acid Ratio	10	8.1	6.5	10.0	10.0	10.0	0.0
Moderation							
Refined Grains	10	6.2	0.8	5.0	10.0	10.0	10.0
Sodium	10	8.9	6.9	7.7	10.0	10.0	6.4
Empty Calories	20	17.6	15.7	20.0	20.0	20.0	18.4
Total Score [a]	100	75.2	56.0	64.9	93.8	88.9	78.9

[a] The Center for Nutrition Policy and Promotion categorizes total scores as poor (less than 51), needs improvement (51–80), and good (greater than 80) [39]. Abbreviations: HEI: Healthy Eating Index; DASH, Dietary Approaches to Stop Hypertension; CACFP, Child and Adult Care Food Program.

To further examine construct validity, broccoli was included in all five sample HFE patterns; broccoli is the only vegetable in the Home-IDEA2 HEI Score database that contributed to the Greens and Beans component. The Highly Processed sample HFE had non-maximum scores for the Greens and Beans component, whereas the Minimally Processed household, DASH household, and CACFP households scored the maximum of 5. This demonstrated that the presence of a single food within the total patterning of a given household may result in a range of scores within a component.

4. Discussion

In this study, a HFE quality score was developed by applying the HEI to the Home-IDEA2, a validated assessment of the HFE. The development process used to produce the Home-IDEA2 HEI Score mirrored those employed for the HEI-2010 [24] and, therefore, utilized a validated method in which an index of dietary quality was quantitatively applied to foods available in the home environment. Because the HFE is a significant target for efforts focused on prevention of childhood obesity, enhancing researchers' ability to measure multiple environmental correlates, including availability, accessibility, and quality of foods, is critical to understanding children's food behaviors and dietary intake.

Having a comprehensive measure of HFE overall quality in addition to dietary intake quality provides a more complete picture of how the HFE may impact dietary intake at the pattern level, thus aligning HFE research with current trends in dietary intake research examining dietary patterning in addition to individual food groups or nutrients [51–54]. Further, having a validated Home-IDEA2 HEI Score provides several important opportunities for researchers. The Home-IDEA2 HEI Score can be used not only to easily summarize food quality in the home, but to measure the overall quality of the home food environment as an intervention target. Similarly, the score could be used in a larger cohort study for assessing the associations between the quality of the HFE and health outcomes.

Extensive steps were taken to validate the Home-IDEA2 HEI Score at each step of the development process. Examining the relative percent change of individual foods to component and total scores confirmed that the vast majority of representative foods had negligible impact on the total score when considered individually. Because the HEI is designed to measure overall patterning, this was critical, as it demonstrated that no individual food had the power to significantly impact the total score. It should be noted that changes in the presence or absence of foods may reflect changes in the overall categorization of a home's Home-IDEA2 HEI Score as poor (less than 51), needs improvement (51–80), or good (greater than 80) [39]. For example, as Ramen induced a 3.4% change to the total score, it is feasible that a home's overall Home-IDEA2 HEI Score might move above or below these prescribed categories. Construct validity was demonstrated through testing of five sample HFEs, which revealed both total and component scores in the expected directions. Similarly, this analysis resulted in a range of total scores for each of the five sample HFEs (56.0–93.8), indicating that scores ranged from nearly all three standardized HEI rating quality categories: poor, needs improvement, and good [39].

The process of applying the HEI algorithm to the Home-IDEA2 revealed opportunities for improvement of the checklist. First, the Home-IDEA2 was not designed with the HEI in mind, thus, the retrospective application of the HEI identified gaps in the food items included in the checklist. The Home-IDEA2 was unbalanced, with a greater variety and higher number of more healthful foods feeding into the HEI components that make up the adequacy score, compared with fewer options for less healthful/processed food items that contribute to the HEI components contributing to the moderation score. This is highlighted by the Home-IDEA HEI score (Table 5) of 75.2 (out of 100) when all foods were checked as present in the home. Ideally, when both healthful (adequacy) and unhealthful (moderation) foods are adequately represented, the total HEI score should be lower. Future iterations of the checklist should include more options of moderation foods. Similarly, future versions of the Home-IDEA should be designed with the HEI in mind and include multiple food types that represent HEI components (so that the presence of one food, like broccoli, does not create a perfect component score). Further understanding of how the presence or absence of these foods in the home might affect the Home-IDEA2 HEI Score, and whether or not equal representation is given to all food components of the HEI, is warranted.

While the HEI is designed to measure adherence to the U.S. Dietary Guidelines, algorithms for other dietary patterns, such as the DASH diet, the Mediterranean diet, the Alternative HEI, and country/region specific dietary guidelines, could be applied in a similar manner as the HEI to the Home-IDEA2. The process of applying a dietary pattern algorithm to the HFE to develop a quality score has the potential to be replicated to encompass culturally specific eating patterns, or could be used to compare and contrast HFE across countries/regions. Culturally tailoring the Home-IDEA2 or the application of the dietary pattern algorithms to different HFE assessment tools would require content, criterion, and construct validity testing to ensure that the tool and the algorithm were reflecting the intent of the dietary pattern appropriately.

There were limitations and strengths to this study. As mentioned, the predetermined list of foods reduced participant and researcher burden, but the Home-IDEA2 is not all-inclusive and may place limits on capturing the full diversity of foods in the home. The Home-IDEA2 is similar to a single dietary recall for one person, and as such, is subject to the same limitations, such as substantial day-to-day variability. While the checklist has been validated and successfully used in low-income, multi-ethnic families with young children [43,44], food items cover a large portion of foods frequently consumed by all Americans, and future research with other audiences is warranted. The food categories of the Home-IDEA2 were assigned representative foods for nutrient content and food amount using the FoodAPS database, a nationally representative database of U.S. households. However, it should be noted that the selection of representative foods (face validity) was completed by the experts in nutrition and psychometric testing, and, therefore, the subjectivity of these selections is a limitation. Finally, the development and validation procedures for the Home-IDEA2 HEI Score were modeled after USDA recommendations. Extensive validation procedures and psychometric testing were used to ensure that the Home-IDEA2 HEI Score was functioning as intended.

5. Conclusions

The ability to assess the quality of the foods in the home holistically via the application of an HEI score allows for a more complete view of the HFE, and provides a useful form of measurement to future observational and intervention studies working to gain a fuller understanding of the HFE. Previous literature has shown the importance of understanding and measuring the HFE, because of the predictive ability of the availability of food in the home to the types of foods that children eat [16–18]. This study adds to the literature a psychometrically tested and thoroughly validated measure. While this study used an existing instrument, future modifications to the Home-IDEA2 are needed to address the aforementioned limitations, to improve sensitivity and enhance the ability to accurately measure the overall quality of the HFE with a constrained number of food items. The ability to quantify HFE quality in a valid way provides researchers with a methodology to holistically assess families and children's food environments, which may contribute to a greater understanding of dietary intake and, ultimately, health outcomes.

Author Contributions: Conceptualization, S.K.H.-S., R.E.B., S.L.J., and L.L.B.; Methodology, S.K.H.-S., R.E.B., S.L.J., M.L.M., S.H., L.L.B.; Formal Analysis, S.K.H.-S.; Writing—original draft preparation, S.K.H.-S., M.L.M., S.H., L.L.B.; Writing—review and editing, S.K.H.-S., R.E.B., S.L.J., M.L.M., S.H., L.L.B.; Project Administration, S.K.H.-S., R.E.B., L.L.B.; Funding Acquisition, L.L.B., S.L.J., R.E.B.

Acknowledgments: The authors would like to acknowledge John Hurdle and Philip Brewster at the University of Utah for their guidance in the development of the Home-IDEA2 HEI Score.

References

1. Altman, M.; Cahill Holland, J.; Lundeen, D.; Kolko, R.P.; Stein, R.I.; Saelens, B.E.; Welch, R.R.; Perri, M.G.; Schechtman, K.B.; Epstein, L.H.; et al. Reduction in food away from home is associated with improved child relative weight and body composition outcomes and this relation is mediated by changes in diet quality. *J. Acad. Nutr. Diet.* **2015**, *115*, 1400–1407. [CrossRef] [PubMed]
2. Kant, A.K.; Whitley, M.I.; Graubard, B.I. Away from home meals: Associations with biomarkers of chronic disease and dietary intake in American adults, NHANES 2005–2010. *Int. J. Obes. (Lond.)* **2015**, *39*, 820–827. [CrossRef] [PubMed]
3. Couch, S.C.; Glanz, K.; Zhou, C.; Sallis, J.F.; Saelens, B.E. Home food environment in relation to children's diet quality and weight status. *J. Acad. Nutr. Diet.* **2014**, *114*, 1569–1579. [CrossRef] [PubMed]
4. Kirkpatrick, S.I.; Reedy, J.; Kahle, L.L.; Harris, J.L.; Ohri-Vachaspati, P.; Krebs-Smith, S.M. Fast-food menu offerings vary in dietary quality, but are consistently poor. *Public Health Nutr.* **2013**, *17*, 924–931. [CrossRef] [PubMed]
5. Powell, L.M.; Nguyen, B.T. Fast-food and full-service restaurant consumption among children and adolescents: Effect on energy, beverage, and nutrient intake. *JAMA Pediatr.* **2013**, *167*, 14–20. [CrossRef] [PubMed]
6. Stern, D.; Ng, S.W.; Popkin, B.M. The nutrient content of US household food purchases by store type. *Am. J. Prev. Med.* **2016**, *50*, 180–190. [CrossRef] [PubMed]
7. Cavanaugh, E.; Mallya, G.; Brensinger, C.; Tierney, A.; Glanz, K. Nutrition environments in corner stores in Philadelphia. *Prev. Med.* **2013**, *56*, 149–151. [CrossRef]

8. Caspi, C.E.; Pelletier, J.E.; Harnack, L.; Erickson, D.J.; Laska, M.N. Differences in healthy food supply and stocking practices between small grocery stores, gas-marts, pharmacies and dollar stores. *Public Health Nutr.* **2016**, *19*, 540–547. [CrossRef]
9. Aggarwal, A.; Monsivais, P.; Cook, A.J.; Drewnowski, A. Positive attitude toward healthy eating predicts higher diet quality at all cost levels of supermarkets. *J. Acad. Nutr. Diet.* **2014**, *114*, 266–272. [CrossRef]
10. Driessen, C.E.; Cameron, A.J.; Thornton, L.E.; Lai, S.K.; Barnett, L.M. Effect of changes to the school food environment on eating behaviours and/or body weight in children: A systematic review. *Obes. Rev.* **2014**, *15*, 968–982. [CrossRef]
11. Drewnowski, A.; Rehm, C.D. Energy intakes of US children and adults by food purchase location and by specific food source. *Nutr. J.* **2013**, *12*, 59. [CrossRef] [PubMed]
12. Poti, J.M.; Slining, M.M.; Popkin, B.M. Where are kids getting their empty calories? Stores, schools, and fast-food restaurants each played an important role in empty calorie intake among US children during 2009–2010. *J. Acad. Nutr. Diet.* **2014**, *114*, 908–917. [CrossRef] [PubMed]
13. Rosenkranz, R.R.; Dzewaltowski, D.A. Model of the home food environment pertaining to childhood obesity. *Nutr. Rev.* **2008**, *66*, 123–140. [CrossRef] [PubMed]
14. Boles, R.E.; Yun, L.; Hambidge, S.J.; Davidson, A. Influencing the Home Food and Activity Environment of Families of Preschool Children Receiving Home-Based Treatment for Obesity. *Clin. Pediatr.* **2015**, *54*, 1387–1390. [CrossRef] [PubMed]
15. Bekelman, T.A.; Bellows, L.L.; Johnson, S.L. Are Family Routines Modifiable Determinants of Preschool Children's Eating, Dietary Intake, and Growth? A Review of Intervention Studies. *Curr. Nutr. Rep.* **2017**, *6*, 1–19. [CrossRef]
16. Gebremariam, M.K.; Vaqué-Crusellas, C.; Andersen, L.F.; Stok, F.M.; Stelmach-Mardas, M.; Brug, J.; Lien, N. Measurement of availability and accessibility of food among youth: A systematic review of methodological studies. *Int. J. Behav. Nutr. Phys. Act.* **2017**, *14*, 22. [CrossRef] [PubMed]
17. Pearson, N.; Biddle, S.J.; Gorely, T. Family correlates of fruit and vegetable consumption in children and adolescents: A systematic review. *Public Health Nutr.* **2009**, *12*, 267–283. [CrossRef] [PubMed]
18. Neumark-Sztainer, D.; Wall, M.; Perry, C.; Story, M. Correlates of fruit and vegetable intake among adolescents: Findings from Project EAT. *Prev. Med.* **2003**, *37*, 198–208. [CrossRef]
19. Cullen, K.W.; Baranowski, T.; Owens, E.; Marsh, T.; Rittenberry, L.; Moor, C.D. Availability, Accessibility, and Preferences for Fruit, 100% Fruit Juice, and Vegetables Influence Children's Dietary Behavior. *Health. Educ. Behav.* **2003**, *30*, 615–626. [CrossRef]
20. Santiago-Torres, M.; Adams, A.K.; Carrel, A.L.; LaRowe, T.L.; Schoeller, D.A. Home food availability, parental dietary intake, and familial eating habits influence the diet quality of urban Hispanic children. *Child. Obes.* **2014**, *10*, 408–415. [CrossRef]
21. Pinard, C.A.; Yaroch, A.L.; Hart, M.H.; Serrano, E.L.; McFerren, M.M.; Estabrooks, P.A. Measures of the home environment related to childhood obesity: A systematic review. *Public Health Nutr.* **2012**, *15*, 97–109. [CrossRef] [PubMed]
22. Boles, R.E.; Burdell, A.; Johnson, S.L.; Gavin, W.J.; Davies, P.L.; Bellows, L.L. Home food and activity assessment. Development and validation of an instrument for diverse families of young children. *Appetite* **2014**, *80*, 23–27. [CrossRef] [PubMed]
23. Guenther, P.M.; Casavale, K.O.; Reedy, J.; Kirkpatrick, S.I.; Hiza, H.A.; Kuczynski, K.J.; Kahle, L.L.; Krebs-Smith, S.M. Update of the Healthy Eating Index: HEI-2010. *J. Acad. Nutr. Diet.* **2013**, *113*, 569–580. [CrossRef] [PubMed]
24. Guenther, P.M.; Kirkpatrick, S.I.; Reedy, J.; Krebs-Smith, S.M.; Buckman, D.W.; Dodd, K.W.; Casavale, K.O.; Carroll, R.J. The Healthy Eating Index-2010 is a valid and reliable measure of diet quality according to the 2010 Dietary Guidelines for Americans. *J. Nutr.* **2014**, *144*, 399–407. [CrossRef] [PubMed]
25. Miller, P.E.; Reedy, J.; Kirkpatrick, S.I.; Krebs-Smith, S.M. The United States Food Supply Is Not Consistent with Dietary Guidance: Evidence from an Evaluation Using the Healthy Eating Index-2010. *J. Acad. Nutr. Diet.* **2015**, *115*, 95–100. [CrossRef] [PubMed]
26. Byker, C.; Smith, T. Food assistance programs for children afford mixed dietary quality based on HEI-2010. *Nutr. Res.* **2015**, *35*, 35–40. [CrossRef] [PubMed]

27. Jahns, L.; Scheett, A.J.; Johnson, L.K.; Krebs-Smith, S.M.; Payne, C.R.; Whigham, L.D.; Hoverson, B.S.; Kranz, S. Diet Quality of Items Advertised in Supermarket Sales Circulars Compared to Diets of the US Population, as Assessed by the Healthy Eating Index-2010. *J. Acad. Nutr. Diet.* **2016**, *116*, 115–122. [CrossRef] [PubMed]
28. He, M.; Tucker, P.; Irwin, J.D.; Gilliland, J.; Larsen, K.; Hess, P. Obesogenic neighbourhoods: The impact of neighbourhood restaurants and convenience stores on adolescents' food consumption behaviours. *Public Health Nutr.* **2012**, *15*, 2331–2339. [CrossRef] [PubMed]
29. Appelhans, B.M.; French, S.A.; Tangney, C.C.; Powell, L.M.; Wang, Y. To what extent do food purchases reflect shoppers' diet quality and nutrient intake? *Int. J. Behav. Nutr. Phys. Act.* **2017**, *14*, 46. [CrossRef]
30. Wilson, M.; Krebs-Smith, S.; Reedy, J.; Story, M.; Britten, P.; Juan, W. Diet Quality, Measured Using the Healthy Eating Index-2010, Varies by Source Where Food is Obtained in the United States. *FASEB J.* **2016**, *30*, 409.6.
31. Rehm, C.D.; Monsivais, P.; Drewnowski, A. Relation between diet cost and Healthy Eating Index 2010 scores among adults in the United States 2007–2010. *Prev. Med.* **2015**, *73*, 70–75. [CrossRef]
32. Clarys, P.; Deliens, T.; Huybrechts, I.; Deriemaeker, P.; Vanaelst, B.; De Keyzer, W.; Hebbelinck, M.; Mullie, P. Comparison of Nutritional Quality of the Vegan, Vegetarian, Semi-Vegetarian, Pesco-Vegetarian and Omnivorous Diet. *Nutrients* **2014**, *6*, 1318. [CrossRef] [PubMed]
33. Wang, D.D.; Leung, C.W.; Li, Y.; Ding, E.L.; Chiuve, S.E.; Hu, F.B.; Willett, W.C. Trends in dietary quality among adults in the united states, 1999 through 2010. *JAMA Intern. Med.* **2014**, *174*, 1587–1595. [CrossRef] [PubMed]
34. Harmon, B.E.; Boushey, C.J.; Shvetsov, Y.B.; Ettienne, R.; Reedy, J.; Wilkens, L.R.; Le Marchand, L.; Henderson, B.E.; Kolonel, L.N. Associations of key diet-quality indexes with mortality in the Multiethnic Cohort: The Dietary Patterns Methods Project. *Am. J. Clin. Nutr.* **2015**, *101*, 587–597. [CrossRef] [PubMed]
35. Liese, A.D.; Krebs-Smith, S.M.; Subar, A.F.; George, S.M.; Harmon, B.E.; Neuhouser, M.L.; Boushey, C.J.; Schap, T.E.; Reedy, J. The Dietary Patterns Methods Project: Synthesis of Findings across Cohorts and Relevance to Dietary Guidance. *J. Nutr.* **2015**, *145*, 93–402. [CrossRef] [PubMed]
36. Reedy, J.; Krebs-Smith, S.M.; Miller, P.E.; Liese, A.D.; Kahle, L.L.; Park, Y.; Subar, A.F. Higher Diet Quality Is Associated with Decreased Risk of All-Cause, Cardiovascular Disease, and Cancer Mortality among Older Adults. *J. Nutr.* **2014**, *144*, 881–889. [CrossRef] [PubMed]
37. Kong, A.; Schiffer, L.; Antonic, M.; Braunschweig, C.; Odoms-Young, A.; Fitzgibbon, M. The relationship between home-and individual-level diet quality among African American and Hispanic/Latino households with young children. *Int. J. Behav. Nutr. Phys. Act.* **2018**, *15*, 5. [CrossRef] [PubMed]
38. U.S. Department of Health & Human Services and U.S. Department of Agriculture. Dietary Guidelines for Americans: 2015–2020. Available online: http://health.gov/dietaryguidelines/2015/guidelines/ (accessed on 27 September 2017).
39. Basiotis, P.P.; Carlson, A.; Gerrior, S.A.; Juan, W.Y.; Lino, M. The Healthy Eating Index: 1999–2000. U.S. Department of Agriculture, Center for Nutrition Policy and Promotion, 2002. Available online: https://www.cnpp.usda.gov/sites/default/files/healthy_eating_index/HEI99-00report.pdf (accessed on 7 February 2019).
40. National Institutes for Health and National Cancer Institute: HEI Tools for Researchers. Available online: https://epi.grants.cancer.gov/hei/calculating-hei-scores.html (accessed on 11 February 2019).
41. National Institutes for Health and National Cancer Institute: Developing the Healthy Eating Index. Available online: https://epi.grants.cancer.gov/hei/developing.html#f1a (accessed on 11 February 2019).
42. Guenther, P.M.; Reedy, J.; Krebs-Smith, S.M.; Reeve, B.B.; Basiotis, P.P. Development and evaluation of the healthy eating index-2005. *J. Am. Diet. Assoc.* **2008**, *108*, 1896–1901. [CrossRef] [PubMed]
43. Boles, R.E.; Johnson, S.L.; Burdell, A.; Davies, P.L.; Gavin, W.J.; Bellows, L.L. Home food availability and child intake among rural families identified to be at-risk for health disparities. *Appetite* **2019**, *34*, 135–141. [CrossRef] [PubMed]
44. Bellows, L.L.; Boles, R.E.; Hibbs-Shipp, S.K.; Burdell, A.; Johnson, S.L. Development of a Comprehensive Checklist to Capture Food, Physical Activity and Sedentary Devices in the Home Environment: The Home Inventory Describing Eating and Activity (Home-IDEA2). *J. Nutr. Educ. Behav.* **2019**, in press. [CrossRef] [PubMed]

45. National Institutes for Health and National Cancer Institute: Research Uses of the HEI; HEI Scoring Illustration. Available online: https://epi.grants.cancer.gov/hei/uses.html#differentlevels (accessed on 11 February 2019).
46. United States Department of Agriculture and Economic Research Service. FoodAPS: National Household Food Acquisition and Purchase Survey. Available online: https://www.ers.usda.gov/foodaps (accessed on 26 April 2017).
47. National Institutes for Health and National Cancer Institute: Healthy Eating Index SAS Code. Available online: https://epi.grants.cancer.gov/hei/tools.html (accessed on 11 February 2019).
48. National Institutes for Health and National Cancer Institute: ASA24 Researcher Website. Available online: https://asa24.nci.nih.gov/researchersite/ (accessed on 11 February 2019).
49. Dash Diet Eating Plan. The Dash Diet Eating Plan, Dash Diet Recipes. Available online: https://www.nhlbi.nih.gov/files/docs/public/heart/new_dash.pdf (accessed on 6 October 2017).
50. U.S. Department of Health and Human Services and U.S. Department of Agriculture. 2010–2015. Dietary Guidelines for Americans. December 2010. Available online: https://health.gov/dietaryguidelines/2010/ (accessed on 30 January 2019).
51. Hu, F.B. Dietary pattern analysis: A new direction in nutritional epidemiology. *Curr. Opin. Lipidol.* **2002**, *13*, 3–9. [CrossRef] [PubMed]
52. Jacobs, D.R.; Steffen, L.M. Nutrients, foods, and dietary patterns as exposures in research: A framework for food synergy. *Am. J. Clin. Nutr.* **2003**, *78*, 508S–513S. [CrossRef] [PubMed]
53. Jannasch, F.; Kröger, J.; Schulze, M.B. Dietary Patterns and Type 2 Diabetes: A Systematic Literature Review and Meta-Analysis of Prospective Studies. *J. Nutr.* **2017**, *147*, 1174–1182. [CrossRef] [PubMed]
54. Cespedes, E.M.; Hu, F.B.; Tinker, L.; Rosner, B.; Redline, S.; Garcia, L.; Hingle, M.; Van Horn, L.; Howard, B.V.; Levitan, E.B.; et al. Multiple healthful dietary patterns and type 2 diabetes in the Women's Health Initiative. *Am. J. Epidemiol.* **2016**, *183*, 622–633. [CrossRef] [PubMed]

4

Socioeconomic Disparities in Diet Vary According to Migration Status among Adolescents in Belgium

Manon Rouche [1,*], Bart de Clercq [2], Thérésa Lebacq [1,3], Maxim Dierckens [2], Nathalie Moreau [1,3], Lucille Desbouys [1], Isabelle Godin [4] and Katia Castetbon [1,3]

1 Research Center in Epidemiology, Biostatistics and Clinical Research, School of Public Health, Université libre de Bruxelles (ULB), 1040 Brussels, Belgium; theresa.lebacq@ulb.ac.be (T.L.); nathalie.moreau@ulb.ac.be (N.M.); lucille.desbouys@ulb.ac.be (L.D.); katia.castetbon@ulb.ac.be (K.C.)

2 Department of Public Health and Primary Care, Ghent University (UGent), 9000 Ghent, Belgium; b.declercq@ugent.be (B.d.C.); maxim.dierckens@ugent.be (M.D.)

3 Service d'Information Promotion Education Santé (SIPES), School of Public Health, Université libre de Bruxelles (ULB), 1040 Brussels, Belgium

4 Research Centre in Social Approaches to Health, School of Public Health, Université libre de Bruxelles (ULB), 1040 Brussels, Belgium; isabelle.godin@ulb.ac.be

* Correspondence: manon.rouche@ulb.ac.be

Abstract: Little information concerning social disparities in adolescent dietary habits is currently available, especially regarding migration status. The aim of the present study was to estimate socioeconomic disparities in dietary habits of school adolescents from different migration backgrounds. In the 2014 cross-sectional "Health Behavior in School-Aged Children" survey in Belgium, food consumption was estimated using a self-administrated short food frequency questionnaire. In total, 19,172 school adolescents aged 10–19 years were included in analyses. Multilevel multiple binary and multinomial logistic regressions were performed, stratified by migration status (natives, 2nd- and 1st-generation immigrants). Overall, immigrants more frequently consumed both healthy and unhealthy foods. Indeed, 32.4% of 1st-generation immigrants, 26.5% of 2nd-generation immigrants, and 16.7% of natives consumed fish ≥two days a week. Compared to those having a high family affluence scale (FAS), adolescents with a low FAS were more likely to consume chips and fries ≥once a day (vs. <once a day: Natives aRRR = 1.39 (95%CI: 1.12–1.73); NS in immigrants). Immigrants at schools in Flanders were less likely than those in Brussels to consume sugar-sweetened beverages 2–6 days a week (vs. ≤once a week: Natives aRRR = 1.86 (95%CI: 1.32–2.62); 2nd-generation immigrants aRRR = 1.52 (1.11–2.09); NS in 1st-generation immigrants). The migration gradient observed here underlines a process of acculturation. Narrower socioeconomic disparities in immigrant dietary habits compared with natives suggest that such habits are primarily defined by culture of origin. Nutrition interventions should thus include cultural components of dietary habits.

Keywords: migration status; dietary habits; food frequency questionnaire; socioeconomic disparities; adolescents

---

1. Introduction

High consumption of foods such as chips and fries [1] and sugar-sweetened beverages (SSB) [2] might be associated with increased noncommunicable diseases (NCD); by contrast, adequate consumption of fruits, vegetables [2,3], fish [2], and dairy products [4] might reduce NCD and all-cause mortality. Furthermore, it has been estimated that up to two-thirds of NCD social inequalities may be explained by dietary disparities [5,6].

In addition, evidence indicates that dietary habits during adolescence may continue into adulthood [7–9]. To implement effective prevention of NCD throughout the lifetime, disparities in adolescent eating behavior warrant elucidation. However, information on this topic is scarce in Western countries. Although several studies have pointed out the association between dietary habits and socioeconomic status (SES) among adolescents [10,11], SES may not explain all observed variations.

Among other determinants of dietary habits, migration status may play a role [12,13]; however, published studies are rare, even among adults, and are often oriented towards a specific ethnic group [12,13]. Studies on health related to migration have revealed a mortality advantage in immigrants compared to natives, despite the lower SES of most immigrants [14]. This paradox could be explained by the "healthy-migrant effect", i.e., positive self-selection, and an unhealthy return-migration effect, also known as the "salmon-bias hypothesis" [14]. However, these selection processes are subject to caution; "beneficial cultural and behavioral factors", like dietary habits, may be the most plausible explanation for this paradox [14]. The immigrant health advantage may also tend to wear off with length of stay in the host country, mostly due to an acculturation process [15,16], wherein foreign individuals partially integrate behaviors and cultural aspects of the host population while maintaining their roots [17]. This has been highlighted in some adult dietary studies and suggests gradual adaptation to the natives' eating habits according to years spent in the host country [18]. In adolescents, dietary habits varying according to migration status (including a gradient across migration generations) might also be expected, but such investigations have thus far been limited [19,20].

An effect modification between migration status and socioeconomic characteristics was emphasized in a previous study on adult self-rated health: A gradient was revealed across social classes in natives, which was not the case for immigrants from poor countries [21]. Similarly, in adolescents, a clear gradient throughout family affluence categories was observed for health-related quality of life in natives but not in immigrants [22]. Therefore, a possible effect modification of migration status on socioeconomic characteristics should be considered when evaluating disparities in dietary habits.

The aim of this study was to estimate socioeconomic disparities in dietary habits of school adolescents from different migration backgrounds. We first hypothesized that adolescent immigrants have healthier dietary habits than natives and that food consumption frequencies increase or decrease gradually according to the migration generation, related to an acculturation process. Secondly, we assumed that migration status might modify the association between socioeconomic characteristics and dietary habits in adolescents.

2. Materials and Methods

Research was carried out using data from the "Health Behavior in School-Aged Children" (HBSC) survey conducted in 2014 in Belgium. The cross-national HBSC survey takes place every four years in around 40 countries in Europe and North America under the aegis of the World Health Organization (WHO) Regional Office for Europe. Its goal is to produce comprehensive indicators supporting implementation of health prevention and promotion policies and interventions. Questionnaires are self-administrated in the classroom, and anonymity and data confidentiality are guaranteed [23].

Belgium has a regionalized administration in which wide demographic variations are observed, including those concerning migration. In 2014 in Belgium, this study was carried out separately in French- and Dutch-speaking schools covering the three regions, Wallonia, Flanders, and Brussels, with the latter including both French- and Dutch-speaking schools.

This survey was carried out according to guidelines articulated in the Declaration of Helsinki. For French-speaking schools, the survey was approved by school authorities. This protocol was not submitted to a medical ethics committee in view of the topics and methods used for data collection (Belgian law of May 7, 2004 and Advisory Committee on Bioethics of Belgium, opinion n°40, 12/2/2007). For Dutch-speaking schools, the study was approved by the ethics review committee of the University Hospital of Ghent (project EC/2013/1145). Following advice from school authorities, no written consent was requested for French-speaking schools; for the Dutch-speaking schools, consent was passive. Adolescents were clearly informed about survey content and about their full right to refuse to fill out the questionnaire or answer specific questions. All procedures used during data collection enabled confidentiality and anonymity.

2.1. Sampling

The French- and Dutch-speaking surveys were conducted on a random sample stratified proportionally with the school networks and included public and private schools. In addition, in the French-speaking part, the sample was stratified proportionally with the province ($n = 6$); in the Dutch-speaking part, it was stratified proportionally with the form of education (ordinary, general, technical, vocational, art secondary education, and non-native newcomer classes).

In all regions, schools were first randomly selected based on an official list. Next, classes from fifth grade elementary school (corresponding to adolescents aged $\pm$ 10 years) to the final grade of the secondary school (corresponding to adolescents aged $\pm$ 18 years) were selected in each grade among the schools that agreed to participate in the study. All adolescents from selected classes were invited to participate on a voluntary basis. In French-speaking schools, classes were randomly selected. In Dutch-speaking schools, distributions of gender, grade, and form of education from the previous survey were used as temporary proxies to select classes.

In 2014, 781 schools in the French-speaking schools and 208 schools in the Dutch-speaking schools were invited to participate. Among these schools, 168 in the French- and 98 in the Dutch-speaking areas actually participated, corresponding, respectively, to a participation rate of 21.5% and 47.1%.

In total, 23,552 questionnaires were collected (Figure 1). Since, in Dutch-speaking schools, adolescents aged 20 or over were not questioned, only adolescents 10 to 19 years old were included in the joint database ($n = 23{,}031$). The basis sample included all participants who responded to all covariates and to the food consumption variable that was most frequently filled in, i.e., fruits. Thus, the maximum number of adolescents included in the analyses was 19,172 (Figure 1). For food consumption other than fruits, the sample size was slightly lower.

2.2. Measures

Food Frequency Questionnaire. Food data were collected using a validated short food frequency questionnaire (FFQ) [24,25] that included a total of 22 food groups (17 in the Dutch part, 18 in the French part, including 13 in common). Seven answer categories were proposed: "more than once a day"; "once a day"; "5–6 days a week"; "2–4 days a week"; "once a week"; "less than once a week"; and "never".

Migration status. Adolescents born abroad and whose parents were not both born in Belgium were considered "1st-generation immigrants". Adolescents born in Belgium and who had at least one parent born abroad were considered "2nd-generation immigrants". Adolescents whose parents were born in Belgium were considered to be "natives".

Geographical area of origin. Based on countries of origin of adolescents for 1st-generation immigrants and of parents for 2nd-generation immigrants, five categories were defined for complementary analyses: (1) Europe; (2) America; (3) Asia; (4) Middle East and North Africa; (5) Sub-Saharan Africa. For 2nd-generation immigrants, in the particular case where the parents were from two different geographical areas, the category was randomly chosen between the mother's and the father's area of origin.

Family affluence. The family affluence scale (FAS) is composed of six items and has been validated in Europe [26]. The FAS score ranged from 0 to 13 and was divided into three categories after ridit analysis transformation—"low", "medium", and "high"—corresponding, in the national sample, to the 20% of adolescents with the lowest FAS scores, the 60% of adolescents with the intermediate score, and the 20% of adolescents with the highest FAS scores, respectively.

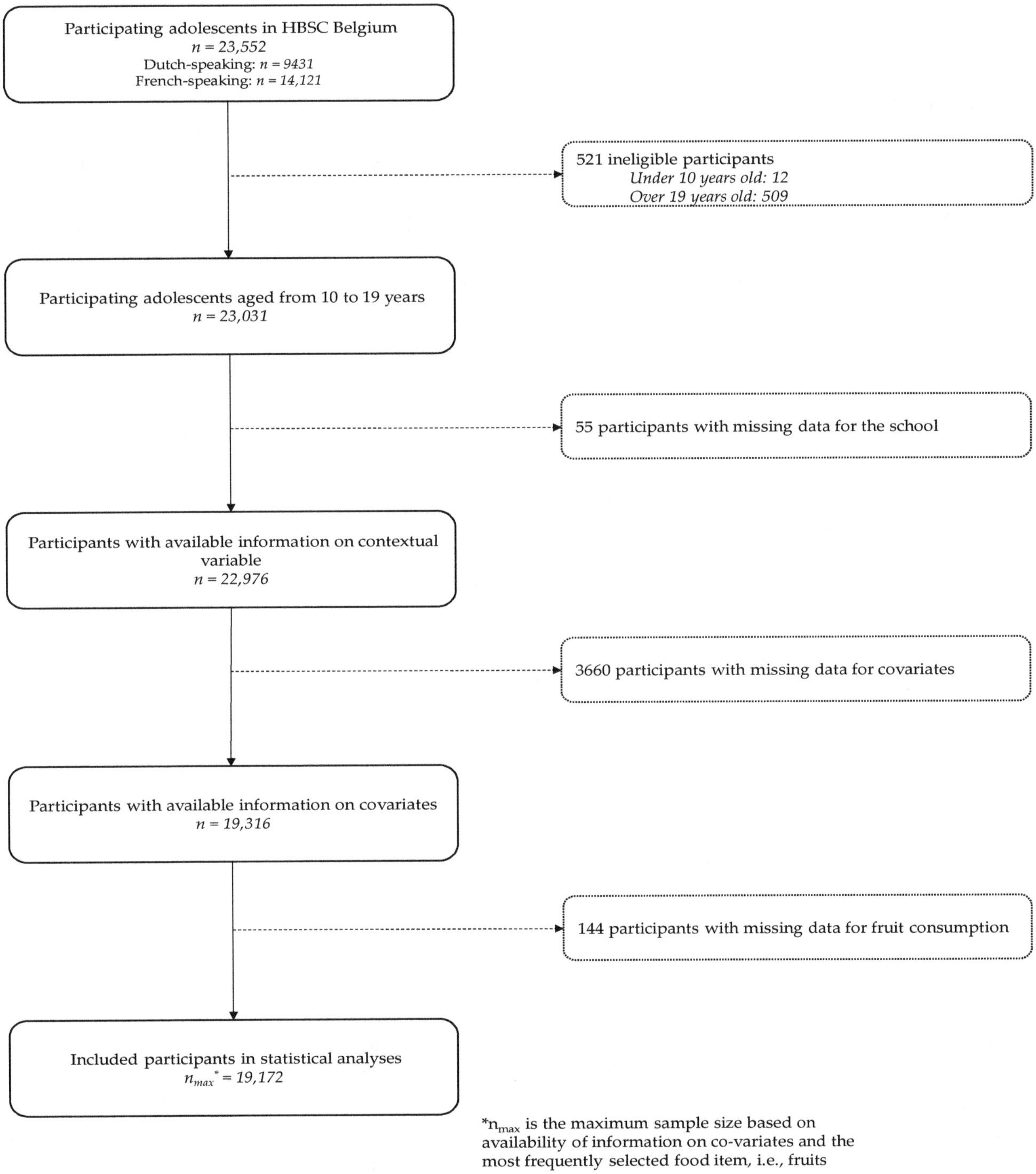

Figure 1. Inclusion diagram of adolescents in Belgium, "Health Behavior in School-Aged Children" (HBSC), 2014.

Parental working status. Based on parental employment and reason for parental unemployment, four categories were defined: (1) Adolescents with both parents working; (2) adolescents with parent(s) not working (those with a parent not working and without a second parent were placed in this category (n = 365)); (3) adolescents with one working parent and the other at home (housewife/husband, pre-retired, disabled or student); (4) adolescents with one working parent and the other "absent" from home (seeking a job, or adolescent not living with the second parent).

In addition, gender, age, family structure, siblings, and school region were taken into account in the analyses.

2.3. *Statistical Analyses*

2.3.1. Reprocessing Data

For all food items, categorization was defined so as to correspond as closely as possible to Belgian nutritional policies [27] but was also determined by the original answer modalities. Food consumption was first divided into three categories: A category corresponding as closely as possible to the Belgian nutritional policies, a category further removed from Belgian nutritional policies, and an intermediate category. If the intermediate category did not provide additional information, categorization was reduced to two categories. Frequency of *fruit and vegetable consumption* was classified into three categories: ">once a day", "5–7 days a week" (low frequency), and "<5 days a week" (very low frequency). Frequency of *fish consumption* was classified into: "≥two days a week" and "<two days a week" (low frequency). Milk (whole and semi-skimmed/skimmed), cheese, and other dairy product frequencies were transformed into consumption per month of 30 days and added up to obtain frequency of *dairy consumption*; this was then divided into total consumption of 31 days or more, which corresponded to consumption ">once a day", or else to consumption "≤once a day" (low frequency). Consumption of chips and fries and SSB was similarly processed. Frequency of *chips and fries* consumption was classified into: "<once a day", strictly corresponding to consumption under 25 days, and "≥once a day" (high frequency). Frequency of *SSB consumption* was classified into: "≤once a week", corresponding to total consumption under 5 days, "2–6 days a week" (high frequency) and "≥once a day" (very high frequency), corresponding to a total of 25 days or more.

2.3.2. Modeling

Due to a significant effect modification of migration status on several covariates for each food group analyzed, analyses were stratified by migration status. Since individuals were nested within schools, multilevel models were used. In each model for each food group, the school effect was controlled and estimated. The "null" model referred to the estimation of the school effect. Associations between covariates and a given food consumption were then evaluated by univariate regression, corresponding to "model 1". Multilevel binary logistic regression was performed for food groups with consumption frequencies in two categories (odds ratio (OR) and 95% CI); multilevel multinomial logistic regression was used for food groups with consumption frequencies falling into three categories (relative risk ratio (RRR) and 95%CI). The reference category was assumed to be the most favorable category in terms of health. All covariates with a p value < 0.20 were included in the initial multivariable regression model. Manual backward stepwise selection was used to determine the final model: It consisted of iteratively removing the predictor with the highest p value, and higher than 0.05. Following removal, confounding was evaluated with a tolerance threshold for variation of OR and RRR set at 10%. If variation was greater than 10%, the variable was then retained in the model. In order to facilitate comparisons between migration strata, a predictor significantly associated with food consumption in a given migration status group was retained for all other migration status groups. The results of the regressions are graphically presented and available as supplementary tables (Supplementary Tables S1–S6).

In order to estimate the role of the immigrants' geographical area of origin on socioeconomic and sociodemographic disparities, the same modeling was carried out only in immigrant adolescents and adjusted for the geographical area of origin.

Colinearity and fitting of models were verified. Statistical significance of tests was set at 0.05. All analyses were performed using Stata/IC 14® (StataCorp, College Station, TX, USA).

3. Results

The sample of 19,172 school participants included 69.6% natives, 22.0% 2nd-generation immigrants, and 8.4% 1st-generation immigrants. In univariate analyses, differences in sociodemographic and socioeconomic characteristics were observed according to migration status (Table 1).

Table 1. Sociodemographic and socioeconomic characteristics of the sample overall and by migration status—HBSC, Belgium, 2014.

Variables	Sample (n = 19,172) %	Natives (n = 13,353) %	2nd-Generation Immigrants (n = 4214) %	1st-Generation Immigrants (n = 1605) %	p value
Gender					<0.001 †
Boys	50.6	51.5	47.5	51.7	
Girls	49.4	48.5	52.5	48.3	
Age					<0.001 ¥
10–12 years	28.8	29.6	28.7	22.5	
13–16 years	50.2	49.9	50.6	51.4	
17–19 years	21.0	20.5	20.7	26.1	
Family structure [a]					<0.001
Two parents	66.4	66.1	67.9	65.0	
Blended family	14.1	15.8	9.9	12.0	
Single-parent family	19.5	18.1	22.2	23.0	
Family Affluence Scale [a]					<0.001
High	19.4	20.6	17.0	16.4	
Medium	63.7	66.1	59.8	53.6	
Low	16.9	13.3	23.2	30.0	
Parental working status [a]					<0.001
Both parents working	68.4	76.1	51.9	47.0	
One working, the other at home	17.4	13.4	27.8	23.7	
One working, the other not at home	8.1	7.2	8.5	14.0	
None working	6.1	3.3	11.8	15.3	
Siblings					<0.001 †
Single child	9.3	9.8	7.5	10.5	
Siblings	90.7	90.2	92.5	89.5	
School Region					<0.001
Brussels-Capital	11.4	3.4	29.2	31.7	
Wallonia	46.6	48.7	43.0	38.2	
Flanders	42.0	47.9	27.8	30.1	
Geographical area of origin					<0.001 *
Europe			43.7	59.8	
America			3.0	6.7	
Asia			7.3	7.7	
Middle East and South Africa			36.0	13.1	
Sub-Saharan Africa			10.0	12.7	

[a] For details, see *Methods* section, † Nonsignificant difference between natives and 1st-generation immigrants, ¥ Nonsignificant difference between natives and 2nd-generation immigrants, * Comparison between 1st- and 2nd-generation immigrants.

Irrespective of migration status, one adolescent out of five ate fruits (17.2%) or vegetables (18.8%) >once a day and fish ≥two days a week (20.2%) (data not tabulated). Eight pupils out of ten (79.6%) ate dairy products >once a day. Nearly half of the adolescents (43.7%) drank SSB ≥once a day; fewer than one-eighth (12.2%) ate chips and fries ≥once a day (data not tabulated).

Immigrants significantly more often ate fruits (>once a day and 5–7 days a week), vegetables (>once a day) and fish (≥two days a week) than did natives (Figure 2). In addition, immigrants significantly more often consumed SSB (≥once a day), and chips and fries (≥once a day) than natives. Moreover, the proportion of 2nd-generation immigrants having low or very low intake of vegetables, fish, chips and fries was significantly at an intermediate level, i.e., higher (or lower) than that of natives, and lower (or higher) than that of 1st-generation immigrants. However, a significant difference in dairy product consumption was observed only between 2nd-generation immigrants and natives (Figure 2).

In immigrants only, and compared with immigrants from a European country, statistically significant differences in food consumption frequencies were found in those from the Middle East and North Africa areas, and from sub-Saharan Africa, for vegetable, fish, dairy, chips and fries, and SSB (Supplementary Table S7). Immigrants from America also slightly differed regarding SSB and chips and fries consumption, and those from Asia for chips and fries consumption. Overall, estimates of the SES characteristics were not modified by the addition of origins in the modeling except only for siblings in 1st-generation immigrants for chips and fries consumption (data not shown).

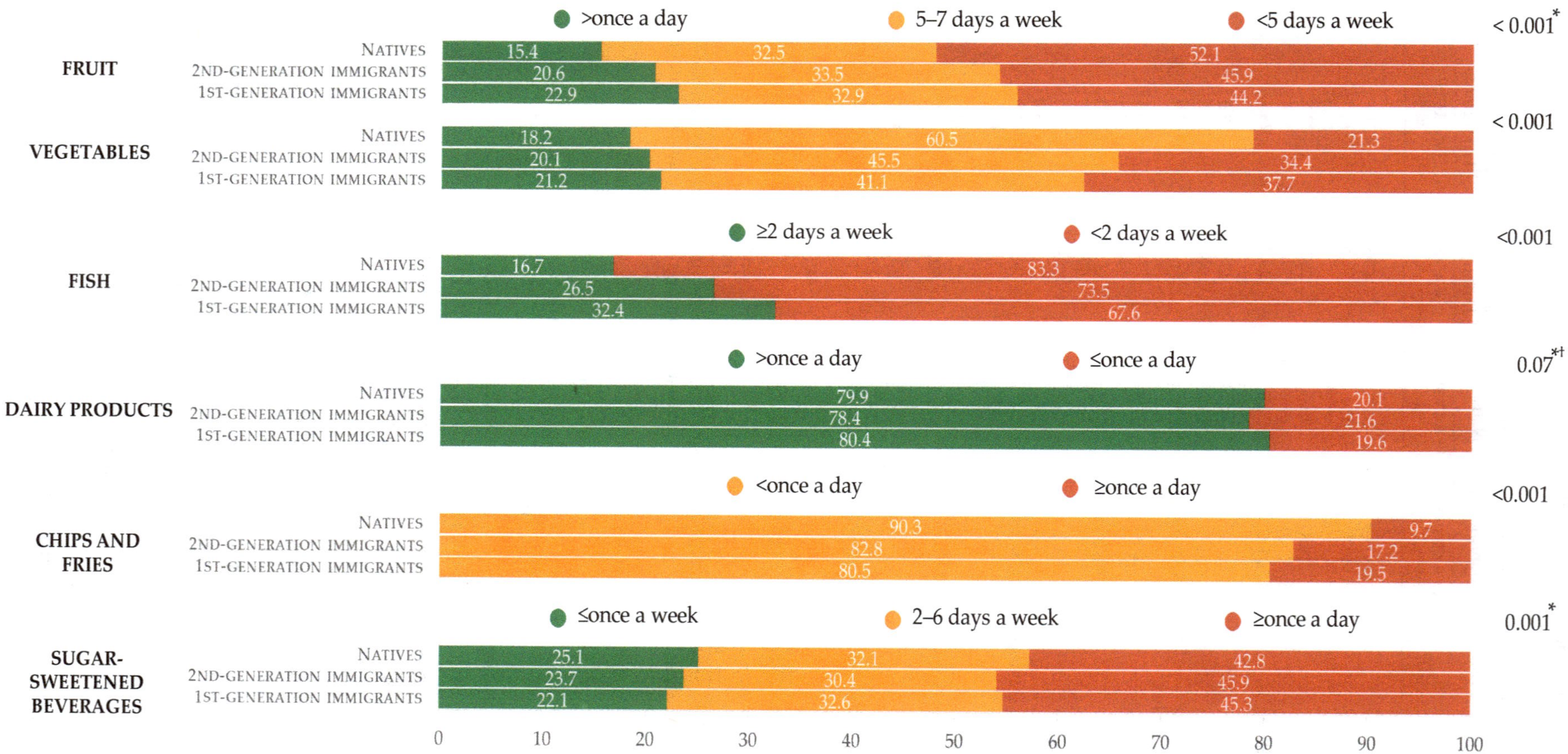

Figure 2. Distribution of food consumption frequencies by migration status in the sample, HBSC, Belgium, 2014. Favorable, moderately favorable, and unfavorable behaviors are represented, respectively, in green, orange, and red. * Nonsignificant difference between 2nd- and 1st-generation immigrants, † nonsignificant difference between natives and 1st-generation immigrants.

3.1. *Fruit Consumption (Reference Category: >Once a Day)*

In all migration strata, the likelihood of very low fruit consumption frequency (<5 days a week) significantly decreased with the FAS (except in 1st-generation immigrants: NS for medium FAS vs. high FAS) (Figure 3). In addition, natives having a medium FAS were more likely to eat fruits 5–7 days a week (low frequency) than those with a high FAS. Native adolescents in blended families were more likely to declare very low or low fruit consumption compared to adolescents with two parents; native adolescents in single-parent families also had greater odds of very low frequency. There was no significant association with parental working status. In all migration strata, adolescents in Flanders were significantly more likely to declare low or very low fruit consumption than adolescents in Brussels-Capital (Figure 3).

Moreover, age was significantly associated with fruit consumption frequency in all migration strata (Figure 3). This was also the case for gender in natives and 2nd-generation immigrants, whereas the existence of siblings was associated with fruit consumption frequency only in natives. The school effect upon the very low fruit consumption of all migration groups was significant, as was its effect upon the low frequency found in natives (Figure 3).

3.2. *Vegetable Consumption (Reference Category: >Once a Day)*

In natives and 1st-generation immigrants only, the odds of very low vegetable consumption frequency (<5 days a week) decreased with FAS (Figure 4). The same applied to low frequency (5–7 days a week) in natives. In 2nd-generation immigrants, adolescents having a medium FAS were more likely to declare very low or low vegetable consumption than those with a high FAS; in addition, adolescents having a low FAS were more likely to eat vegetables <5 days a week.

Compared with adolescents with two parents, native adolescents from a single-parent family were at greater odds of consuming vegetables <5 days a week (Figure 4). Native adolescents with two working parents were more likely to declare a low frequency than adolescents with one parent who worked and the other who stayed at home. Moreover, 2nd-generation immigrants with both working parents were less likely to declare a very low frequency. Compared with adolescents in Brussels-Capital, adolescents in Flanders were more likely to eat vegetables 5–7 days a week in all migration strata; in addition, immigrants in Flanders were more likely to declare a very low frequency, whereas 2nd-generation immigrants in Wallonia were less likely to do so (Figure 4).

Gender was significantly associated with vegetable consumption frequency in all migration strata. This was also the case for age in natives and 2nd-generation immigrants, while the existence of siblings was associated only in natives. The school effect was significant only in natives (Figure 4).

3.3. *Fish Consumption (Reference Category: ≥Two Days a Week)*

In natives and 2nd-generation immigrants, the likelihood of eating fish at low frequency (<two days a week) decreased with FAS. Moreover, low fish consumption was more frequent in adolescents from blended families than in those having two parents (Figure 5). Compared with adolescents with one working parent and the other who stayed at home, 2nd-generation immigrants with no working parents were less likely to eat fish at low frequency. In 1st-generation immigrants, adolescents whose parents both worked were more likely to declare low fish-eating frequency. For all migration strata, compared with Brussels-Capital, adolescents in Flanders and Wallonia were significantly more likely to declare low frequency (Figure 5).

In addition, gender was significantly associated with fish consumption frequency in natives and 2nd-generation immigrants. The school effect was significant in natives and 2nd-generation immigrants.

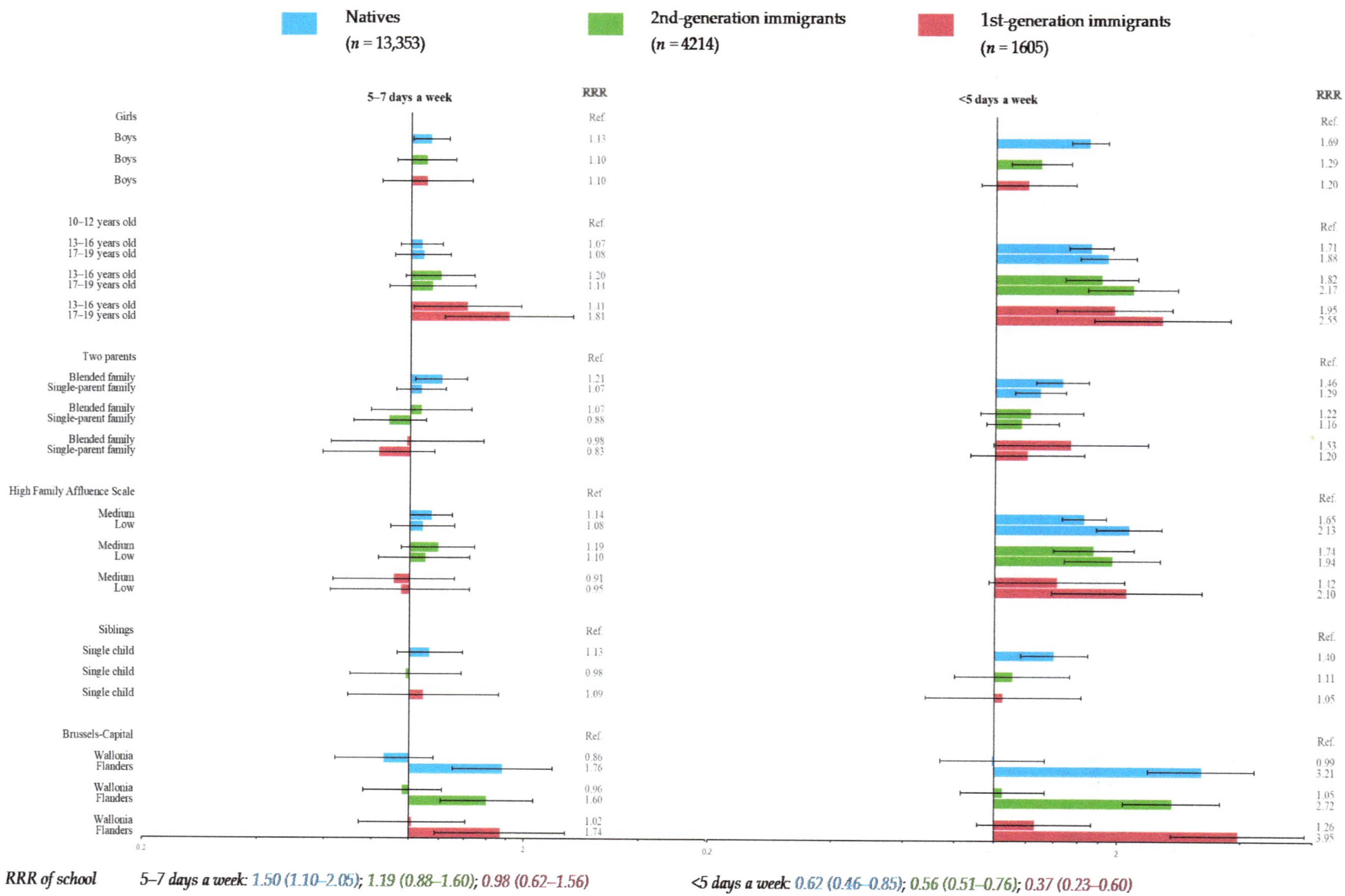

Figure 3. Multiple multilevel multinomial regression* for fruit consumption (reference category: >once a day) stratified by migration status—HBSC, Belgium, 2014 (n = 19,172). * RRR < 1: More favorable for health; RRR > 1: Less favorable for health.

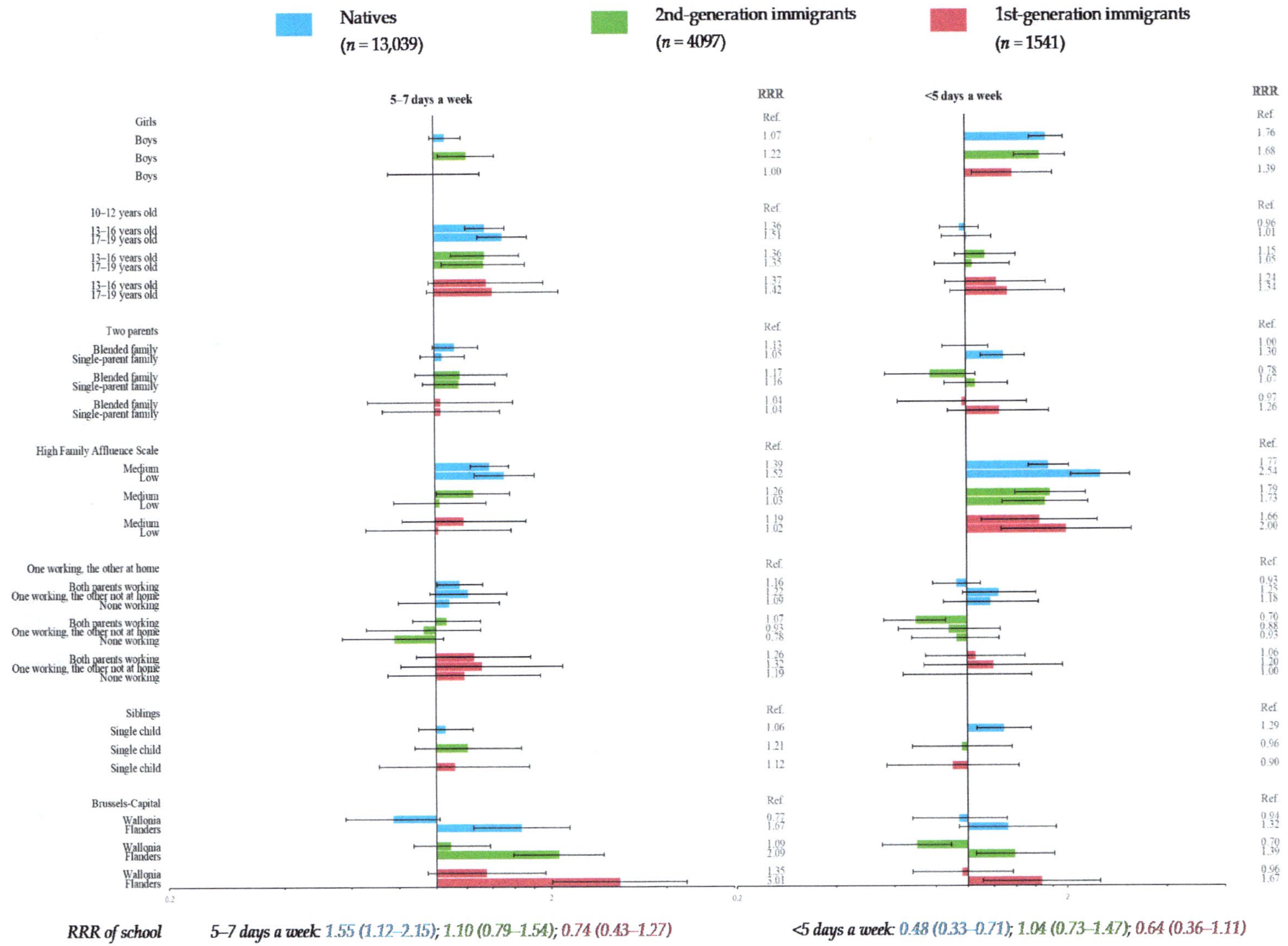

Figure 4. Multiple multilevel multinomial regression* for vegetable consumption (reference category: >once a day) stratified by migration status—HBSC, Belgium, 2014 (n = 18,974). * RRR < 1: More favorable for health; RRR > 1: Less favorable for health.

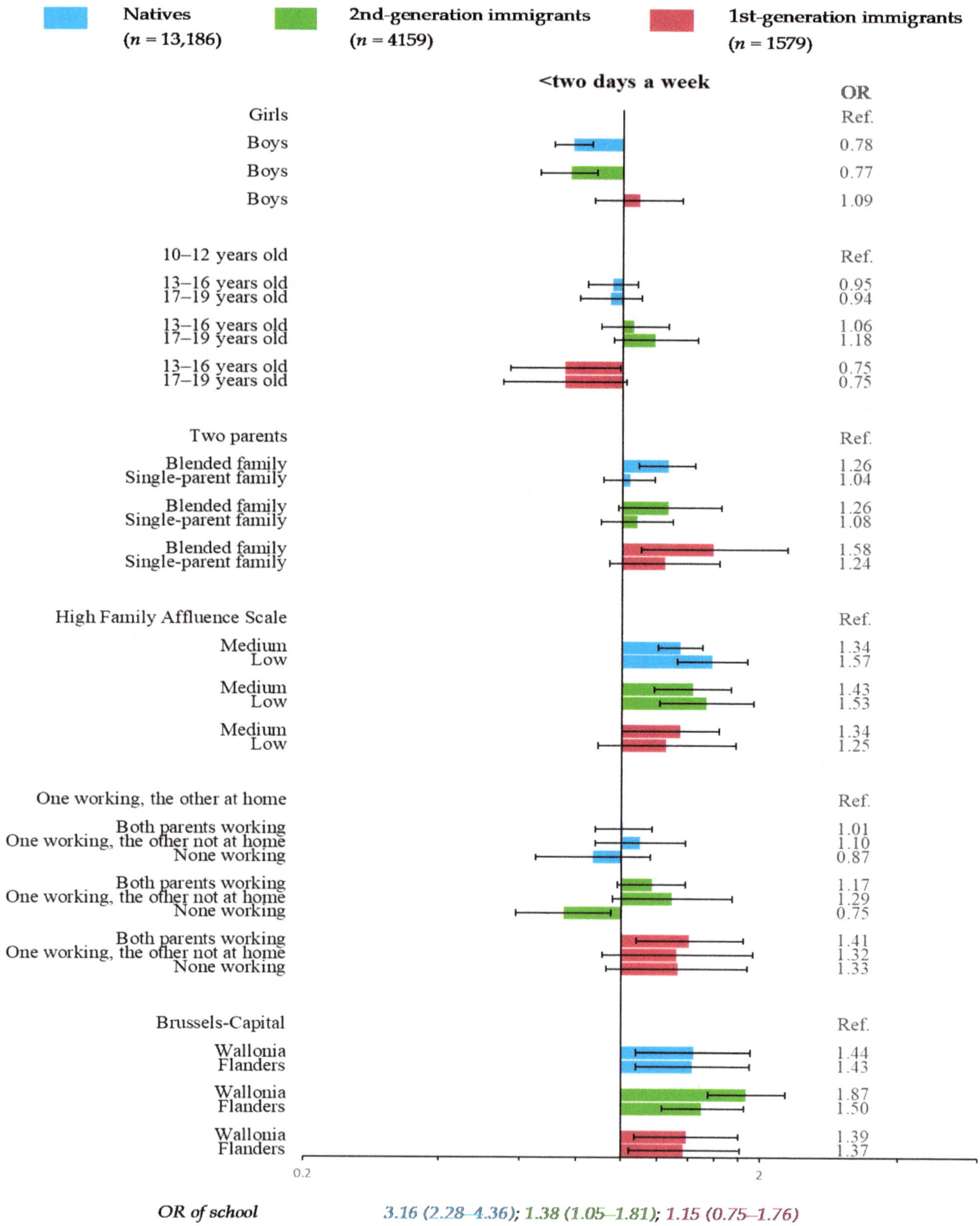

Figure 5. Multiple multilevel logistic regression* for fish consumption (reference category: ≥two days a week) stratified by migration status—HBSC, Belgium, 2014 (n = 18,924). * OR < 1: More favorable for health; OR > 1: Less favorable for health.

3.4. Dairy Product Consumption (Reference Category: >Once a Day)

For all migration situations, neither FAS nor family structure nor parental working status was significantly associated with dairy consumption (Figure 6). Compared with Brussels-Capital, natives and 2nd-generation immigrants in Flanders were at significantly lower odds of consuming dairy foods ≤once a day (Figure 6).

In addition, dairy consumption frequency was significantly associated with gender in all migration strata and with age in natives and 2nd-generation immigrants, whereas the presence of siblings was significant only in natives. The school effect was significant in all migration strata (Figure 6).

3.5. Chips and Fries Consumption (Reference Category: <Once a Day)

Compared with those having a high FAS, natives with a low FAS were significantly more likely to declare frequent eating of chips and fries (≥once a day) (Figure 7). High frequency was also more likely in natives from blended or single-parent families than in those with two parents. Compared with adolescents having one working parent and the other who stayed at home, adolescents with two working parents were less likely to consume chips and fries ≥once a day whatever their migration status. In natives and 2nd-generation immigrants with no working parents, high frequency was more likely. In Flanders, compared to Brussels-Capital, adolescents among all migration groups were significantly less likely to declare high consumption of chips and fries; in Wallonia, this was also the case for 2nd- and 1st-generation immigrants (Figure 7).

In addition, frequent eating of chips and fries was significantly associated with gender in all migration strata, and with age in natives and 2nd-generation immigrants. Sibling presence was significantly associated only in 1st-generation immigrants. The school effect was significant in all migration strata (Figure 7).

3.6. Sugar-Sweetened Beverages (Reference Category: ≤Once a Week)

In natives and 2nd-generation immigrants, the odds of declaring very high SSB consumption (≥once a day) decreased with FAS (Figure 8). For all migration strata, adolescents from blended families were significantly more likely to declare very high frequency. In addition, natives from blended families were more likely to consume SSB at high frequency (2–6 days a week). In natives and 2nd-generation immigrants, very high SSB frequency was more often seen in adolescents from single-parent families (vs. two-parent families) and in adolescents with nonworking parents (vs. one working parent and the other at home) and was less likely in adolescents with both parents working. In 2nd-generation immigrants only, very high SSB frequency was also less likely in adolescents with one parent working and the other absent from the home. In Flanders, compared with Brussels-Capital, natives and 2nd-generation immigrants were more likely to consume SSB 2–6 days a week.

In addition, "gender and age" was significantly associated with SSB frequency in all migration strata, whereas "siblings" was significant only in natives. The school effect was significant only in natives (Figure 8).

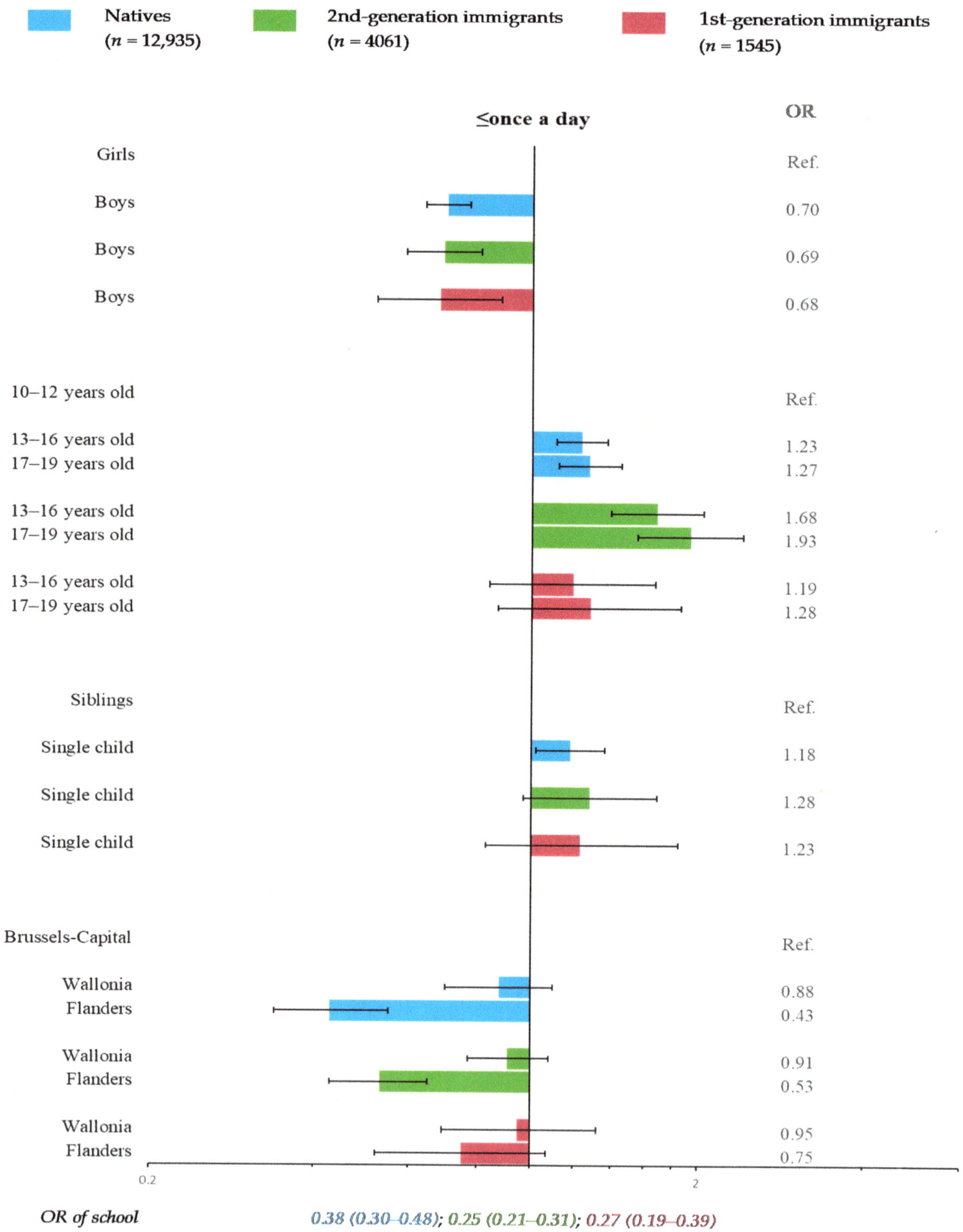

Figure 6. Multiple multilevel logistic regression* for dairy product consumption (reference category: >once a day) stratified by migration status—HBSC, Belgium, 2014 (n = 18,541). * OR < 1: More favorable for health; OR > 1: Less favorable for health.

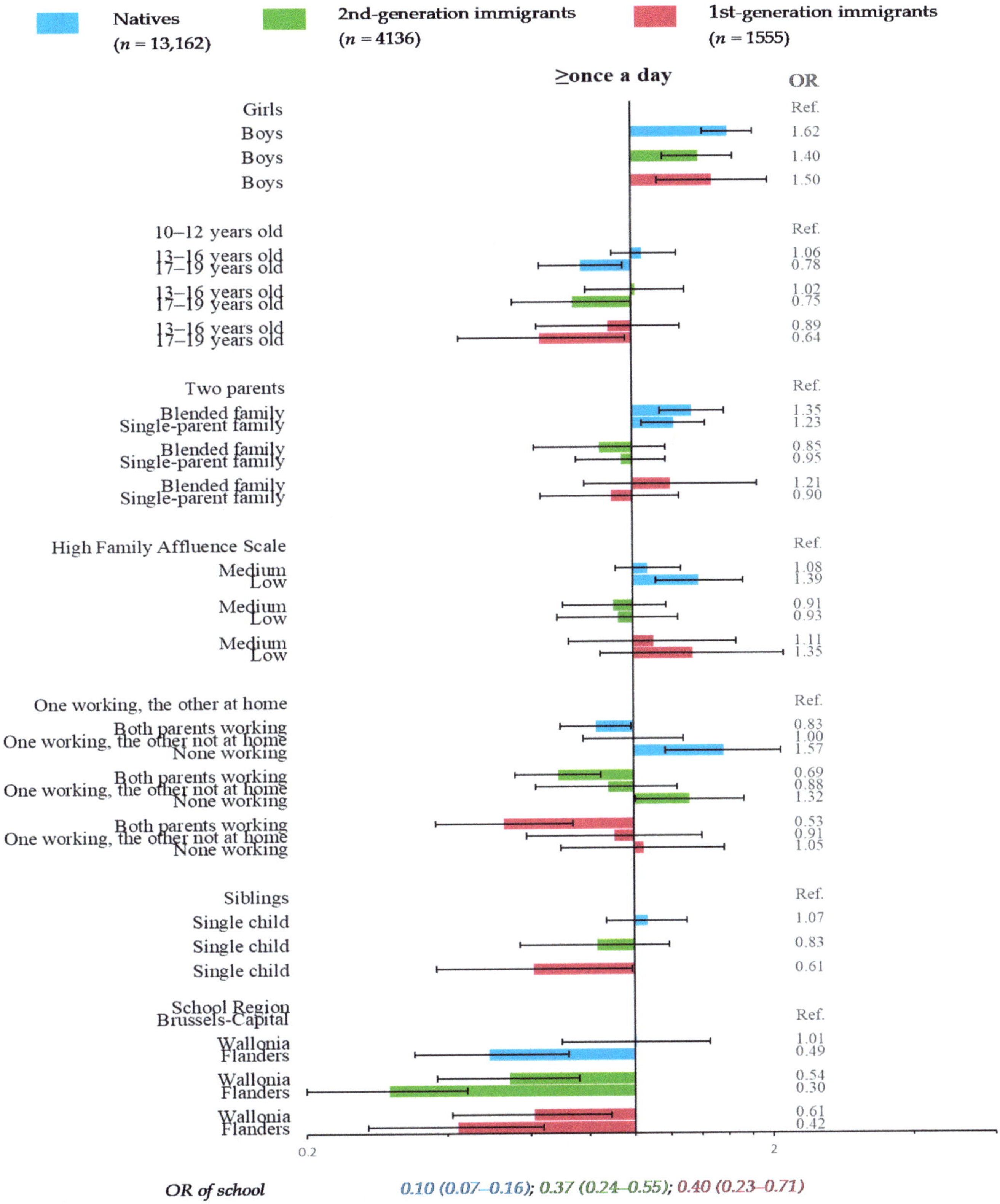

Figure 7. Multiple multilevel logistic regression* for chips and fries consumption (reference category: <once a day) stratified by migration status—HBSC, Belgium, 2014 (n = 18,853). * OR < 1: More favorable for health; OR > 1: Less favorable for health.

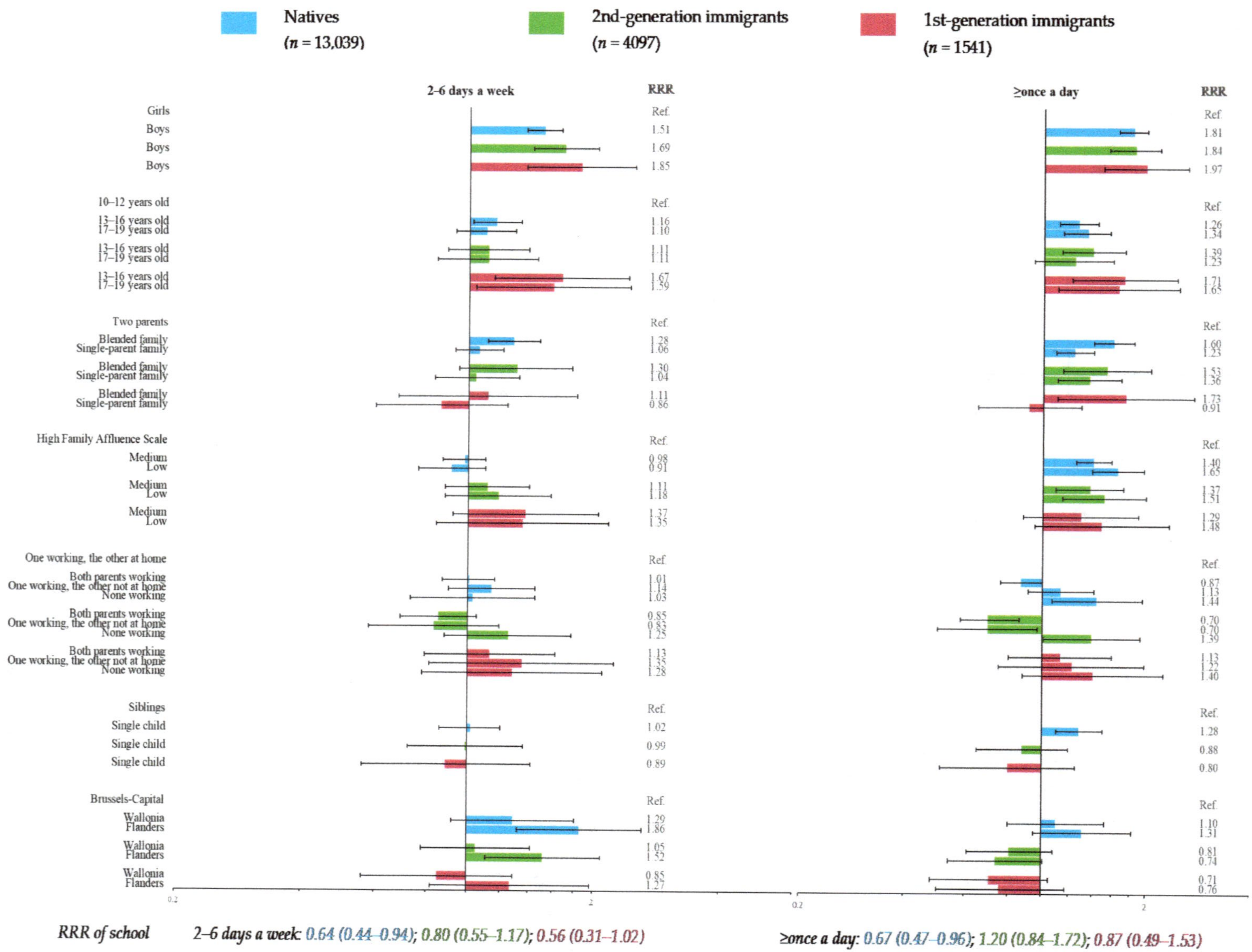

Figure 8. Multiple multilevel multinomial regression* for sugar-sweetened beverages consumption (reference category: ≤once a week) stratified by migration status—HBSC, Belgium, 2014 (n = 18,642). * RRR < 1: More favorable for health; RRR > 1: Less favorable for health.

4. Discussion

The aim of the present study was to estimate socioeconomic disparities in dietary habits of school adolescents in Belgium from different migration backgrounds. Our results emphasize that the migration component that was rarely considered in previous studies is fundamental regarding dietary behavior at these ages. Indeed, dietary habits differed according to migration strata. Furthermore, socioeconomic disparities varied amongst the migration groups: For all food groups, disparities were particularly wide in natives and more limited in 1st-generation immigrants. Overall, the sociodemographic and socioeconomic disparities observed in immigrants did not change after adjusting for their geographical area of origin. By food group, the widest socioeconomic and cultural disparities were observed for SSB and vegetables, and the least for dairy foods. Such findings provide interesting and original hypotheses that could further support the development of health promotion interventions in the future.

4.1. Dietary Acculturation

In descriptive analyses, immigrant adolescents, whether of the 1st or 2nd generation, were more likely to frequently consume both healthy (fruits, vegetables, and fish, but not dairy products) and unhealthy foods (chips and fries, SSB). In addition, a migration gradient in food frequencies was underlined for vegetables, fish, and chips and fries: Consumption gradually increased (for healthy food) or decreased (for unhealthy food) from natives to 2nd-generation immigrants, and from 2nd-generation immigrants to 1st-generation immigrants. However, no significant differences were found between 1st- and 2nd-generation immigrants regarding consumption of fruits, dairy products, and SSB.

The situation of 2nd-generation immigrants in terms of food consumption, intermediate between natives and 1st-generation immigrants, suggests ongoing acculturation. The interplay of host behavior and culture with that of immigrants may lead to a mixture of healthy and unhealthy dietary habits. Indeed, at a given age, 2nd-generation immigrants have probably been in Belgium much longer than 1st-generation immigrants and are therefore more likely to be further engaged in the process of integration of culinary habits of the host country and partial substitution of family roots, as reported for adults in different countries [18]. In addition to the migration generation, the region of origin may play differently in the acquisition of European dietary habits for immigrants. Indeed, differences in dietary habits were of lower size between European, American, and Asian, than between European and African and Middle-East immigrants. Nevertheless, the results could not be precisely interpreted due to the cultural heterogeneity remaining in this categorization by the geographical area of origin.

The acculturation process may depend on factors such as accessibility and affordability, acting as an "external push", and on individual factors such as curiosity, acting as an "internal pull" [28], which might encourage the adding of novel foods to the traditional diet, thus offering wider diversity. Such diversity could result in greater intake via gradual adaptation to new food products [29]. This may also explain why immigrants more frequently ate almost each food group studied. Maintaining traditional food habits implies the availability and accessibility of such food; when this is not the case, then people of foreign culture might progressively abandon their diet in favor of the host diet [30]. The acculturation process should also be further studied by considering the age of arrival in Belgium of the 1st-generation immigrants, unavailable in this survey.

4.2. Socioeconomic Disparities in Dietary Habits

Our results emphasize several socioeconomic disparities in dietary habits in adolescents, mainly in natives and 2nd-generation immigrants. Indeed, adolescents with lower FAS less frequently ate healthy foods like fruits and more frequently consumed unhealthy foods like SSB, consistent with previous studies [10,11]. These disparities may be explained by a lower level of familiarity or adoption of dietary recommendations by parents [31], and by the affordability of healthy foods [32].

Some disparities related to family structure were also revealed, mainly in natives and 2nd-generation immigrants. In line with previous studies [33,34], adolescents from blended or single-parent families more frequently ate chips and fries and SSB and less frequently ate fruits, vegetables and fish. Single-parent families often have fewer financial resources, thereby impairing their access to healthy foods [32]. Indeed, in our sample, 30.8% of adolescents belonging to a single-parent family were in a low FAS compared to 14.0% of adolescents from two-parent families and 15.7% of adolescents from blended families (data not shown). In addition, single parents may also have less time for monitoring meals compared to dual-parent families [33,35]. Adolescents from blended families also tended to have less healthy food habits than adolescents from two-parent families. Indeed, stepparents may have fewer opportunities for active involvement in their stepchildren's education and health [33].

Moreover, parental work status disparities were observed, mainly in natives and 2nd-generation immigrants. In our study, parental working status was mainly related to the socioeconomic condition: 10.2% of adolescents with both parents working had a low FAS, while 51.8% of adolescents with no parents working fell into this category ($p < 0.001$; 24.1% in those with one parent working and one at home, 31.5% for one parent working and the other "absent" from home). After adjustment for FAS and other covariates, our results related to parental working status were mixed. Indeed, compared to adolescents with both parents working, those with no working parents were more likely to frequently eat vegetables and fish, but they also more frequently ate chips and fries and SSB (data not shown). These results might appear surprising if we assume that parental working status is related only to socioeconomic conditions. However, they suggest an interplay between free time and work. Indeed, parental working status might also indicate that fully employed parents have less time to cook [36].

For all migration strata, eating habits varied according to the school region. Numerous differences were found in consumption frequencies between adolescents attending schools in Flanders, mainly Dutch-speaking, and those in Brussels and Wallonia, both primarily French-speaking. Another study indicating similar regional linguistic specificities in consumption of vegetables, dairy products, fish, and SSB in Switzerland hypothesized a possible influence of culture and eating habits of neighboring countries [37], which might also apply to Belgium: Culinary customs in Flanders may be strongly influenced by the Netherlands, while those in Brussels, although they do not border, and in Wallonia, may be influenced by France, which shares the same language, i.e., French. Further, several differences were pointed out between Brussels and Wallonia, mainly concerning 1st- and 2nd-generation immigrants. In 2011, nearly half of the inhabitants of the Brussels-Capital Region (42.4%) were born outside of Belgium, compared to 10.2% in Flanders and 14.1% in Wallonia [38]. Since the Brussels-Capital region is multicultural, this vast proportion of immigrants might contribute to slowing down the acculturation process; indeed, immigrants are usually surrounded by other immigrants [17]. By contrast, in Wallonia, such a process may have been accelerated, meaning that food habits in immigrants would differ from those of immigrants in Brussels.

Socioeconomic disparities were measurable in all food groups, except for dairy products, for which disparities were statistically significant only for the school region. The absence of socioeconomic disparities in consumption of dairy foods (milk, cheese, and other) could be explained by the diversity of these products and their overall affordability.

4.3. Sociodemographic Disparities in Dietary Habits

Our results underlined gender disparities in food consumption in almost all migration strata. Compared to boys, girls were more likely to more frequently eat fruits and vegetables, which could be explained by taste preferences [39,40], health beliefs, and greater concern about weight [41].

After adjustment for other covariates, sibling disparities continued to be unfavorable to the single child (except for chips and fries in 1st-generation immigrants). The sibling role in food consumption might be explained by two opposite phenomena: "Modeling" leads to imitation of the model (i.e., of the sibling), whereas "de-identification" leads to differentiation from the sibling [42]. The absence of sibling disparities in immigrants could be explained by the manner in which society views sibling relationships and their respective roles [43]. Thus, immigrants in our study might come from countries that do not promote sibling relationships. However, the sibling role has rarely been examined in dietary studies irrespective of migration status [44], thus preventing interpretation. Certain psychologists have suggested that older siblings may influence health behavior [45]; thus, birth order should be considered when evaluating the association between diet and siblings.

4.4. Strengths and Limitations

Due to the cross-sectional design of the HBSC survey and use of self-administrated questionnaires, a substantial sample size was obtained in each region of Belgium, along with a wide range of topics addressed. Although both Dutch- and French-speaking surveys were conducted separately and in different languages, standardization of the questionnaires according to the international HBSC protocol made it possible to combine data sets [23]. However, the two surveys were not identical. For instance, they were differently stratified in order to reach the representativeness of the linguistic regions. Therefore, the generalization of the results to the school population in Belgium should be interpreted cautiously. A second point related to the independence of studies is the use of reverse order categorization for food frequencies ("never" to ">once a day" for the Dutch-speaking survey versus ">once a day" to "never" for the French-speaking survey) may have contributed to lower frequencies of fruit and vegetable consumption in Flanders compared to Wallonia, since initial responses may have been chosen more frequently. This discrepancy could explain why we obtained results differing from the final national food consumption survey (based on 24-h recall) [46]. The short HBSC FFQ might also lead to inaccuracies due to use of large food group names rather than exact food names, and to the overestimation of consumption frequencies [25]. However, it has been validated in Belgium through a comparison with a seven-day record [24,25]. The conclusion was that it can be considered reliable for "ranking subjects according to consumption of the individual food items" [25]. In addition, we can only conclude about frequencies and the results must be interpreted as such given that a more frequent consumption does not necessarily imply—nor rules out—a higher food amount or a higher energy intake.

A significant strength of the current study was the use of multilevel analyses controlling for the school effect and, therefore, cluster bias. Nevertheless, further interpreting the school effect is difficult given that food-related school characteristics were unavailable in this study. To better understand such effects, further studies should simultaneously consider contextual characteristics of the schools, such as implementation of nutritional actions and canteen use. For some food groups (fruits, vegetables, and SSB), categorization was in three instead of two, as is the case in numerous studies using categorization and FFQ. Although disparities were narrower for the intermediate category and, therefore, little difference from the reference category was observed, intermediate categories provided new information in certain cases. Indeed, in natives and 2nd-generation immigrants, age-related disparities existed for vegetables 5–7 days a week but not for vegetables <5 days a week; in addition, school-region-related disparities existed for SSB consumption 2–6 days a week but not for SSB $\geq$once a day. Although difficult to interpret, the school effect for natives might be a protective factor for fruits 5–7 days a week and a risk factor for fruits <5 days a week.

Another limitation was the rather small sample size of 1st-generation immigrants (n_{max} = 1605), leading to fewer participants in some categories (n_{min} = 159) and resulting in loss of statistical power. However, confidence intervals of OR and RRR (Figures 3–8) suggested that nonsignificant results in 1st-generation immigrants were mainly due to fewer disparities rather than a lack of precision.

This rather small sample size was also restrictive for in-depth analysis stratified by countries or continental regions of origin. To get around the small sample, results were subsequently adjusted for geographical areas of origin. Nevertheless, some cultural heterogeneity remained in this categorization and did not help to precisely interpret the findings.

Several biases could also be highlighted. First, adolescents may have overreported consumption of healthy foods and underreported consumption of unhealthy products due to social pressure [47]. Second, we observed differential distribution of fish and SSB consumption and of several covariates (migration status, gender, family structure, FAS, parental working status, and school region) between included participants and eligible participants not included in analyses due to missing data (Supplementary Table S8), leading to selection bias. Interpretation of results should thus be approached with caution, although some differences in percentages were slight, and statistical significance was mainly due to the large sample size. The generalization of the results is limited to the school adolescents, especially for the eldest beyond the legal school age (18 years of age in Belgium). It should also be interpreted cautiously due to the relatively low participation rate of schools.

5. Conclusions

Overall, rather poor adolescent dietary habits indicate that efforts should be made to improve knowledge and further prevent NCD in adulthood. The process of acculturation of dietary habits pointed out here warrants confirmation, taking into consideration the number of years in the host country and the age of arrival in that country. Narrower socioeconomic disparities in dietary habits among 2nd- and 1st-generation immigrants compared to natives suggest the prevailing role of culture in immigrant dietary habits with respect to socioeconomic conditions. Finally, our study reveals that interventions aimed at improving dietary habits in adolescents must take into account the cultural component of dietary habits, especially in immigrant adolescents. However, further research is needed to better understand the role of culture and its interaction with socioeconomic components in dietary habits.

Supplementary Materials:
Table S1: Multilevel multinomial regressions for fruit consumption (reference category: >once a day) stratified by migration status—HBSC, Belgium, 2014 (n = 19,172), Table S2: Multilevel multinomial regressions for vegetable consumption (reference category: >once a day) stratified by migration status—HBSC, Belgium, 2014 (n = 18,974), Table S3: Multilevel logistic regressions for fish consumption (reference category: ≥two days a week) stratified by migration status—HBSC, Belgium, 2014 (n = 18,924), Table S4: Multilevel logistic regressions for dairy product consumption (reference category: >once a day) stratified by migration status—HBSC, Belgium, 2014 (n = 18,541), Table S5: Multilevel logistic regressions for chips and fries consumption (reference category: <once a day) stratified by migration status—HBSC, Belgium, 2014 (n = 18,853), Table S6: Multilevel multinomial regressions for sugar-sweetened beverages consumption (reference category: ≤once a week) stratified by migration status—HBSC, Belgium, 2014 (n = 18,642), Table S7: Multilevel logistic regressions* for food consumption stratified by migration status—HBSC, Belgium, 2014, Table S8: Comparisons of food consumptions, cultural, and sociodemographic characteristics between participants included in the analyses and those excluded due to missing data.

Author Contributions: Conceptualization, M.R. and K.C.; methodology, M.R. and K.C.; formal analysis, M.R.; investigation, M.R.; resources, B.d.C., N.M. and I.G.; data curation, B.d.C., N.M. and I.G.; writing—original draft preparation, M.R. and K.C.; writing—review and editing, B.d.C., T.L., M.D., N.M., L.D. and I.G.; visualization, M.R.; supervision, K.C.; project administration, K.C..; funding acquisition, I.G., K.C. and B.d.C.

Acknowledgments: The authors thank the schools and students for their participation in the French-speaking and Dutch-speaking Belgian HBSC surveys. They also thank the HBSC International Coordination Center (University of St Andrews, United Kingdom) and the HBSC data Management Center (University of Bergen, Norway) for their scientific support, as well as Maud Dujeu, Camille Pedroni and Patrick De Smet (SIPES, Université libre de Bruxelles, Belgium) for their collaboration in data cleaning and management, and Jerry Bram for editing reviewing.

References

1. Grootveld, M.; Percival, B.C.; Grootveld, K. Chronic Non-Communicable Disease Risks Presented by Lipid Oxidation Products in Fried Foods. *HepatoBiliary Surg. Nutr.* **2018**, *7*, 305–312. [CrossRef] [PubMed]
2. Schwingshackl, L.; Schwedhelm, C.; Hoffmann, G.; Lampousi, A.-M.; Knuppel, S.; Iqbal, K.; Bechthold, A.; Schlesinger, S.; Boeing, H. Food groups and risk of all-cause mortality: A systematic review and meta-analysis of prospective studies. *Am. J. Clin. Nutr.* **2017**, *105*, 1462–1473. [CrossRef] [PubMed]
3. Aune, D.; Giovannucci, E.; Boffetta, P.; Fadnes, L.T.; Keum, N.; Norat, T.; Greenwood, D.C.; Riboli, E.; Vatten, L.J.; Tonstad, S. Fruit and vegetable intake and the risk of cardiovascular disease, total cancer and all-cause mortality—A systematic review and dose-response meta-analysis of prospective studies. *Int. J. Epidemiol.* **2017**, *46*, 1029–1056. [CrossRef]
4. Fardet, A.; Rock, E. In vitro and in vivo antioxidant potential of milks, yoghurts, fermented milks and cheeses: A narrative review of evidence. *Nutr. Res. Rev.* **2018**, *31*, 52–70. [CrossRef] [PubMed]
5. Stringhini, S.; Dugravot, A.; Shipley, M.; Goldberg, M.; Zins, M.; Kivimäki, M.; Marmot, M.; Sabia, S.; Singh-Manoux, A. Health behaviours, socioeconomic status, and mortality: Further analyses of the British Whitehall II and the French GAZEL prospective cohorts. *PLoS Med.* **2011**, *8*, e1000419. [CrossRef]
6. Méjean, C.; Droomers, M.; Van Der Schouw, Y.T.; Sluijs, I.; Czernichow, S.; Grobbee, D.E.; Bueno-de-Mesquita, H.B.; Beulens, J.W.J. The contribution of diet and lifestyle to socioeconomic inequalities in cardiovascular morbidity and mortality. *Int. J. Cardiol.* **2013**, *168*, 5190–5195. [CrossRef]
7. Lien, N.; Jacobs, D.R.; Klepp, K.-I. Exploring predictors of eating behaviour among adolescents by gender and socio-economic status. *Public Health Nutr.* **2002**, *5*, 671–681. [CrossRef] [PubMed]
8. Kelder, S.H.; Perry, C.L.; Klepp, K.I.; Lytle, L.L. Longitudinal tracking of adolescent smoking, physical activity, and food choice behaviors. *Am. J. Public Health* **1994**, *84*, 1121–1126. [CrossRef] [PubMed]
9. Lake, A.A.; Mathers, J.C.; Rugg-Gunn, A.J.; Adamson, A.J. Longitudinal change in food habits between adolescence (11–12 years) and adulthood (32–33 years): The ASH30 Study. *J. Public Health* **2006**, *28*, 10–16. [CrossRef]
10. Drouillet-Pinard, P.; Dubuisson, C.; Bordes, I.; Margaritis, I.; Lioret, S.; Volatier, J.-L. Socio-economic disparities in the diet of French children and adolescents: A multidimensional issue. *Public Health Nutr.* **2017**, *20*, 870–882. [CrossRef]
11. Béghin, L.; Dauchet, L.; de Vriendt, T.; Cuenca-García, M.; Manios, Y.; Toti, E.; Plada, M.; Widhalm, K.; Repasy, J.; Huybrechts, I.; et al. Influence of parental socio-economic status on diet quality of European adolescents: Results from the HELENA study. *Br. J. Nutr.* **2014**, *111*, 1303–1312. [CrossRef]
12. Allen, M.L.; Elliott, M.N.; Morales, L.S.; Diamant, A.L.; Hambarsoomian, K.; Schuster, M.A. Adolescent participation in preventive health behaviors, physical activity, and nutrition: Differences across immigrant generations for Asians and Latinos compared with Whites. *Am. J. Public Health* **2007**, *97*, 337–343. [CrossRef]
13. Brown, A.G.M.; Houser, R.F.; Mattei, J.; Rehm, C.D.; Mozaffarian, D.; Lichtenstein, A.H.; Folta, S.C. Diet quality among US-born and foreign-born non-Hispanic blacks: NHANES 2003-2012 data. *Am. J. Clin. Nutr.* **2018**, *107*, 695–706. [CrossRef]
14. Deboosere, P.; Gadeyne, S. Adult Migrant Mortality Advantage in Belgium: Evidence Using Census and Register Data. *Population* **2005**, 655–698. [CrossRef]
15. Neuman, S. Are immigrants healthier than native residents? *IZA World Labor* **2014**. [CrossRef]
16. Vandenheede, H.; Willaert, D.; de Grande, H.; Simoens, S.; Vanroelen, C. Mortality in adult immigrants in the 2000s in Belgium: A test of the 'healthy-migrant' and the 'migration-as-rapid-health-transition' hypotheses. *Trop. Med. Int. Health* **2015**, *20*, 1832–1845. [CrossRef]
17. Barker, G.G. Choosing the best of both worlds: The acculturation process revisited. *Int. J. Intercult. Relat.* **2015**, *45*, 56–69. [CrossRef]
18. Méjean, C.; Traissac, P.; Eymard-Duvernay, S.; Delpeuch, F.; Maire, B. Influence of acculturation among Tunisian migrants in France and their past/present exposure to the home country on diet and physical activity. *Public Health Nutr.* **2009**, *12*, 832–841. [CrossRef]
19. Llull, R.; Bibiloni, M.; Pons, A.; Tur, J.A. Food consumption patterns of Balearic Islands' adolescents depending on their origin. *J. Immigr. Minor Health* **2015**, *17*, 358–366. [CrossRef]

20. Te Velde, S.J.; Wind, M.; van Lenthe, F.J.; Klepp, K.-I.; Brug, J. Differences in fruit and vegetable intake and determinants of intakes between children of Dutch origin and non-Western ethnic minority children in the Netherlands—A cross sectional study. *Int. J. Behav. Nutr. Phys. Act.* **2006**, *3*, 31. [CrossRef]
21. Malmusi, D.; Borrell, C.; Benach, J. Migration-related health inequalities: Showing the complex interactions between gender, social class and place of origin. *Soc. Sci. Med.* **2010**, *71*, 1610–1619. [CrossRef]
22. Pantzer, K.; Rajmil, L.; Tebé, C.; Codina, F.; Serra-Sutton, V.; Ferrer, M.; Ravens-Sieberer, U.; Simeoni, M.-C.; Alonso, J. Health related quality of life in immigrants and native school aged adolescents in Spain. *J. Epidemiol. Community Health* **2006**, *60*, 694–698. [CrossRef]
23. Currie, C.; Griebler, R.; Inchley, J.; Theunissen, A.; Molcho, M.; Samdal, O.; Dür, W. *Health Behaviour in School-Aged Children (HBSC) Study Protocol: Background, Methodology and Mandatory Items for the 2009/10 Survey*; CAHRU: St Andrews, Hong Kong, China, 2010.
24. Vereecken, C.A.; Maes, L. A Belgian study on the reliability and relative validity of the Health Behaviour in School-Aged Children food-frequency questionnaire. *Public Health Nutr.* **2003**, *6*, 581–588. [CrossRef]
25. Vereecken, C.A.; Rossi, S.; Giacchi, M.V.; Maes, L. Comparison of a short food-frequency questionnaire and derived indices with a seven-day diet record in Belgian and Italian children. *Int. J. Public Health* **2008**, *53*, 297–305. [CrossRef]
26. Torsheim, T.; Cavallo, F.; Levin, K.A.; Schnohr, C.; Mazur, J.; Niclasen, B.; Currie, C. Psychometric Validation of the Revised Family Affluence Scale: A Latent Variable Approach. *Child. Indic. Res.* **2016**, *9*, 771–784. [CrossRef]
27. Conseil Supérieur de la Santé. *Recommandations Nutritionnelles pour la Belgique 2016. Avis n°9285*; Conseil Supérieur de la Santé: Bruxelles, Belgium, 2016.
28. Hartwell, H.J.; Edwards, J.S.A.; Brown, L. Acculturation and food habits: Lessons to be learned. *Br. Food J.* **2011**, *113*, 1393–1405. [CrossRef]
29. Raynor, H.A.; Vadiveloo, M. Understanding the Relationship Between Food Variety, Food Intake, and Energy Balance. *Curr. Obes. Rep.* **2018**, *7*, 68–75. [CrossRef]
30. Papadaki, S.; Mavrikaki, E. Greek adolescents and the Mediterranean diet: Factors affecting quality and adherence. *Nutrition* **2015**, *31*, 345–349. [CrossRef]
31. Skårdal, M.; Western, I.M.; Ask, A.M.S.; Øverby, N.C. Socioeconomic differences in selected dietary habits among Norwegian 13–14 year-olds: A cross-sectional study. *Food Nutr. Res.* **2014**, *58*. [CrossRef]
32. Morris, M.A.; Hulme, C.; Clarke, G.P.; Edwards, K.L.; Cade, J.E. What is the cost of a healthy diet? Using diet data from the UK Women's Cohort Study. *J. Epidemiol. Community Health* **2014**, *68*, 1043–1049. [CrossRef]
33. Stewart, S.D.; Menning, C.L. Family structure, nonresident father involvement, and adolescent eating patterns. *J. Adolesc. Health* **2009**, *45*, 193–201. [CrossRef]
34. Baek, Y.J.; Paik, H.Y.; Shim, J.E. Association between family structure and food group intake in children. *Nutr. Res. Pract.* **2014**, *8*, 463–468. [CrossRef]
35. Reicks, M.; Banna, J.; Cluskey, M.; Gunther, C.; Hongu, N.; Richards, R.; Topham, G.; Wong, S.S. Influence of Parenting Practices on Eating Behaviors of Early Adolescents during Independent Eating Occasions: Implications for Obesity Prevention. *Nutrients* **2015**, *7*, 8783–8801. [CrossRef]
36. Bauer, K.W.; Hearst, M.O.; Escoto, K.; Berge, J.M.; Neumark-Sztainer, D. Parental employment and work-family stress: Associations with family food environments. *Soc. Sci. Med.* **2012**, *75*, 496–504. [CrossRef]
37. Chatelan, A.; Beer-Borst, S.; Randriamiharisoa, A.; Pasquier, J.; Blanco, J.M.; Siegenthaler, S.; Paccaud, F.; Slimani, N.; Nicolas, G.; Camenzind-Frey, E.; et al. Major Differences in Diet across Three Linguistic Regions of Switzerland: Results from the First National Nutrition Survey menuCH. *Nutrients* **2017**, *9*, 1163. [CrossRef]
38. Census/Statbel. Population par Lieu de Résidence (Province), Sexe, Position dans le Ménage (C), État Civil, Situation sur le Marché de L'emploi (A) et Lieu de Naissance (A). Available online: http://census2011.fgov.be/censusselection/selectionFR.html (accessed on 16 July 2018).
39. Bere, E.; Brug, J.; Klepp, K.-I. Why do boys eat less fruit and vegetables than girls? *Public Health Nutr.* **2008**, *11*, 321–325. [CrossRef]
40. Caine-Bish, N.L.; Scheule, B. Gender differences in food preferences of school-aged children and adolescents. *J. Sch. Health* **2009**, *79*, 532–540. [CrossRef]
41. Wardle, J.; Haase, A.M.; Steptoe, A.; Nillapun, M.; Jonwutiwes, K.; Bellisle, F. Gender differences in food choice: The contribution of health beliefs and dieting. *Ann. Behav. Med.* **2004**, *27*, 107–116. [CrossRef]

42. Salvy, S.-J.; Vartanian, L.R.; Coelho, J.S.; Jarrin, D.; Pliner, P.P. The role of familiarity on modeling of eating and food consumption in children. *Appetite* **2008**, *50*, 514–518. [CrossRef]
43. McHale, S.M.; Updegraff, K.A.; Whiteman, S.D. Sibling Relationships and Influences in Childhood and Adolescence. *J. Marriage Fam.* **2012**, *74*, 913–930. [CrossRef]
44. Berge, J.M.; Meyer, C.; Maclehose, R.F.; Crichlow, R.; Neumark-Sztainer, D. All in the Family: Correlations between Parents' and Adolescent Siblings' Weight and Weight-related Behaviors. *Obesity* **2015**, *23*, 833–839. [CrossRef]
45. Senguttuvan, U.; Whiteman, S.D.; Jensen, A.C. Family Relationships and Adolescents' Health Attitudes and Weight: The Understudied Role of Sibling Relationships. *Fam. Relat.* **2014**, *63*, 384–396. [CrossRef]
46. De Ridder, K.; Bel, S.; Brocatus, L.; Cuypers, K.; Lebacq, T.; Moyersoen, I.; Ost, C.; Teppers, E. Enquête de Consommation Alimentaire 2014-2015: Rapport 4: La Consommation Alimentaire. Available online: https://fcs.wiv-isp.be/nl/Gedeelde%20%20documenten/FRANS/Rapport%204/Resume_rapport_4_finaal_finaal.pdf (accessed on 13 August 2018).
47. Moore, G.F.; Tapper, K.; Moore, L.; Murphy, S. Cognitive, behavioral, and social factors are associated with bias in dietary questionnaire self-reports by schoolchildren aged 9 to 11 years. *J. Am. Diet. Assoc.* **2008**, *108*, 1865–1873. [CrossRef]

5

Parents' Reports of Preschoolers' Diets: Relative Validity of a Food Frequency Questionnaire and Dietary Patterns

Liisa Korkalo [1,†], Henna Vepsäläinen [1,*,†], Carola Ray [2], Essi Skaffari [1], Reetta Lehto [2], Helena Henrietta Hauta-alus [3], Kaija Nissinen [4], Jelena Meinilä [2,5], Eva Roos [2,6] and Maijaliisa Erkkola [1]

1 Department of Food and Nutrition, University of Helsinki, P.O. Box 66, 00014 Helsinki, Finland; liisa.korkalo@helsinki.fi (L.K.); essi.skaffari@helsinki.fi (E.S.); maijaliisa.erkkola@helsinki.fi (M.E.)
2 Folkhälsan Research Center, Topeliuksenkatu 20, 00250 Helsinki, Finland; carola.ray@folkhalsan.fi (C.R.); reetta.lehto@folkhalsan.fi (R.L.); jelena.meinila@helsinki.fi (J.M.); eva.roos@folkhalsan.fi (E.R.)
3 Children's Hospital, Pediatric Research Center, University of Helsinki and Helsinki University Hospital, Biomedicum 2 C, P.O. Box 705, 00020 HUS Helsinki, Finland; helena.hauta-alus@helsinki.fi
4 Seinäjoki University of Applied Sciences, Kampusranta 11, 60101 Seinäjoki, Finland; kaija.nissinen@seamk.fi
5 Department of Obstetrics and Gynecology, University of Helsinki and Helsinki University Hospital, P.O. Box 22, 00014 Helsinki, Finland
6 Department of Public Health, University of Helsinki, P.O. Box 20, 00014 Helsinki, Finland
* Correspondence: henna.vepsalainen@helsinki.fi
† These authors contributed equally to this work.

Abstract: The accurate assessment of food consumption is crucial in nutritional studies. Since modern nutrition science has become more interested in diet as a whole, studies validating food frequency questionnaires (FFQs) and exploratory dietary patterns are needed. We aimed at examining the relative validity of a 47-item FFQ against three-day food records among three- to six-year-old Finnish children, as well as investigating the consistency of the dietary patterns derived using the principal component analysis (PCA), with food record and FFQ data as inputs. We conducted the PCA without forcing the food record data to match the FFQ items. Altogether, 75% or more of the participants were classified into the same or adjacent quarter of vegetables and fruits as well as sugary food consumption. Furthermore, the intake of folate and vitamin C increased linearly in the quarters of vegetable and fruit consumption, as did the intake of sucrose in quarters of sugary food consumption. Three fairly similar dietary patterns were identified from food records and FFQ data. Concerning the patterns, more than 70% of the participants were classified into the same or adjacent quarter. However, the Spearman correlation coefficients between the respective pattern scores were low (0.25–0.33). The FFQ showed acceptable validity when ranking food group consumption compared to food records. Additionally, the FFQ-derived dietary patterns were consistent with those derived using food record data.

Keywords: validation study; dietary assessment methods; food diary; cross-classification; children; whole diet; preschool; DAGIS Study

---

1. Introduction

As food consumption cannot be measured objectively, researchers must rely on self-reported methods, such as food records, dietary recalls, or food frequency questionnaires (FFQs). FFQs are often used in large, epidemiological studies because of their cost-effectiveness and relatively low respondent burden [1,2]. Children under the age of 7 years are not able to report their own food consumption, and thus, the acquisition of dietary information is dependent on parents, other guardians, or early childhood educators, for instance [3]. Therefore, the accuracy of dietary assessment in children is dependent on the adults' ability to reliably and validly report the children's food consumption. The relative validity of an FFQ can be investigated by comparing the food consumption data obtained using an FFQ with the data obtained using a separate dietary assessment method. Food records are a good method for estimating the relative validity of an FFQ, because the two methods do not share the main sources of errors [4], but other reference methods, such as 24-hour recalls or plasma biomarkers, have also been used in studies validating FFQs among children [5].

Traditionally, validation studies have compared the consumption frequency of certain foods or food groups (e.g., fruits and vegetables, or beverages) or calculated nutrient intakes (e.g., calcium or energy intake) derived using two separate methods (see, for example, [6–10]). However, data-driven dietary patterns that are indicative of a person's whole diet have become popular in nutritional epidemiology [11]. One of the most frequently used methods to derive dietary patterns is principal component analysis (PCA), which is based on intercorrelations between food items [12,13]. The extraction of dietary patterns using PCA requires, however, multiple subjective decisions, such as the selection of dietary variables, to be included in the analysis [14]. Furthermore, the dietary assessment method used to measure food consumption may affect the extracted patterns. Thus, the validation of PCA-derived dietary patterns is beneficial.

Data-driven dietary patterns are thought to reflect the usual food consumption of the participants. Thus, FFQs, which also describe food consumption in general, have mostly been used as inputs in the dietary pattern analysis. Since the late 1990s, several studies have compared FFQ-based dietary patterns with patterns derived from food record data among adults [15–21]. Only two studies have compared FFQ- and food-record-based patterns among children [22,23]. However, the studies have matched each food in the food records with an FFQ item, possibly resulting in artificially increased correlation coefficients [20].

The objective of the current study was two-fold, namely: (1) to study the relative validity of a non-quantitative 47-item FFQ against a three-day food record (reference method) of preschool children by evaluating the ability of the FFQ to rank individuals in the same order according to food consumption as compared to the reference method, and (2) to study the consistency of the data-driven dietary patterns derived by PCA using two sources (food record and FFQ) of data. Our study broadly looked at the validity by examining both the direct (comparison of food consumption to food consumption) and indirect (comparison of food consumption to nutrient intake) validity of the FFQ, as well as the relative validity of the dietary patterns. However, we only measured food consumption outside of preschool.

2. Materials and Methods

2.1. Study Participants

Increased Health and Wellbeing in Preschools (DAGIS) is a research project that aims to diminish socio-economic differences in preschool children's energy balance-related behaviors in Finland (www.dagis.fi). As a part of the larger project, a cross-sectional study was conducted between September 2015 and April 2016, and the details of the sampling process are described in open access format [24]. In short, the cross-sectional study was conducted in eight municipalities. Altogether, 86 communal preschools (56% of those invited) consented to participate. These preschools operated from Monday to Friday and served three meals per day—breakfast, lunch, and an afternoon snack. Preschools operating 24 hours per day were not included in the sample. From the consenting preschools, all of the children in the target age of three to six years (n = 3592) and their families were invited to participate through an invitation letter. Children in preschools with a low participation rate (≤30% in each of the preschool groups for three to six year-olds) were excluded. The final sample consisted of 864 children (24% of those invited) from 66 preschools. A parent or legal guardian of each participating child provided written informed consent. The University of Helsinki Ethical review board in humanities and social and behavioral sciences reviewed the study on 24 February 2015, and found the study ethically acceptable (Statement 6/2015).

2.2. FFQ

We designed a short FFQ for measuring children's food consumption during the previous week outside of preschool hours. The FFQ was developed to assess the children's dietary quality in general, and specific attention was paid to capturing the consumption patterns of vegetables and fruits as well as sugary foods and beverages. The FFQ included 47 food items divided under seven headings, as follows: vegetables, fruits, and berries; dairy products; fish; meat and eggs; cereal products; drinks; and others (i.e., sweets and snacks). The questionnaire was available in both official languages of Finland (Finnish and Swedish) and in English; the English version of the FFQ is available online [25]. A shortened, 25-item version of the FFQ has been tested for reproducibility with mostly moderate or good intraclass correlation coefficients [26].

The participating families received a letter including the FFQ, a three-day food record, and detailed instructions by post. The instructions were to fill in the FFQ first and the three-day food record later, on pre-set dates. The time between the two methods was roughly one week. In the FFQ, the respondent (parent or legal guardian) reported how many times during the past week the child had consumed different foods outside preschool. We intentionally restricted the FFQ to not cover foods and drinks consumed during the preschool hours because the parents would not have been able to reliably report these foods. The time spent at preschool may vary from child to child as well as from day to day, and therefore, we did not specify which meals should be included or excluded in the FFQ. The FFQ included the following three answer columns: "not at all", 'times per week", and "times per day". The instruction was to either tick the "not at all" box or to write a number in one of the other columns. If two or more FFQ items were missing, nutritionists contacted the families and the missing items were completed if possible.

2.3. Three-Day Food Record Data

The study group assigned the exact dates (two weekdays and one weekend day) for each family to fill in the food record. These three days were not always consecutive days. In some cases, when the pre-set dates were unsuitable for the family, the parents contacted the study group and the dates were renegotiated. The instruction was to record all of the foods and beverages consumed by the child during the three days, except for consumption at preschool. We provided the families with a children's food picture book, specifically designed for use in this project, to assist in portion size estimation [27,28]. The parents estimated portion sizes by using the food picture book or household measures, by weighing, or from package labels. The instruction was to list all of the ingredients of the composite dishes. For prepacked products, the exact brand and product name was to be given. Preschool personnel filled in a separate food record during preschool hours, but these data were not used in the analyses of this paper.

The larger DAGIS project had a specific focus on vegetables and fruits as well as sugary food consumption [29]; therefore, these food groups were given special attention in the food record checking process. Nutritionists checked all of the food records. If there were shortcomings in the information concerning vegetables, fruits, and berries, or sugar-containing foods or beverages, the nutritionists made follow-up phone calls or emailed the parents to complete missing details of these foods. As an example, if the parent had forgotten to record the type of yoghurt product, we asked if it was a natural yoghurt or sugar-sweetened yoghurt. Nutritionists entered the food record data using AivoDiet dietary software (version 2.2.0.0, Aivo Oy, Turku, Finland). AivoDiet software included the Fineli Food Composition Database Release 16 (2013). New food items were added into the database when necessary. The database includes recipes for typical Finnish mixed dishes. For each individual meal, the nutritionists either used a suitable recipe found in the database or created a new recipe according to parents' reports. During data entry, each meal was tagged with a code indicating the place of consumption, which enabled us to remove the foods eaten at preschool from the analyses.

To compare the food consumption frequencies during the three-day food record period with the food consumption frequencies reported in the FFQ, we listed every food code used in the food record data and assigned them to the corresponding FFQ row(s). The food record data used in the analyses of this paper included a total of 2421 individual food codes (food items or mixed dishes). Each mixed dish food code was assigned to no more than three rows, according to the main ingredients. For example, a meat soup, which included carrots and potatoes, was assigned to the rows "red meat", "potatoes", and "cooked and canned vegetables". Out of the 2421 food codes, 1714 codes were assigned to one FFQ row, 228 codes to two FFQ rows, and 96 codes to three FFQ rows. The rest (i.e., 383 codes) represented foods not covered by the FFQ, and these were not assigned to any FFQ rows. These codes included, for example, spices, savory pastries, and fat spreads.

2.4. Comparison of the FFQs and Food Records

For the comparison of the FFQs and food records, we used data from all of the children with their FFQs filled in with no more than six missing rows out of the 47 rows, and three days of complete data in the food record ($n = 756$). The number of families who filled in the FFQs for these children was 674; 594 families had one child in the sample, 78 families had two children in the sample, and two families had three children in the sample. The majority ($n = 747$; 99%) of these children were in the target age group of three to six years old, but seven children were two years old and two were seven years old. The differences in the age and sex distribution between the children included in the analysis and the children excluded from the analysis because of missing food consumption information ($n = 108$) were tested using the Student's t-test and Chi-Squared test.

To test how well the FFQ was able to rank individuals in the same categories of food consumption frequency when compared to the reference method (food record), each child was assigned to one of four categories created according to the quartiles of the distribution. Note that we only considered food consumption outside of preschool hours. The categories were cross-tabulated, and the percentages in the same, same or adjacent, and opposite quarters were calculated. We also calculated the proportions of non-consumers and the weekly and daily consumers according to the FFQ. For foods with a high proportion of non-consumers, the majority of the participants were automatically assigned to the first category and the data were assigned into only two or three categories in total. This was true for both methods. Thus, some cells in the cross-tabulations remained empty.

To evaluate whether the food consumption frequency, as measured by the FFQ, was associated with the intake of key nutrients, as calculated from the three-day food records that indicate the consumption of specific types of foods, the mean intakes of selected nutrients were computed according to the consumption categories of selected food groups from the FFQs. We selected the food groups that the DAGIS project has a specific focus on (i.e., vegetables and fruit, and sugary foods and beverages). The consumption frequency was evaluated against the folate and vitamin C (vegetable and fruit consumption) and sucrose intake (sugary foods and beverages). In addition, we evaluated milk, which is typically consumed daily by Finnish preschoolers, against calcium intake. The food group frequency categories were created by summing the responses of the selected FFQ rows. Missing values were treated as zeros when summing the responses. We then categorized the food group consumption frequencies into quarters. Trend analysis was performed using linear regression. The food consumption frequency quarter was treated as a continuous predictor variable, and the nutrient intakes were square root transformed.

2.5. Comparison of Dietary Patterns

In order to identify the existing dietary patterns in the sample, we conducted separate PCAs using (1) the FFQ food groups and (2) food record data (all of the items consumed outside preschool) as inputs. All of the children with complete FFQ data ($n = 758$; 88% of all of the DAGIS participants) were included in the FFQ-based PCA, in which all of the 47 FFQ food items were used as input variables (see [30] for more details). For the food-record-based analysis, the food record codes were collapsed into 64 food groups based on the nutritional similarity of the foods. All of the children with food record data from three days and with no more than six missing FFQ rows (n = 756) were included in the analysis. Of these food groups, we excluded 17 because of low consumption (mean consumption less than 10 g in three days). Due to having no nutritional value and inconsistencies in reporting, we further excluded water from the analysis. Similarly, a mixed group containing foods that could not easily be classified into any of the existing food groups (e.g., spices, spice sauces, meal replacement products, and other miscellaneous foods) was excluded. Thus, the consumption of 45 food groups (g/day) were used as inputs in the food-record-based PCA (see Supplementary Table S1 for included and excluded food groups). IBM SPSS Statistics versions 22 (IBM Corp., Armonk, NY, USA) and 25 (IBM Corp., Armonk, NY, USA) were used in the PCA.

Based on the eigenvalues (minimum value of at least 1.5), scree plots, and interpretability of the components, we chose three components for the FFQ-based analysis and five components for the food-record-based analysis. The analyses were then rerun with forced three- or five-component solutions, respectively. The components were rotated with an orthogonal Varimax transformation, and standardized component scores for all of the components were calculated for each participant. Thus, the obtained component scores represented how closely the food consumption of each participant mirrored each of the empirically derived dietary patterns. The children with complete data for both methods (n = 705; 93% of those included in the comparison of FFQs and food records) were included in the dietary pattern analysis comparison. We used Spearman correlation coefficients to compare the FFQ- and food-record-based dietary pattern scores. In addition, we categorized the FFQ- and food-record-based dietary pattern scores into quarters and calculated the proportion of participants classified into the same quarter, same or adjacent quarter, or grossly misclassified into opposite quarters.

3. Results

The majority of the children (n = 742; 98%) had food record data for two weekdays and one weekend day, as planned. The rest (n = 14; 2%) had food record data for one weekday and two weekend days. A preschool day was defined as a day when the child ate at least one meal at preschool, and most children had food record data for two preschool days (n = 621; 82%). Others had either one (n = 108; 14%) or no preschool days (n = 27; 4%) included in the three-day food record. The children included in the current analysis did not differ from the excluded children in terms of age (Student's t-test p = 0.89) or gender (Chi-Squared test p = 0.51).

3.1. Comparison of FFQs and Food Records

Table 1 shows the proportions of participants classified into same, same or adjacent, and opposite quarters, using the two dietary assessment methods. Depending on the FFQ food item, 60%–96% of the participants were classified into the same or adjacent quarter. The proportion of participants classified into the same or adjacent quarter were 72%–80% for vegetables and fruits (fresh fruit; fresh vegetables; cooked and canned vegetables; peas, beans, lentils, and soya). The respective proportions for sugary treats (ice cream; chocolate; sweets; cakes, cupcakes, sweet rolls, Danish pastries, pies, and other sweet pastries; sweet biscuits and cereals bars) were 70–81%, whereas the consumption of sugary everyday foods (flavored yoghurt; puddings; sugar-sweetened cereals and muesli; berry, fruit, and chocolate porridge with added sugar; berry and fruit soups with added sugar) were classified into the same or adjacent quarter in 71%–87% of participants. Regarding the consumption of sugary beverages (soft drinks; flavored and sweetened milk- and plant-based drinks; sugar-sweetened juice drinks), 69%–78% of the participants were classified into the same or adjacent quarter. The proportion of participants grossly misclassified was 10% or less for vegetables and fruits as well as for sugary foods. Of the individual food items, flavored nuts, almonds, and seeds; whole milk and sour milk; berry, fruit, and chocolate porridge; and reduced-sugar soft juices and soft drinks were most similarly reported, with 85% or more of the participants classified into the same quarter. Canned and frozen fruits, eggs, reduced-sugar soft juices and soft drinks, and dried fruit and berries were the least accurately classified, with 15%–22% of the participants grossly misclassified into opposite quarters.

Table 1. Comparison of food consumption frequencies of foods eaten outside preschool measured with a seven-day food frequency questionnaire (FFQ) and a three-day food record in the Increased Health and Wellbeing in Preschools (DAGIS) study (2015–2016, n = 756).

		Consumption Frequency according to FFQ, % of Participants			**Comparison of the Two Methods, % of Participants**		
Food Item	n	**Not at All**	**Less than Daily**	**Daily**	**In the Same Quarter**	**In the Same or Adjacent Quarter**	**Grossly Misclassified Into Opposite Quarters**
Vegetables, fruit and berries							
Fresh vegetables	754	2	29	69	35	76	7
Cooked and canned vegetables [1]	753	25	59	16	35	73	9
Potatoes (in all its forms)	755	3	85	13	30	72	6
Peas, beans, lentils, and soya	754	70	29	1	68	72	13
Fresh fruit	756	2	47	51	38	80	3
Canned and frozen fruit	754	80	20	0.4	78	78	22
Berries	752	30	63	7	41	70	7
Dried fruit and berries	756	58	41	1	61	64	15
Commercial baby foods and smoothies (no added sugar)	755	75	23	1	75	77	14
Berry and fruit soups (with added sugar)	754	64	34	2	66	71	10
Dairy products							
Skimmed milk and sour milk	752	51	6	43	71	96	0.9
1% fat milk, semi-skimmed milk, and sour milk	755	46	8	46	63	94	0.3
Whole milk and sour milk	753	89	7	4	90	90	10
Low-fat cheese (less than 20% fat)	751	60	26	14	59	71	10
High-fat cheese (20% or more fat)	755	33	40	27	50	81	5
Flavored and sweetened milk- and plant-based drinks	755	55	38	7	60	76	12
Natural yoghurt and quark (also plant-based products)	755	63	33	3	67	72	14
Flavored yoghurt and quark (also plant-based products)	754	23	61	16	49	83	3
Puddings	755	67	32	1	69	72	14
Ice cream	754	41	58	1	37	81	10
Fish, meat, and eggs							
Fish dishes and fish products	754	20	79	0.4	29	73	6
Red meat (beef, pork, lamb and mutton, and game)	754	3	91	6	33	65	12
White meat (poultry)	756	13	84	3	35	70	7
Cold cuts	750	35	46	20	43	74	9
Sausages, frankfurters, and luncheon meats	754	23	71	6	31	72	8
Eggs	755	39	60	1	47	71	21
Cereal products							
Brown rice and pasta	755	39	59	2	45	70	12
White rice and pasta	755	30	69	2	33	70	9
Rye bread, crispbread, and thin rye crackers	755	13	55	32	45	75	9
Multigrain bread and wholemeal bread	754	18	59	24	36	74	8
White bread	755	67	28	5	58	63	12
Sugar-sweetened cereals and muesli	754	52	44	3	52	74	10
Berry, fruit, and chocolate porridge (with added sugar)	756	91	9	1	87	87	13
Wholegrain porridge and cereals (no added sugar)	756	31	54	15	46	82	5
Sweet biscuits and cereal bars	755	29	69	2	35	70	9
Sweet pastries [2]	755	22	77	0.3	27	71	6
Drinks							
Sugar-sweetened juice drinks	752	24	68	8	37	69	8
Fruit juice (no added sugar)	754	54	39	6	58	79	9
Soft drinks (with added sugar)	756	72	28	0.1	72	78	7
Reduced sugar juices and soft drinks	755	87	12	1	85	85	15

Table 1. *Cont.*

Food Item	n	Consumption Frequency according to FFQ, % of Participants			Comparison of the Two Methods, % of Participants		
		Not at All	Less than Daily	Daily	In the Same Quarter	In the Same or Adjacent Quarter	Grossly Misclassified Into Opposite Quarters
Others							
Chocolate	754	35	64	1	33	78	13
Sweets	756	16	83	1	20	78	14
Added sugar, honey, or syrup [3]	754	59	35	6	62	69	9
Jams, marmalades, and sweetened spreads	755	67	30	3	66	73	9
Plain nuts, almonds, and seeds	754	72	25	3	78	80	11
Flavored nuts, almonds, and seeds (e.g., salted nuts)	755	91	9	0	91	91	9
Crisps and popcorn	756	48	52	0.4	45	60	10

Items in the table are in the same order as in the FFQ (available at https://helda.helsinki.fi/handle/10138/235382). [1] As a side dish or as an ingredient in a dish. [2] Cakes, cupcakes, sweet rolls, Danish pastries, pies, and other sweet pastries. [3] for example, in porridge, tea, berries, yoghurt, or quark.

The calculated mean daily vitamin C and folate intakes increased linearly in the quarters of vegetable and fruit consumption (Table 2). Similarly, calcium intake was positively associated with milk consumption frequency, whereas sucrose intake increased in the quarters of sugary treats, sugary everyday foods, and sugary beverage consumption.

Table 2. Mean daily nutrient intake from foods consumed outside of preschool (three-day food record) according to categories of food group consumption (FFQ) in the DAGIS study (2015–2016, $n = 756$).

	Quarter of Food Group Consumption Frequency according to FFQ				p-Value for Trend [1]
	First	Second	Third	Fourth	
Vitamin C (mg) intake according to vegetable and fruit [2] consumption	35	47	54	61	<0.001
Folate intake (µg) according of vegetable and fruit [2] consumption	88	91	104	109	<0.001
Calcium intake (mg) according to milk [3] consumption	503	610	724	770	<0.001
Sucrose intake (g) according to sugary treats [4] consumption	26	29	29	34	<0.001
Sucrose intake (g) according to sugary everyday food [5] consumption	25	28	31	35	<0.001
Sucrose intake (g) according to sugary beverage [6] consumption	26	28	29	36	<0.001

[1] Linear regression with food consumption frequency category as a continuous predictor variable; nutrient intakes were square root transformed. [2] Sum of the FFQ rows "fresh vegetables", "cooked and canned vegetables", "peas, beans, lentils, and soya", and "fresh fruit'. [3] Sum of the FFQ rows "skimmed milk and sour milk", "1% fat milk, semi-skimmed milk, and sour milk", and "whole milk and sour milk'. [4] Sum of the FFQ rows "ice cream", "sweet biscuits and cereal bars", "cakes, cupcakes, sweet rolls, Danish pastries, pies, and other sweet pastries", "chocolate", and "sweets". [5] Sum of the FFQ rows "flavored yoghurt and quark", "puddings", "sugar-sweetened cereals and muesli", "berry, fruit and chocolate porridge (with added sugar)", and "berry and fruit soups (with added sugar)". [6] Sum of the FFQ rows "flavored and sweetened milk- and plant-based drinks", "sugar-sweetened juice drinks", and "soft drinks (with added sugar)".

3.2. *Comparison of Dietary Patterns*

The five food-record-based components explained altogether 19.7% of the variance in the sample (Supplementary Table S2), whereas the corresponding percentage in the FFQ-based analysis was 16.7% (for more details regarding the FFQ-based dietary patterns, please see [30]). Supplementary Table S2 also shows the loadings of foods into the components, percentage of variance explained by each component, and the eigenvalues in the food-record-based PCA. The food-record-based patterns were labelled "health-conscious", "sandwich", "sweets-and-treats", "milk, potatoes, and minced meat", and "pasta, minced meat, and fruit", based on the foods loading positively to each component. The FFQ-based patterns were named "sweets-and-treats", "health-conscious", and "vegetables-and-processed meats", and have been reported in more detail elsewhere [30]. The three strongest patterns identified using the two methods were very similar to each other, and there were relatively low, positive correlations between the pattern scores (Table 3). Regarding each of the dietary pattern scores, over 70% of the participants were classified into the same or adjacent quarter, whereas the proportion of participants classified into opposite quarters was 6%–9% for the three patterns (Table 4).

Table 3. Spearman correlation coefficients between the FFQ- and food-record-based dietary pattern scores (strongest positive correlation shown in bold).

	Food-Record-Based Dietary Patterns				
	Health-Conscious	Sandwich	Sweets-and-Treats	Milk, Potatoes and Minced Meat	Pasta, Minced Meat and Fruit
FFQ-based dietary patterns					
Sweets-and-treats	−0.19 [1]	−0.18 [1]	**0.27** [1]	0.22 [1]	−0.10 [1]
Health-conscious	**0.33** [1]	−0.05	−0.30 [1]	−0.16 [1]	0.08 [2]
Vegetables-and-processed meats	0.19 [1]	**0.25** [1]	0.16 [1]	0.08 [2]	0.11 [1]

[1] $p \leq 0.01$. [2] $p \leq 0.05$.

Table 4. The proportion of participants classified into the same, same or adjacent, or opposite quarters using the FFQ- and food-record-based dietary pattern scores.

	% of Participants Classified into the Same Quarter	% of Participants Classified into the Same or Adjacent Quarters	% of Participants Grossly Misclassified into Opposite Quarters
Sweets-and-treats patterns	34	72	7
Health-conscious patterns	35	73	6
Vegetables-and-processed meats/sandwich patterns	35	73	9

4. Discussion

The aim of the current study was to compare the food consumption frequencies and empirical dietary patterns derived with the following two methods: food records and FFQs. Regarding consumption frequencies, the percentage of participants classified into the same or adjacent quarter as measured with FFQs and food-records was 60%–96%. Considering vegetable and fruit consumption, 72%–80% of the participants were classified into the same or adjacent quarter in the current study, whereas the corresponding percentages for sugar-containing foods were 69%–87%. Furthermore, the calculated nutrient intakes for key nutrients increased linearly in the quarters of vegetable and fruit, and sugar-containing food consumption. In addition, we found dietary patterns of the same kind using FFQ and food-record food groups as input variables. To our knowledge, this is the first study to perform PCA separately based on FFQs and food records without forcing the food record food codes to match the FFQ rows, which could lead to overestimated correlation coefficients [20].

4.1. Relative Validity of the DAGIS FFQ

The percentages of participants classified into the same or adjacent quarter were the greatest for skimmed milk and sour milk (96%); 1% fat milk, semi-skimmed milk, and sour milk (94%); flavored nuts, almonds, and seeds (91%); and whole milk and sour milk (90%). In general, the food items that were used only by a small percentage of participants (less than 20% according to the FFQ) had the largest proportions of participants classified into the same or adjacent quarter. Among food items that were used by more than 20% of the participants at least once according to the FFQs, commercial baby foods and smoothies with no added sugar; plain almonds, nuts, and seeds; and soft drinks with added sugar were most similarly reported, as 77%–80% of the participants were classified into the same or adjacent quarter as measured with the FFQs and food records. By contrast, the relative validity of our FFQ to assess the consumption frequency of canned and frozen fruit, eggs, reduced sugar juices and soft drinks, and dried fruit and berries could partly be criticized, because 15%–22% of the participants were grossly misclassified into opposite quarters by the two methods. The difference in time spans (three days vs. seven days) might at least partly explain these misclassifications. In the future, it would be advisable to rephrase these items or to incorporate the foods into FFQ rows with a lower proportion of misclassification (for example, canned and frozen fruit could be incorporated into fresh fruit).

Our first aim was to compare the consumption frequencies reported using food records and FFQs. Considering vegetable and fruit consumption, 35%–68% of the participants were classified into the same quarter in the current study, whereas previous studies reported respective percentages ranging from 35%–49% for vegetable and fruit FFQ items [6,8,9]. The fact that the calculated intakes of vitamin C and folate increased linearly through the quarters of vegetable and fruit consumption frequency (Table 2) gives additional support to our finding that, compared to food records, the FFQ is able to rank the children acceptably according to food group consumption. Using a somewhat similar approach, Flood et al. reported an increasing trend in the calculated vitamin C intake for vegetable consumption, but not for fruit consumption [7].

Regarding sugary foods, the percentages of participants classified into the same quarter varied depending on the type of foods. The lowest percentages were observed for sugary treats (ice cream 37%; sweet biscuits and cereal bars 35%; sweet pastries 27%; sweets 20%; chocolate 33%). These are typically foods that are not consumed daily, and thus, their habitual consumption frequency may have been more accurately captured by the FFQ. On the other hand, as keeping a food record is known to affect food behavior [1], it may be that the parents withheld sugary treats during the three days the food records were kept. Previous studies have reported corresponding percentages ranging from 32%–37% [6,8,9]. However, the wide variation in food groupings between the studies limits the comparison. In the current study, 49%–87% of the participants were classified into the same quarter with regard to sugary everyday foods (berry and fruit soups; flavored yoghurt and quark; puddings; sugar-sweetened cereals and muesli; berry, fruit, and chocolate porridge), whereas the corresponding range for sugary beverages (flavored and sweetened milk- and plant-based drinks; sugar-sweetened juice drinks; soft drinks) was 37%–72%. The calculated sucrose intake increased linearly in the quarters of sugary treats, sugary everyday foods, and sugary beverages, suggesting a good indirect validity.

4.2. Relative Validity of the Dietary Patterns

Currently, explorative or data-driven dietary patterns are used frequently in modern nutrition science [11]. The dietary pattern approach has many advantages. First, the patterns provide us with a broader conception of food consumption and can add to our understanding of dietary behavior [31]. Second, the pattern approach is free of a priori assumptions concerning, for example, healthful diets, and describes the actual parallel presence of different patterns in the diets of the participants [12]. PCA is one of the most frequently used methods for dietary pattern analysis, and usually FFQ data are used as inputs for the analysis. The validity of the FFQs used to derive dietary patterns is often under study, but only a few studies have investigated the relative validity of the resulting dietary patterns among children [22,23].

To our knowledge, this is the first study to compare dietary patterns derived using two dietary assessment methods, without forcing the input variables to be similar (i.e., matching the foods from the food records into FFQ rows). The matching of the food items has resulted in the exclusion of a large number of foods that cannot be matched to each of the FFQ rows. For example, in a sample of middle-aged and elderly Swedish women, as much as 54% of the foods in the food records were excluded from the analyses [18]. Using this approach, the validity of the patterns is likely to be better than the actual validity [20].

In the present study, we found three quite similar dietary patterns using two dietary assessment methods (FFQs and food records). The pattern scores were correlated as statistically significantly, but the correlation coefficients were relatively low (0.25–0.33) [32]. Previous studies have reported correlations ranging from 0.32–0.74 among adults [15–20], and the correlations have been of the same order among adolescents [22] and toddlers [23]. Our lower correlation coefficients are probably due to not matching the foods from the food records to the FFQ rows. Instead, we conducted the PCA separately, using FFQ rows and food record data as inputs. Thus, we believe that the correlation coefficients in this study reflect the validity of the dietary patterns more realistically. However, more than 70% of the participants were classified into the same or adjacent quarter, according to the dietary pattern scores. Hence, it seems that despite the low correlation coefficients, the two dietary assessment methods can provide fairly similar dietary patterns and rank the participants similarly based on the dietary pattern scores.

4.3. Strengths and Limitations

The present study had several strengths. First, we had a large sample size of preschool-aged children and their parents as participants. Second, we used both direct (cross-classification) and indirect (calculated nutrient intakes) measures to assess the validity of the DAGIS FFQ. Furthermore, we investigated the relative validity of the dietary patterns using both food record data and FFQ rows as inputs. As we did not match the foods in the food records to the FFQ rows for this analysis, we were able to examine the similarity of the derived patterns without artificially overestimating the correlation coefficients. We believe that our approach provided us a more realistic and comprehensive view of the validity of the FFQ.

Our study used food records as the reference method for dietary assessment. However, it is crucial to consider the design of the study critically. FFQs are designed to measure the usual consumption of foods, whereas food records capture only the foods eaten during a few days [1]. Thus, three-day food records may underestimate the consumption of certain foods, such as sugar-containing treats or fish, and FFQs may be able to assess the consumption of these foods more accurately. As dietary patterns are thought to reflect the usual consumption of foods and beverages, FFQs could be thought of as a more accurate assessment method for less frequently used foods. In the present study, the FFQ measured food consumption during the previous week. Thus, the time span did not vary considerably between the two methods (seven days vs. three days), suggesting that the two methods can be meaningfully compared. As our FFQ only measured foods eaten outside of preschool hours, it does not represent the whole diet of the children. Thus, to make the two methods comparable, we excluded foods eaten at preschool from the reference method (three-day food record). However, should the FFQ be used in other studies, it must be noted that the relative validity has only been investigated concerning the foods eaten outside of preschool hours.

As measuring food consumption is not straightforward and every method has its own pitfalls, our measurements were not free of error. It is possible that some foods are most accurately measured using food records, whereas for other foods, the most accurate method might be FFQ. Thus, it must be kept in mind that whenever we are "validating" an FFQ, we are, in fact, just comparing it with another, equally (although differently) biased dietary assessment method, and not the true food consumption, which we unfortunately are unable to assess. Furthermore, the participating families in the DAGIS study were highly educated (in nearly 70% of the families, the highest educational level was bachelor's degree or higher [24]). As the socio-economic status of the family may be associated with misreporting [33], the results of this study may have to be generalized with caution.

5. Conclusions

The FFQ designed for the DAGIS study can rank participants acceptably. Special attention was paid to vegetables and fruits, and sugar-containing foods. The indirect measures of validity (mean intake of selected nutrients in quarters of the consumption) supported the aforementioned conclusion. In addition, three fairly similar dietary patterns were identified using both food-record and FFQ data as inputs, and the percentage of participants classified into the same or adjacent quarters were acceptable. Thus, we conclude that the DAGIS FFQ is a valid measure for vegetable and fruit as well as sugary food consumption. In addition, the DAGIS FFQ can be used to derive dietary patterns that are consistent with those derived using food record data.

Supplementary Materials:

Table S1: Food groups included and excluded in the food-record-based analysis and their mean consumption among 3–6 year-olds in the DAGIS study (2015–2016, $n = 756$); Table S2: Characteristics of the five food-record-based dietary patterns identified among 3–6 year-olds in the DAGIS study (2015–2016).

Author Contributions: Conceptualization, L.K., H.V., E.R. and M.E.; methodology, L.K., H.V., C.R., R.L., H.H.H.-a., K.N., J.M., E.R. and M.E.; formal analysis, L.K. and H.V.; investigation, C.R., E.S., R.L. and K.N.; data curation, L.K., H.V., E.S., R.L. and K.N.; writing (original draft preparation), L.K. and H.V.; writing (review and editing), C.R., E.S., R.L., H.H.H.-a., K.N., J.M., E.R. and M.E.; visualization, L.K. and H.V.; supervision, E.R. and M.E.; project administration, M.E.; funding acquisition, E.R. and M.E.

Acknowledgments: The authors thank the preschools, the preschool personnel, and the families for their participation in the DAGIS study, as well as the staff for data collection.

References

1. Slimani, N.; Freisling, H.; Illner, A.; Huybrechts, I. Methods to determine dietary intake. In *Nutrition Research Methodologies*, 1st ed.; Lovegrove, J.A., Hodson, L., Sharma, S., Lanham-New, S.A., Eds.; John Wiley & Sons Ltd.: Chichester, UK, 2015.
2. Willett, W. Food frequency methods. In *Nutritional Epidemiology*, 3rd ed.; Willett, W., Ed.; Oxford University Press: New York, NY, USA, 2013.
3. Livingstone, M.B.E.; Robson, P.J. Measurement of dietary intake in children. *Proc. Nutr. Soc.* **2000**, *59*, 279–293. [CrossRef] [PubMed]
4. Willett, W.; Lenart, E. Reproducibility and validity of food frequency questionnaires. In *Nutritional Epidemiology*, 3rd ed.; Willett, W., Ed.; Oxford University Press: New York, NY, USA, 2013.
5. Kolodziejczyk, J.; Merchant, G.; Norman, G. Reliability and validity of child/adolescent food frequency questionnaires that assess foods and/or food groups. *J. Pediatr. Gastroenterol. Nutr.* **2012**, *55*, 4–13. [CrossRef] [PubMed]
6. Buch-Andersen, T.; Pérez-Cueto, F.J.A.; Toft, U. Relative validity and reproducibility of a parent-administered semi-quantitative FFQ for assessing food intake in Danish children aged 3-9 years. *Public Health Nutr.* **2016**, *19*, 1184–1194. [CrossRef] [PubMed]
7. Flood, V.M.; Wen, L.M.; Hardy, L.L.; Rissel, C.; Simpson, J.M.; Baur, L.A. Reliability and validity of a short FFQ for assessing the dietary habits of 2-5-year-old children, Sydney, Australia. *Public Health Nutr.* **2014**, *17*, 498–509. [CrossRef] [PubMed]
8. Huybrechts, I.; De Backer, G.; De Bacquer, D.; Maes, L.; De Henauw, S. Relative validity and reproducibility of a food-frequency questionnaire for estimating food intakes among Flemish preschoolers. *Int. J. Environ. Res. Public Health* **2009**, *6*, 382–399. [CrossRef] [PubMed]
9. Klohe, D.M.; Clarke, K.K.; George, G.C.; Milani, T.J.; Hanss-Nuss, H.; Freeland-Graves, J. Relative validity and reliability of a food frequency questionnaire for a triethnic population of 1-year-old to 3-year-old children from low-income families. *J. Am. Diet Assoc.* **2005**, *105*, 727–734. [CrossRef] [PubMed]

10. Marshall, T.A.; Eichenberger, G.J.M.; Broffitt, B.; Stumbo, P.J.; Levy, S.M. Relative validity of the Iowa Fluoride Study targeted nutrient semi-quantitative questionnaire and the block kids' food questionnaire for estimating beverage, calcium, and vitamin D intakes by children. *J. Am. Diet Assoc.* **2008**, *108*, 465–472. [CrossRef]
11. Mozaffarian, D.; Rosenberg, I.; Uauy, R. History of modern nutrition science—Implications for current research, dietary guidelines, and food policy. *BMJ* **2018**, *361*, k2392. [CrossRef]
12. Newby, P.K.; Tucker, K.L. Empirically derived eating patterns using factor or cluster analysis: A review. *Nutr. Rev.* **2004**, *62*, 177–203. [CrossRef]
13. Willett, W. Issues in analysis and presentation of dietary data. In *Nutritional Epidemiology*, 3rd ed.; Willett, W., Ed.; Oxford University Press: New York, NY, USA, 2013.
14. Martínez, M.E.; Marshall, J.R.; Sechrest, L. Invited commentary: Factor analysis and the search for objectivity. *Am. J. Epidemiol.* **1998**, *148*, 17–19. [CrossRef]
15. Beck, K.L.; Kruger, R.; Conlon, C.A.; Heath, A.M.; Coad, J.; Matthys, C.; Jones, B.; Stonehouse, W. The relative validity and reproducibility of an iron food frequency questionnaire for identifying iron-related dietary patterns in young women. *J. Acad. Nutr. Diet* **2012**, *112*, 1177–1187. [CrossRef]
16. Crozier, S.R.; Inskip, H.M.; Godfrey, K.M.; Robinson, S.M. Dietary patterns in pregnant women: A comparison of food-frequency questionnaires and 4 d prospective diaries. *Br. J. Nutr.* **2008**, *99*, 869–875. [CrossRef] [PubMed]
17. Hu, F.B.; Rimm, E.; Smith-Warner, S.A.; Feskanich, D.; Stampfer, M.J.; Ascherio, A.; Sampson, L.; Willett, W.C. Reproducibility and validity of dietary patterns assessed with a food-frequency questionnaire. *Am. J. Clin. Nutr.* **1999**, *69*, 243. [CrossRef] [PubMed]
18. Khani, B.R.; Ye, W.; Terry, P.; Wolk, A. Reproducibility and validity of major dietary patterns among Swedish women assessed with a food-frequency questionnaire. *J. Nutr.* **2004**, *134*, 1541–1545. [CrossRef] [PubMed]
19. Nanri, A.; Shimazu, T.; Ishihara, J.; Takachi, R.; Mizoue, T.; Inoue, M.; Tsuqane, S. Reproducibility and validity of dietary patterns assessed by a food frequency questionnaire used in the 5-year follow-up survey of the Japan Public Health Center-Based Prospective Study. *J. Epidemiol.* **2012**, *22*, 205–215. [CrossRef] [PubMed]
20. Okubo, H.; Murakami, K.; Sasaki, S.; Kim, M.K.; Hirota, N.; Notsu, A.; Fukui, M.; Date, C. Relative validity of dietary patterns derived from a self-administered diet history questionnaire using factor analysis among Japanese adults. *Public Health Nutr.* **2010**, *13*, 1080–1089. [CrossRef] [PubMed]
21. Togo, P.; Heitmann, B.L.; Sørensen, T.I.; Osler, M. Consistency of food intake factors by different dietary assessment methods and population groups. *Br. J. Nutr.* **2003**, *90*, 667–678. [CrossRef]
22. Ambrosini, G.L.; O'Sullivan, T.A.; de Klerk, N.H.; Mori, T.A.; Beilin, L.J.; Oddy, W.H. Relative validity of adolescent dietary patterns: A comparison of a FFQ and 3 d food record. *Br. J. Nutr.* **2011**, *105*, 625–633. [CrossRef] [PubMed]
23. Mills, V.C.; Skidmore, P.M.; Watson, E.O.; Taylor, R.W.; Fleming, E.A.; Heath, A.L. Relative validity and reproducibility of a food frequency questionnaire for identifying the dietary patterns of toddlers in New Zealand. *J. Acad. Nutr. Diet* **2015**, *115*, 551–558. [CrossRef] [PubMed]
24. Lehto, E.; Ray, C.; Vepsäläinen, H.; Korkalo, L.; Lehto, R.; Kaukonen, R.; Suhonen, E.; Nislin, M.; Nissinen, K.; Skaffari, E.; et al. Increased Health and Wellbeing in Preschools (DAGIS) Study—differences in children's energy balance-related behaviors (EBRBs) and in long-term stress by parental educational level. *Int. J. Environ. Res. Public Health* **2018**, *15*, 2313. [CrossRef] [PubMed]
25. Vepsäläinen, H. Food Environment and Whole-Diet in Children—Studies on Parental Role Modelling and Food Availability. Ph.D. Thesis, University of Helsinki, Helsinki, Finland, June 2018.
26. Määttä, S.; Vepsäläinen, H.; Lehto, R.; Erkkola, M.; Roos, E.; Ray, C. Reproducibility of preschool and guardian reports on energy balance-related behaviors and their correlates in Finnish preschool children. *Children* **2018**, *5*, 144. [CrossRef] [PubMed]
27. Nissinen, K.; Sillanpää, H.; Korkalo, L.; Roos, E.; Erkkola, M. *Annoskuvakirja Lasten Ruokamäärien Arvioinnin Avuksi*, 1st ed.; Unigrafia: Helsinki, Finland, 2016.

28. Nissinen, K.; Korkalo, L.; Vepsäläinen, H.; Mäkiranta, P.; Koivusilta, L.; Roos, E.; Erkkola, M. Accuracy in the estimation of children's food portion sizes against the food picture book: Do parents and early educators estimate portions with similar accuracy? *J. Nutr. Sci.* **2018**, *7*, e35. [CrossRef] [PubMed]
29. Määttä, S.; Lehto, R.; Nislin, M.; Ray, C.; Erkkola, M.; Sajaniemi, N.; Roos, E. Increased health and well-being in preschools (DAGIS): Rationale and design for a randomized controlled trial. *BMC Public Health* **2015**, *15*, 402. [CrossRef] [PubMed]
30. Vepsäläinen, H.; Korkalo, L.; Mikkilä, V.; Lehto, R.; Ray, C.; Nissinen, K.; Skaffari, E.; Fogelholm, M.; Koivusilta, L.; Roos, E.; et al. Dietary patterns and their associations with home food availability among Finnish pre-school children: A cross-sectional study. *Public Health Nutr.* **2018**, *21*, 1232–1242. [CrossRef] [PubMed]
31. Hu, F.B. Dietary pattern analysis: A new direction in nutritional epidemiology. *Curr. Opin. Lipidol.* **2002**, *13*, 3–9. [CrossRef] [PubMed]
32. Hinkle, D.E.; Jurs, S.G.; Wiersma, W. *Applied Statistics for the Behavioral Sciences*, 5th ed.; Houghton Mifflin Company: Boston, MA, USA, 2003.
33. Börnhorst, C.; Huybrecths, I.; Ahrens, W.; Eiben, G.; Michels, N.; Pala, V.; Molnár, D.; Russo, P.; Barba, G.; Bel-Serrat, S.; et al. Prevalence and determinants of misreporting among European children in proxy-reported 24 h dietary recalls. *Br. J. Nutr.* **2013**, *109*, 1257–1265. [CrossRef] [PubMed]

6

Dietary Patterns of European Children and their Parents in Association with Family Food Environment: Results from the I.Family Study

Antje Hebestreit [1,*,†], Timm Intemann [1,†], Alfonso Siani [2], Stefaan De Henauw [3], Gabriele Eiben [4], Yiannis A. Kourides [5], Eva Kovacs [6,7], Luis A. Moreno [8], Toomas Veidebaum [9], Vittorio Krogh [10], Valeria Pala [10], Leonie H. Bogl [1,11,12], Monica Hunsberger [4], Claudia Börnhorst [1] and Iris Pigeot [1]

1 Leibniz-Institute for Prevention Research and Epidemiology—BIPS, 28359 Bremen, Germany; intemann@leibniz-bips.de (T.I.); leonie-helen.bogl@helsinki.fi (L.H.B.); boern@leibniz-bips.de (C.B.); pigeot@leibniz-bips.de (I.P.)

2 Institute of Food Sciences, National Research Council, 83100 Avellino, Italy; asiani@isa.cnr.it

3 Department of Public Health, Ghent University, 9000 Ghent, Belgium; stefaan.dehenauw@ugent.be

4 Department of Public Health and Community Medicine, University of Gothenburg, 40530 Gothenburg, Sweden; gabriele.eiben@medfak.gu.se (G.E.); monica.hunsberger@gu.se (M.H.)

5 Research and Education Institute of Child Health, 2035 Strovolos, Cyprus; kourides@cytanet.com.cy

6 Institute for Medical Information Processing, Biometrics and Epidemiology, Ludwig-Maximilians-Universität München, 81377 Munich, Germany; eva.kovacs@med.uni-muenchen.de

7 German Center for Vertigo and Balance Disorders, Ludwig-Maximilians-Universität München, 81377 Munich, Germany

8 GENUD (Growth, Exercise, Nutrition and Development) Research Group, Instituto Agroalimentario de Aragón (IA2), Instituto de Investigación Sanitaria Aragón (IIS Aragón), Centro de Investigación Biomédica en Red Fisiopatología de la Obesidad y Nutrición (CIBERObn), University of Zaragoza, 50009 Zaragoza, Spain; lmoreno@unizar.es

9 Department of Chronic Diseases, National Institute for Health Development, 11619 Tallinn, Estonia; toomas.veidebaum@tai.ee

10 Department of Preventive and Predictive Medicine, Fondazione IRCCS Istituto Nazionale dei Tumori, 20133 Milan, Italy; Vittorio.Krogh@istitutotumori.mi.it (V.K.); Valeria.Pala@istitutotumori.mi.it (V.P.)

11 Department of Public Health, University of Helsinki, 00014 Helsinki, Finland

12 Finnish Institute of Molecular Medicine, University of Helsinki, 00014 Helsinki, Finland

* Correspondence: hebestr@leibniz-bips.de

† Shared first authorship.

Abstract: The aim of this study was to determine whether an association exists between children's and parental dietary patterns (DP), and whether the number of shared meals or soft drink availability during meals strengthens this association. In 2013/2014 the I.Family study cross-sectionally assessed the dietary intakes of families from eight European countries using 24-h dietary recalls. Usual energy and food intakes from six- to 16-year-old children and their parents were estimated based on the NCI Method. A total of 1662 child–mother and 789 child–father dyads were included; DP were derived using cluster analysis. We investigated the association between children's and parental DP and whether the number of shared meals or soft drink availability moderated this association using mixed effects logistic regression models. Three DP comparable in children and parents were obtained: Sweet & Fat, Refined Cereals, and Animal Products. Children were more likely to be allocated to the Sweet & Fat DP when their fathers were allocated to the Sweet & Fat DP and when they shared at least one meal per day (OR 3.18; 95% CI 1.84; 5.47). Being allocated to the Sweet & Fat DP increased when the mother or the father was allocated to the Sweet & Fat DP and when soft drinks were available (OR 2.78; 95% CI 1.80; 4.28 or OR 4.26; 95% CI 2.16; 8.41, respectively). Availability of soft drinks and negative parental role modeling are important predictors of children's dietary patterns.

Keywords: food consumption; family resemblance; cluster analysis; shared meals; soft drink; childhood obesity

1. Introduction

Family members share similar eating habits that are affected by individual factors and the family food environment [1]. Parental role modeling and perception of adequacy of their child's diet are important predictors for the child's current dietary behavior [2] and watching the parents eat raises the children's awareness of their parents' eating behaviors [3,4]. Despite the fact that fathers and mothers were found to influence the child's eating behavior [5,6], the influence differs for mothers compared to fathers [7,8]. Paternal dietary influence was identified for fruit but also for fat-and energy-dense, nutrient-poor foods [9,10], whereas positive child–mother correlations have been reported for fruit and vegetable intake [11] and soft drinks [12]. Thus, parents build their children's food environment by making healthy foods [13] or unhealthy foods [14] available. Accordingly the children's food consumption was associated with healthy foods (so-called core foods, e.g., cereals, dairy, fruit, and vegetables) or with unhealthy non-core foods (e.g., snack foods, fats, and oils) [5]. As an example, adolescents were more likely to consume fruit and vegetables when parents made those foods available [15,16]. It has been observed that the person who prepares the majority of family meals largely influences the consumption of fruit and vegetables but also high-fat foods; this association increases with increasing numbers of shared meals [17].

Previous research has demonstrated that the association between parental and child intake increased with an increasing number of family meals at home [18] and that the number of family meals was positively associated with the consumption of healthier foods [19]. Family mealtimes provide structure and a regular opportunity for developing emotional connections among family members and therefore help children to monitor their mood and learn healthy dietary behaviors [20]. Accordingly, higher family meal frequency was found to be associated with significantly fewer weekly servings of sweets and sugar-sweetened beverages [21]; however, the consumption of those non-core foods (e.g., sugar sweetened beverages) was found to be higher when their home availability was higher [5]. Consumption of sugar-sweetened beverages is one epidemiological key health indicator of the European Core Health Indicators [22] and is frequently used in public health monitoring, especially when addressing socioeconomic determinants of eating behavior in European children and adolescents [23,24]. Investigations in low-income parent–child dyads found that soft drink availability at home was a strong influencing factor for the children's soft drink intake [25], identifying parents as gatekeepers for the family food environment.

Apart from this literature, it is striking that there is little knowledge about the resemblance of entire dietary patterns among children and their parents across Europe, which was described in the present study. The previous literature mainly investigated parental influence on the children's intake of particular food groups such as fruit and vegetables or sugar-sweetened beverages. We therefore aimed at adding knowledge on the influence of the entire parental DP on the children's DP. Besides parental intake, home availability has also been found to predict children's intake of core-food and non-core foods. Thus, we aimed at determining whether the family food environment (operationalized as the number of shared meals and availability of soft drinks during meals) moderated the association between children's DP and parental DP. Understanding to what extent the family food environment, along with the parental DP, influences children's eating behavior has important public health implications, because in this age children and adolescents mostly still live with their parents and potentially eat up to three meals a day at home. Development of intervention strategies to improve children's dietary patterns is likely to be more successful if supported by an understanding not only healthy but also unhealthy food intake.

2. Materials and Methods

2.1. Study Participants

Data from this investigation were obtained from the I.Family cohort. In 2013/2014 the I.Family study cross-sectionally examined children and parents from Sweden, Germany, Hungary, Italy, Cyprus, Spain, Belgium, and Estonia in order to investigate associations between eating habits and lifestyle factors leading to overweight and obesity [26]. For this investigation children and adolescents from six years to approximately 16 years who lived with their families were invited to the examination, together with the person having the care and custody of the child (hereinafter named parents). In the present analysis we included children and parents providing at least one 24HDR ($N = 4816$). In the final mixed effects logistic regression model, we included 1662 child–mother dyads (with 1269 mothers) and 789 child–father dyads (with 566 fathers); of those, 516 families provided information from siblings and 362 families provided information from the mother and father. Information on the availability of soft drinks during meals was provided for 1607 child–mother dyads and 763 child–father dyads.

Parents and children older than 16 years provided written informed consent. Younger children gave oral consent for examinations and sample collection. Study subjects and their parents could consent to single components of the study while abstaining from others. Study participants did not undergo any procedures unless they (and their parents) had given consent for examinations, collection of samples, subsequent analysis, and storage of personal data and collected samples. All applicable institutional and governmental regulations concerning the ethical use of human volunteers were followed during this research. Each participating center obtained ethical approval from the local responsible authorities in accordance with the ethical standards of the 1964 Declaration of Helsinki and its later amendments.

2.2. Questionnaires and Anthropometric Measurements

Questionnaires were developed in English, translated into local languages, and then back-translated to check for translation errors. Parents reported the age and sex of their children and themselves in addition to their highest educational level according to the International Standard Classification of Education (ISCED) [27], which was used as a proxy indicator for the socioeconomic status (SES) of the family. Additionally, parents reported if soft drinks are available at home during meals (answer options: Yes, often or always; No or rarely).

The field methods comprised anthropometric measurements of standing height (cm) using a Seca 225 stadiometer (Seca GmbH & KG, Birmingham, UK) in accordance with international standards for anthropometric assessment and weight (kg) [28]. Body weight was assessed in fasting status using a prototype of the TANITA BC 420 SMA digital scale for children and a TANITA BC 418 MA for adolescents and adults (TANITA Europe GmbH, Sindelfingen, Germany). All measurements were performed in light clothing (e.g., underwear) [29].

The BMI of the participants was calculated by dividing body weight in kilograms by squared body height in meters. The BMI of children was transformed to an age- and sex-specific z-score according to Cole et al. [30]. Weight groups (thin/normal and overweight/obese) of children were categorized using age- and sex-specific cutoff values based on the extended IOTF criteria [31]. Weight groups of adolescents and parents above 18 years were calculated using WHO cutoffs [32]. Even though weight status was not a focus of this investigation, it was calculated for a better characterization of the study population.

2.3. Dietary Information

Dietary intake of the previous 24 h was assessed using an online 24-h dietary recall (24HDR) assessment program, called 'Self-Administered Children, Adolescents and Adult Nutrition Assessment' (SACANA), based on the validated SACINA offline version [33]. The instrument has been validated and results supported the validity of SACANA as a self-reporting instrument for assessing intakes in children (publications in progress).

Children and parents were asked to recall their diet and to enter the type and amount (g) of all drinks and foods consumed during the previous day, starting with the first intake after waking up in the morning. Children under 11 years were advised to ask their parents for help [34]. Study participants above 11 years of age could ask for assistance from a dietician or trained study nurse during the survey examinations, but the majority of participants had no questions since they already participated in the IDEFICS study and were therefore familiar with the recall procedures and software structure used. Standardized photographs were used to assist with accurate estimation of portion size [35]. In the present study, participants were asked to complete at least three 24HDR during the upcoming four weeks. However, the availability of repeated 24HDR varied among individuals from one to four recalls. For 43% of parents (39% of children), three repeated 24HDR were available.

The total number of main meals (breakfast, lunch, and dinner) per participant was calculated. Breakfast was defined as "shared" if the total number of shared breakfasts (parent with child) divided by the number of all reported breakfasts of the respective parent was at least 0.5. Shared lunches and dinners were categorized accordingly. The sum of all shared main meals per parent was calculated and the following categories were derived: (1) <1 shared meal per day and (2) $\geq$1 shared meal per day.

2.4. Dietary Data Analysis

Missing or implausible values for intake of single food items that could not be corrected were imputed by country, food group, and age-specific median intakes (0.15% of the entries). Incomplete 24HDR (recalls that have not been completed throughout) and those with more than four imputed values were excluded from the analysis.

Age- and sex-specific Goldberg cutoffs were applied to classify each recall day as under-reported, plausibly reported, and over-reported energy intake, as described elsewhere [36].

In total, we excluded 955 participants classified as misreporters from the analysis: 484 children and 471 adults; among those 95% and 99% were under-reporters, and 5% and 1% were over-reporters, respectively.

Each food recorded by SACANA was assigned to one of 15 dietary categories: healthy and unhealthy cereals and cereal products, unhealthy sugar and sugar products, healthy and unhealthy fat and fat savory sauces, healthy fruit and vegetables, healthy and unhealthy meat and meat products, healthy meat alternatives, healthy and unhealthy milk and dairy products, healthy and unhealthy non-alcoholic beverages, healthy and unhealthy mixed dishes (Table 1). Foods were categorized as "healthy" when they contained less energy, less sugar, less (unhealthy) fat, or more fiber than the unhealthy food alternative, e.g., table water (healthy beverage) vs. juice (unhealthy beverage), plain yogurt (healthy) vs. full fat and sweetened yogurt (unhealthy). Consumption of unhealthy mixed dishes was so rare that this category was not included in further analysis.

After food categorization, individual usual daily energy intake (EI, kcal/day) and individual usual intakes of dietary categories (kcal/day, healthy non-alcoholic beverages: g/day) were estimated based on the U.S. National Cancer Institute Method [37,38]. This method allows the inclusion of covariates like age and additional food frequency information, accounts for different intake on weekend vs. work days, and corrects for the variance inflation caused by the daily variation in diet. Usual intakes were estimated for children as well as for their parents, stratified by sex (all participants with at least one plausible 24HDR). Age was considered as a covariate in all models. When estimating usual food intakes, the corresponding food consumption frequency obtained from the I.Family food frequency questionnaire was also used as a covariate to improve estimates (except for mixed dishes, as this food group was not queried in the food frequency questionnaire but was a generic category in SACANA food groups). The I.Family food frequency questionnaire was built on the valid and reproducible IDEFICS study food frequency questionnaire, which was described in detail previously [39–41]. The FFQ contained 59 food items comparable to those in the SACANA web tool, thus allowing categorizing the food items according to the 15 dietary categories mentioned above. The answer possibilities in the FFQ were "never/less than once a week", "1–3 times a week", "4–6 times a week", "1 time/day", "2 times a day", "3 times a day", and "I have no idea". All participants were asked to complete one FFQ for the four weeks prior to the survey examination.

Table 1. Food groups and healthy/unhealthy dietary categories.

Food Group	Healthy Alternative	Unhealthy Alternative
Cereals & cereal products	Low sugar content (<15%), low fat content (<20%) and high fiber content (≥5%)	≥15% sugar, ≥20% fat, and <5% fiber content
Sugar & sweets	-	Sugar, sweets, candies, marzipan, chocolate, nut spreads, jam, honey, ice cream, canned/sugared fruit, etc.
Fats & oils	From mainly plant origin, and for sauces <40% fat content	Mainly animal and processed origin and ≥40% fat for sauces
Non-alcoholic beverages	Non-caloric and non-processed beverages such as table water, plain herbal teas, plain coffee	Sweetened and processed beverages: manufactured juices, sodas, ice tea, energy drinks, coffee/tea with milk/sugar, broth
Meat	Containing <10% fat, and meat products with <20% fat from poultry, rabbit or game	Meat from all other origins than poultry, including offal, with ≥10% fat and meat products containing ≥20% fat
Meat alternative	Soy products, meat and dairy substitutes from soy, vegetarian burgers, tempeh, tofu, seitan and lean prepared fish and eggs	-
Milk & dairy products	Low fat and unsweetened	Full fat and sweetened, flavored
Fruit & vegetables	Fresh fruit and vegetables, their fresh juices/smoothies, or lean preparation, without added sugars	-
Mixed dishes	Based on cereals, legumes, vegetables/potatoes with small amounts of fish, egg or dairy, soups, veloutés, mixed salad	Based on meat; fried foods (also fried vegetables), fast food, snack foods (not included in the final cluster analysis)

The individual percentage of energy contribution from all dietary categories was calculated to correct for individual total EI. For children and adults separately, these percentages were transformed into *z*-scores using sample means and sample standard deviations. The *z*-score represents the distance between the percentage of energy contribution and the corresponding population mean in units of the standard deviation. This procedure was not applied for usual EI and usual intake of non-alcoholic beverages (g/day) since EI correction is neither reasonable for EI itself nor for the calorie-free dietary category. Therefore, age-dependent *z*-scores were derived for these variables with the Generalized Additive Models for Location, Scale, and Shape (this procedure is described in detail in Appendix A).

2.5. Statistical Analysis

K-means clustering was applied for children and parents separately to identify distinct clusters of participants with similar dietary patterns. In this procedure the previously derived *z*-scores were taken into account. Details of this procedure are described in Appendix A. As clusters were comparable between children and parents, the same cluster names were used. Three clusters representing the DP (Figure 1) were obtained: Sweet and Fat cluster, Refined Cereals cluster, and Animal Products cluster. Each participant was allocated to exactly one DP and corresponding indicator variables were derived (participant is in the respective cluster versus participant is not in the respective cluster).

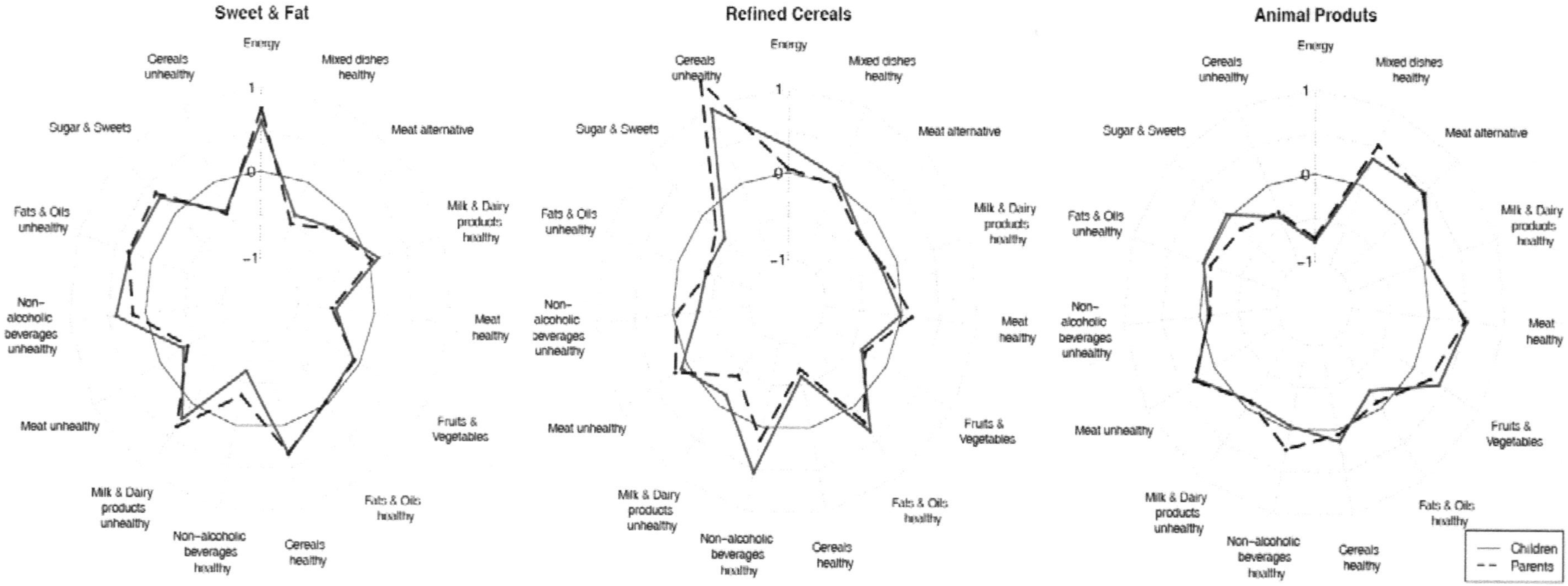

Figure 1. Dietary patterns of children and their parents: Sweet and Fat, Refined Cereals, and Animal Products. Mean *z*-scores of percentage of energy intake of different food groups in the three clusters for children and parents are shown (for details, see Table 2). The scale ranges from −1 to 1 with tick lines for −0.5, 0 (solid line) and 0.5.

Family food environment was operationalized using the number of shared meals (<1 or ≥1 shared meal per day) as an indicator of parental role modeling and the availability of soft drinks during meals as an indicator of home food availability. As a first step, we investigated associations between the outcome children's DP (indicator variable) and the exposure parental DP (indicator variable) and the number of shared meals using mixed effects logistic regression. To examine whether the number of shared meals strengthened the associations between parental and children's DP, an interaction term was included (number of shared meal × parental DP). For each of the three DP, we conducted a regression analysis separately for fathers and mothers (six models). Accordingly, we investigated in a second step the associations between children's DP and the exposure parental DP and availability of soft drinks during meals. To examine whether the availability of soft drinks during meals strengthened the associations between parental DP and children's DP, an interaction term (availability of soft drinks during meals × parental DP) was included. The models were adjusted for sex, age and BMI *z*-score of the children, ISCED, country, and BMI of the respective parent. In order to account for dependencies between siblings, a random effect was added for family membership. Based on the mixed effects logistic regression models, odds ratios (OR) and confidence intervals (95%CI) were calculated for a child being allocated to the DP corresponding to the parental DP depending on the number of shared meals and availability of soft drinks during meals. The analysis was performed using the procedure PROC GLIMMIX of the statistical software SAS (version 9.3; SAS Institute, Cary, NC, USA).

3. Results

The aims of the present study were to investigate the resemblance of children's DP and their parents' DP as well as to determine whether structural conditions of the family food environment moderated the association between children's DP and parental DP.

3.1. Dietary Clusters

Based on dietary categories (Table 1) and usual EI, the three-cluster solutions were derived. For comparable clusters of children and parents, the following labels were assigned: Sweet and Fat ($N = 697$ for children and $N = 728$ for parents), Refined Cereals ($N = 563$ for children and $N = 410$ for parents), and Animal Products ($N = 716$ for children and $N = 747$ for parents).

Table 2 presents the mean *z*-scores and standard deviations of usual intake for all dietary categories in the three clusters for children and parents.

In general, we observed a resemblance of children's dietary patterns to parents' dietary pattern; details of these analyses can be found in Appendix A. The overall agreement between cluster allocation of children and mothers was 52% (for fathers, 53%).

In particular, we observed the following characteristics for the three clusters representing dietary patterns (DP).

Sweet and Fat: Children and adults allocated to this cluster reported higher-than-mean intake of sugar and sweets (children's mean 0.27; parents' mean 0.34), unhealthy fats and oils (children's mean 0.29; parents' mean 0.31), unhealthy (sweetened) non-alcoholic beverages (children's mean 0.39; parents' mean 0.17) and unhealthy milk and dairy products (children's mean 0.22; parents' mean 0.34) (Figure 1). Cereals were categorized as healthy in case of low sugar content and low fat content and high fiber content (Table 1), such as whole-grain breads, plain breakfast cereals, or crispbread (children's mean 0.34; parents' mean 0.33). Family members allocated to this DP reported the highest EI (children's mean 0.60; parents' mean 0.75).

Refined Cereals: Children and parents from this cluster reported higher-than-mean intake of unhealthy cereals (e.g., white breads, refined and/or sugared breakfast cereals, pasta from refined wheat, refined rice, sweet and/or fatty bakery products (biscuits, cakes, fritters, etc.; children's mean 0.96; parents' mean 1.32) and healthy fats and oils (children's mean 0.36; parents' mean 0.23). Both children and parents also consumed more healthy non-alcoholic beverages (children's mean 0.54; parents' mean 0.15).

Table 2. *z*-scores of usual intake in the three clusters for children and for parents (mean values and standard deviations).

Children	Sweet & Fat (*N* = 697; 35%)		Ref. Cereals (*N* = 563; 28%)		Animal Products (*N* = 716; 36%)	
	Mean	SD	Mean	SD	Mean	SD
Energy	0.60 [a]	0.82	0.32	0.83	−0.78 [b]	0.79
Non-alcoholic beverages—healthy	−0.64 [b]	0.89	0.54 [a]	0.81	−0.04	1.01
Non-alcoholic beverages—unhealthy	0.39 [a]	1.24	−0.33 [b]	0.67	−0.12	0.82
Cereals—unhealthy	−0.37	0.7	0.96 [a]	1.06	−0.40 [b]	0.61
Cereals—healthy	0.34 [a]	1.05	−0.61 [b]	0.64	0.14	0.97
Sugar & Sweets	0.27 [a]	0.94	−0.39 [b]	0.94	0.05	1.00
Fats & Oils—unhealthy	0.29 [a]	1.21	−0.38 [b]	0.61	0.02	0.93
Fats & Oils—healthy	−0.03	1.03	0.36 [a]	1.18	−0.25 [b]	0.69
Fruit & Vegetables	−0.09	0.96	−0.37 [b]	0.87	0.39 [a]	1.00
Meat—unhealthy	−0.35 [b]	0.88	0.09	1.02	0.27 [a]	1.00
Meat—healthy	−0.51 [b]	0.73	−0.01	0.96	0.51 [a]	1.01
Milk & Dairy products—unhealthy	0.22 [a]	1.13	−0.15 [b]	0.91	−0.1	0.89
Milk & Dairy products—healthy	0.12 [a]	1.09	−0.22 [b]	0.82	0.05	1.02
Meat alternative	−0.24	0.78	−0.25 [b]	0.71	0.42 [a]	1.22
Mixed dishes—healthy	−0.41 [b]	0.89	0.08	0.97	0.34 [a]	0.98
Parents	**Sweet & Fat (*N* = 728; 39%)**		**Ref. Cereals (*N* = 410; 22%)**		**Animal Products (*N* = 747; 40%)**	
	Mean	**SD**	**Mean**	**SD**	**Mean**	**SD**
Energy	0.75 [a]	0.76	0.05	0.83	−0.73 [b]	0.75
Non-alcoholic beverages—healthy	−0.36 [b]	1.01	0.15	0.87	0.23 [a]	0.96
Non-alcoholic beverages—unhealthy	0.17 [a]	1.12	−0.05	1.03	−0.14 [b]	0.82
Cereals—unhealthy	−0.40 [b]	0.59	1.32	1.09	−0.34	0.55
Cereals—healthy	0.33 [a]	1.02	−0.69 [b]	0.58	0.06	0.97
Sugar & Sweets	0.34 [a]	0.96	−0.24 [b]	0.93	−0.20	0.99
Fats & Oils—unhealthy	0.31 [a]	1.17	−0.41 [b]	0.66	−0.08	0.87
Fats & Oils—healthy	−0.03	1.04	0.23 [a]	1.11	−0.09 [b]	0.87
Fruit & Vegetables	−0.08	0.94	−0.32 [b]	0.95	0.25 [a]	1.02
Meat—unhealthy	−0.41 [b]	0.87	0.18	0.91	0.30 [a]	1.03
Meat—healthy	−0.56 [b]	0.74	0.13	0.84	0.48 [a]	1.03
Milk & Dairy products—unhealthy	0.34 [a]	1.14	−0.42 [b]	0.72	−0.09	0.87
Milk & Dairy products—healthy	0.03	1.02	−0.18 [b]	0.93	0.07 [a]	1.00
Meat alternative	−0.25	0.77	−0.29 [b]	0.65	0.40 [a]	1.21
Mixed dishes—healthy	−0.53 [b]	0.91	−0.01	0.84	0.52 [a]	0.89

[a] The highest mean value within a row; [b] The lowest mean value within a row.

Animal Products: Children and parents who were allocated to this cluster reported higher intake of all types of meat (children's mean for meat unhealthy 0.27, meat healthy 0.51; parents' mean 0.30 and 0.48, respectively) and meat alternatives (children's mean 0.42; parents' mean 0.40) as well as of healthy mixed dishes (children's mean 0.34; parents' mean 0.52). Healthy mixed dishes were mainly based on cereals, legumes, and vegetables/potatoes, with small proportions of fish, egg, or dairy. Children and parents further reported higher-than-mean intakes of fruit and vegetables (children's mean 0.39; parents' mean 0.25). Parents reported a higher-than-mean intake for healthy non-alcoholic beverages (mean 0.23). The energy intake of children and parents was lowest in this DP (children's mean −0.78; parents' mean −0.73).

3.2. Participant Characteristics

The largest proportion of children (36%) and parents (40%) was allocated to the Animal Products cluster (Table 3). The mean age of children (11.4 years) and parents (44.2 years) was highest in the

Refined Cereals cluster. Girls (39%) and mothers (44%) were mainly found in the Sweet and Fat cluster, whereas most boys and men were found in the Animal Products cluster (38% and 44%, respectively).

Table 3. Characteristics of the study population, including plausible reporters stratified by cluster membership and misreporters (number and percentages).

Covariates	Plausible Reporters												Misreporters			
	Children, Adolescents						Parents						Children, Adolescents		Parents	
	Sweet & Fat (N = 697; 35%)		Ref. Cereals (N = 563; 28%)		Animal Products (N = 716; 36%)		Sweet & Fat (N = 728; 39%)		Ref. Cereals (N = 410; 22%)		Animal Products (N = 747; 40%)		(N = 484)		(N = 471)	
Age mean (SD)	10.9 (2.1)		11.4 (2.1)		11.2 (2.1)		41.8 (5.4)		44.2 (5.8)		41.8 (5.4)		12.2 (1.9)		42.3 (5.7)	
Age range (min; max)	6.0; 15.8		6.0; 16.0		6.0; 16.0		28.1; 58.5		30.3; 65.4		27.0; 63.0		6.5; 15.7		27.8; 58.7	
Sex (N, %)																
Male	322	32	311	30	387	38	149	26	173	30	257	44	238	49	139	30
Female	375	39	252	26	329	34	579	44	237	18	490	38	246	51	332	71
Weight group (N, %N) [a]																
Normal weight	588	37	403	25	613	38	428	43	175	18	388	39	310	64	159	34
Overweight	93	32	115	39	84	32	209	34	157	25	255	41	123	25	156	33
Obese	16	20	45	56	19	24	91	33	78	29	104	38	51	11	156	33
ISCED-Level of parents [b] (N, %)																
Low Education	5	12	31	76	5	12	1	3	24	71	9	26	26	5	31	7
Medium Education	200	31	245	38	207	32	185	30	190	31	234	38	227	47	235	50
High Education	482	39	271	22	491	39	529	44	182	15	488	41	226	47	199	42
Missing ISCED [c]	10	26	16	41	13	33	13	30	14	33	16	37	5	1	6	1
County (N, %)																
Italy	8	3	232	85	32	12	14	6	179	77	38	16	59	12	77	16
Estonia	275	50	29	5	246	45	341	56	28	5	244	40	148	31	82	17
Cyprus	28	17	66	39	75	44	33	21	40	26	81	53	27	6	41	9
Belgium	67	44	14	9	73	47	66	55	14	12	39	33	24	5	18	4
Sweden	133	39	120	35	89	26	113	40	58	20	113	40	55	11	66	14
Germany	149	49	40	13	113	37	133	47	39	14	114	40	143	30	147	31
Hungary	29	32	38	42	23	26	11	12	41	45	39	43	17	4	25	5
Spain	8	8	24	25	65	67	17	16	11	10	79	74	11	2	15	3

[a] Weight categories according to Cole et al. [30] for children and according to WHO for adults; [b] International Standard Classification of Education Maximum (ISCED); maximum of both parents (0, 1, 2 = low education; 3, 4 = medium education; 5, 6 = high education); [c] Those individuals with missing ISCED information were excluded from mixed effects logistic regression models.

Most normal weight children were allocated to the Animal Products cluster (38%), whereas most overweight (39%) and obese (56%) children were allocated to the Refined Cereals cluster. Most normal weight adults (43%) were in the Sweet and Fat cluster; most overweight (41%) and obese (38%) adults were found in the Animal Products cluster.

Children and adults from low SES families mainly belonged to the Refined Cereals cluster (76% and 71%, respectively). Children from high SES families were equally allocated to the Sweet and Fat and the Animal Products clusters (both 39%).

In all countries—except Belgium—those cluster memberships with the highest proportion of children and parents were comparable. In Italy and Hungary most children and parents shared the

Refined Cereals cluster; in Estonia, Sweden and Germany most shared the Sweet and Fat cluster; and in Cyprus and Spain most shared the Animal Products cluster. In Belgium 47% of children were found in the Animal Products cluster, but 55% of their parents in the Sweet and Fat cluster.

3.3. Family Food Environment

Shared meals: Resemblance was observed between parental DP and children's DP: the chance of the child being allocated to the Sweet and Fat DP, the Refined Cereals DP, and the Animal Products DP is higher if the mother was allocated to the same DP, independently of the number of shared meals, compared to the chance if the mother was in a different DP (Table 4). Overall, children were more likely to be allocated to the Sweet and Fat DP if the father was allocated to the same DP; the odds ratio increased with an increase in the number of shared meals from <1 to ≥1 (OR 2.30; 95% CI 1.15; 4.57 or OR 3.18; 95% CI 1.84; 5.47, respectively).

Soft drink availability during meals: The child was more likely to be allocated to the Sweet and Fat DP if soft drinks were available during meals, even if the mother was not allocated to the Sweet and Fat DP (OR 1.97; 95% CI 1.20; 3.25, Table 5). The chance of being allocated to the Sweet and Fat DP was highest if the mother was allocated to the Sweet and Fat DP and soft drinks were available during meals (OR 2.78; 95% CI 1.80; 4.28). The child was more likely to be allocated to the Refined Cereals DP or the Animal Products DP if the mother was allocated to the same DPs and if no soft drinks were available during meals (OR 2.48; 95% CI 1.43 and 4.27; OR 2.16;1.59; 2.92, respectively). The child was most likely to be allocated to the Sweet and Fat DP, the Refined Cereals DP, and the Animal Products DP if the father was allocated to the respective DP and if soft drinks were not available during meals (OR 2.48; 95% CI 1.58; 3.87, OR 2.05; 95% CI 1.22; 3.45 and OR 2.48; 95% CI 1.62; 3.79, respectively). The chance of the child sharing the father's Sweet and Fat DP is higher if soft drinks are available during meals (OR 4.26; 95% CI 2.16; 8.41).

Table 4. Odds Ratios (OR) and confidence intervals (CI) for a child being allocated to a dietary pattern depending on parental dietary pattern and number of shared daily meals, given by sex of parents; all models were adjusted for age and BMI *z*-score of child, parental BMI, highest ISCED of family, and country of residence.

Parental Dietary Pattern	Children's Dietary Pattern								
	Sweet & Fat			Ref. Cereals			Animal Products		
	N	OR	95%CI	*N*	OR	95%CI	*N*	OR	95%CI
Maternal dietary pattern (*N* = 1662)									
Different & <1 shared meal (reference)	132	1.00		265	1.00		183	1.00	
Different & ≥1 shared meals	771	0.97	0.59; 1.58	1096	1.20	0.70; 2.07	877	1.06	0.70; 1.60
Identical & <1 shared meal	158	2.12	1.18; 3.81	25	5.70	1.51; 21.48	107	2.18	1.21; 3.92
Identical & ≥1 shared meals	601	1.91	1.17; 3.13	276	2.70	1.34; 5.45	495	2.19	1.41; 3.40
Paternal dietary pattern (*N* = 789)									
Different & <1 shared meal (reference)	149	1.00		153	1.00		112	1.00	
Different & ≥1 shared meals	430	1.31	0.82; 2.09	396	0.83	0.45;1.54	338	0.55	0.32; 0.92
Identical & <1 shared meal	58	2.30	1.15; 4.57	54	1.66	0.68;4.06	95	1.45	0.78; 2.71
Identical & ≥1 shared meals	152	3.18	1.84; 5.47	186	1.99	0.98;4.08	244	1.54	0.91; 2.59

Table 5. Odds Ratios (OR) and confidence intervals (CI) for a child being allocated to a dietary pattern depending on parental dietary pattern and availability of soft drinks during meals, given by sex of parents; all models were adjusted for age and BMI z-score of child, parental BMI, highest ISCED of family, and country of residence.

Parental Dietary Pattern	Children's Dietary Pattern								
	Sweet & Fat			Ref. Cereals			Animal Products		
	N	OR	95%CI	*N*	OR	95%CI	*N*	OR	95%CI
Maternal dietary pattern (*N* = 1607)									
Different & soft drink not available (reference)	742	1.00		1017	1.00		767	1.00	
Different & soft drink is available	138	1.97	1.20; 3.25	294	0.46	0.25; 0.84	256	0.95	0.65; 1.38
Identical & soft drink not available	521	2.04	1.49; 2.80	246	2.48	1.43; 4.27	496	2.16	1.59; 2.92
Identical & soft drink is available	206	2.78	1.80; 4.28	50	1.67	0.66; 4.22	88	1.42	0.82; 2.47
Paternal dietary pattern (*N* = 763)									
Different & soft drink not available (reference)	465	1.00		407	1.00		360	1.00	
Different & soft drink is available	92	1.55	0.90; 2.68	122	0.43	0.18; 1.04	80	0.83	0.45; 1.52
Identical & soft drink not available	151	2.48	1.58; 3.87	209	2.05	1.22; 3.45	256	2.48	1.62; 3.79
Identical & soft drink is available	55	4.26	2.16; 8.41	25	1.97	0.61; 6.39	67	1.80	0.96; 3.36

4. Discussion

The present study suggests important similarities between children's and parental DP. Three DP were obtained in this multi-country study: Animal Products, Refined Cereals, and Sweet and Fat. To our knowledge, this is the first study presenting the resemblance of the DP of pan-European children and their parents using cluster analysis. The study was further able to describe how the family food environment (operationalized as the number of shared meals and the availability of soft drinks during meals) moderated the association between children's DP and parental DP.

Resemblance of dietary patterns between children and parents: Previously, maternal consumption of core foods (e.g., cereals, dairy, fruit, and vegetables) and non-core foods (e.g., snack foods, fats, and oils) has been shown to be associated with a child's higher intake of the same foods [5]. Mothers tend to be the person habitually preparing the family meals [17] and mothers reported greater perceived responsibility for feeding their children [18]. Women are known to exert positive influence on children's food consumption [42] because they are more likely to adhere to dietary guidelines [43]. This is in line with our findings that identified the influencing nature of the maternal Animal Products DP per se and when the mother was eating with the child: in our study the Animal Products DP was characterized through the above-the-mean intake of healthy food alternatives such as fruit vegetables, healthy alternatives for meat, meat substitutes, milk and dairy products, cereals, and mixed dishes (Figure 1). Reported EIs were lowest in the Animal Products DP and we observed the highest proportion of normal weight children in this DP but the highest proportion of overweight parents. Fathers' influence on the child's food choices was highest for the foods of the Sweet and Fat DP including all types of sugar and sweets, unhealthy fats and oils, unhealthy beverages, and unhealthy milk and dairy products. In particular, the z-scores for non-alcoholic unhealthy beverages (including also soft drinks) were highest in the Sweet and Fat DP compared to the other two DP. Likewise, previous studies have reported that fathers have primary influence on the children's intake of non-core foods [8].

Dietary patterns and shared meals: In our study associations were found between children's DP and maternal DP independently of the number of shared meals and in particular between children's DP and fathers' Sweet and Fat DP if $\geq$1 meal was eaten together. Also in previous studies, paternal influence has been found to predict child's food intake in that fathers used pressure tactics whereas mothers praised children for eating certain things [44]. In particular, Robinson et al. [7] observed strong correlations for foods typically eaten at breakfast such as grains and fruit in child–father dyads for families with working mothers, indicating that fathers have breakfast with their children when mothers leave home early. Children and adolescents sharing three or more meals per week with the family had healthier dietary patterns compared to those who share fewer than three family meals [45]. This is in contrast to our findings, where children who eat together with their fathers at least once a day were more likely to share the Sweet and Fat DP with their fathers than sharing the generally healthier Animal Products DP.

Dietary patterns and the availability of soft drinks during meals: Although the mechanisms for how family meals facilitate healthy eating behaviors have not been empirically explained, different approaches are currently discussed. Eating together is an important ritual for interacting with family members and offers opportunities for children to learn about eating by watching others [3]. Also, low availability and consumption of convenient foods or sodas during family meals can contribute to healthy dietary intake patterns [46]. On the other hand, the availability of soft drinks during shared meals and parental soft drink consumption were associated with the child's soft drink consumption (Sweet and Fat DP) in our study. This is in line with earlier findings from U.S. studies where parental food choices [3] and soft drink availability were strong influencing factors for the children's intake [25], identifying parents as gatekeepers for the family food environment and as role models. Those foods (preferred and) consumed by the parents were the foods to which children were routinely exposed and shaped the children's food preferences and consumption [47,48]. It is not surprising that the availability of soft drinks and chips has been observed to be greater in families who frequently consumed fast food during family meals [49]. We therefore suggest that home availability of foods is an important predictor for children's preferences, even more so if parents choose the same foods during meals [50]. Making healthy foods available and also eating those foods may enhance children's understanding and acceptance of a healthy diet [51].

Limitations and Strengths

In the I.Family study dietary information was mainly given by self-respondents. Self-reporting can be susceptible to reporting bias [52]. We therefore followed a rigorous approach in order to reduce errors due to portion size estimation, incomplete recalls, misreporting, or daily variations in intake. Firstly, the development of the SACANA computer-assisted assessment tool with standardized photographs, multiple plausibility checks, and reminding questions facilitated the reporting of accurate portion sizes and complete recall. Secondly, as a first step in the data analysis, the exclusion of incomplete recalls and recalls with implausible energy reporting helped to correct for reporting bias. Individuals with misreported EI (under-reporters: 462 children, 465 adults; over-reporters: 22 children, six adults) were more likely to be female, from medium educated families, and from Estonia or Germany. They were more often overweight and obese (66% of adults; 36% of children) compared to plausible reporters (16% adults, 4% children). In a separate analysis we derived the clusters including the 955 misreporters in order to compare cluster memberships of the plausible reporters sample (1662 child–mother dyads and 789 child–father dyads) with the cluster memberships of the full study sample (2269 child–mother dyads and 1058 child–father dyads). After comparing the cluster membership of the full sample (also including misreporters) with the final study sample (plausible reporters only) we observed that the three DP remained comparable, except that EI was found to be lower in the Animal Products cluster when misreporters were included. As the Animal Products cluster included 58% of misreporting children and 83% of misreporting parents, including misreporters would overestimate intake (particularly in the Animal Product cluster) and underestimate the intake of plausible reporters (particularly in the Refined Cereals and Sweet and Fat clusters), given that we consider the percentage of energy contribution from dietary categories. We therefore decided to exclude the misreporters from the analysis. However, the question of how to handle possibly implausible interviews has not been answered conclusively: the inclusion of misreports may obscure or even inverse diet–disease relationships, as recently reported, and adjustment for the reporting group may also lead to bias [53]. Finally, deriving the usual intake based on the NCI method [37] and accounting for day-to-day variation in intake is a clear strength of this study.

As might be expected, we observed a resemblance between the parental DP and children's DP. These improved relations do not reflect reporting bias (due to proxy-reporting of dietary intake), as reported in other studies [18]. In the present study, participants personally reported dietary intake; thus the strength of association between child–mother dyads and child–father dyads truly reflect the environmental influence of parents on the child's DP and can be seen as an additional strength of this study. In general, the I.Family study allows a deep insight into the resemblance of DP among family members across Europe and the influence of parental DP on their child's DP when eating together or not. The large sample size comprises data from eight European countries; the strictly standardized data assessment, documentation, and data cleaning processing guarantee the highest possible data quality.

5. Conclusions

Using cluster analysis to derive dietary patterns allowed us to compare groups of European children and their parents with different dietary profiles and to examine the effect of daily number of shared meals and soft drink availability during meals on the association between child's and parental DP. The availability of soft drinks during meals and negative parental role modeling are important predictors for intake of sweet and fat foods in children. Intervention strategies should focus on healthy shopping choices. Parents as gatekeepers for home food availability and as role models for children's eating behavior should be counseled in which foods should be consumed on a regular basis and which foods should be avoided at home. Not purchasing unhealthy foods will decrease their availability at home and during meals; thus, their consumption may be hampered and may decline in parents and their children.

Acknowledgments: We gratefully acknowledge the financial support of the European Community within the Seventh RTD Framework Program Contract No. 266044. We thank the I.Family children and their parents for participating in this extensive examination. We are grateful for the support from school boards, headmasters, and communities. The publication of this article was funded by the Open Access Fund of the Leibniz Association.

Author Contributions: The authors' responsibilities were as follows—Antje Hebestreit had the idea for the analysis and wrote the paper; Antje Hebestreit and Timm Intemann had primary responsibility for the final content; Claudia Börnhorst and Timm Intemann performed the data analysis; Alfonso Siani, Stefaan De Henauw, Gabriele Eiben, Yiannis A. Kourides, Eva Kovacs, Luis A. Moreno, Toomas Veidebaum, Vittorio Krogh, Valeria Pala, Leonie H. Bogl, Monica Hunsberger, and Iris Pigeot participated in the coordination of the data collection. All authors were responsible for critical revisions and final approval of the manuscript. This manuscript represents original work that has not been published previously and is not currently being considered by another journal. If accepted, it will not be published elsewhere, including electronically in the same form, in English or in any other language, without the written consent of the copyright holder.

Appendix A

In the appendix we give details on (1) the derivation of z-scores of usual energy intake and z-scores of healthy non-alcoholic beverages and (2) on the clustering procedure. Both were conducted with the statistical software R (version 3.1.0) [54].

Appendix A.1. Derivation of z-Scores

In contrast to the intake of the food groups (measured in kcal/day) the usual energy intake (kcal/day) and usual intake of healthy non-alcoholic beverages (g/day) cannot be reasonably adjusted for total energy intake. Therefore, we decided to adjust energy intake and the percentage of intake contribution from healthy non-alcoholic beverages for age and sex as a surrogate for adjustment for total energy intake, since age and sex are strongly associated with total energy intake. We applied the Generalized Additive Models for Location, Scale, and Shape (GAMLSS) [55] in order to derive sex- and age-specific z-scores for these variables. GAMLSS allows for deriving sex- and age-specific percentile curves. Stratified by sex and separately for children and parents, such curves were estimated. By default, we used a GAMLSS model consisting of Box–Cox power exponential distribution.

The distribution parameters were modeled with penalized B-splines depending on age. If this default model did not converge or provided inadequate results, we used the Box–Cox Cole and Green distribution (BCCG) and/or cubic splines instead: For energy intake in men and intake of healthy non-alcoholic beverages in women, we used the BCCG distribution; for healthy non-alcoholic beverages in boys we used cubic splines. According to the estimated curves, values of usual energy intake and intake of healthy non-alcoholic beverages were transformed into individual *z*-scores.

The interpretation of the *z*-scores derived by GAMLSS differs slightly from the common z-scores of the food groups (measured in kcal/day): For the common *z*-score, a positive (negative) value indicates a value above (below) the mean percentage of energy from the specific food group, whereas for the *z*-scores derived by GAMLSS, a positive (negative) value indicates a value above (below) the sex- and age-specific mean. However, for both types of *z*-scores, the mean is zero and the standard deviation is one.

Appendix A.2. Clustering Procedure

Cluster analysis using the k-means approach by Hartigan and Wong [56] was applied to identify clusters of children and clusters of parents with similar dietary patterns. The usual intake variables (sex- and age-adjusted *z*-scores and energy-adjusted *z*-scores) were used in the cluster analysis to find clusters of children and adults with distinct dietary patterns.

Since the true number of clusters is unknown and k-means only converge to a local minimum, the k-means algorithm was applied with 50 random starts for each number of clusters from two to eight. Accordingly, out of these 50 solutions the one with the lowest total within cluster sum of squares was chosen. For these solutions the convergence criterion was reached in fewer than nine iterations. To decide on the appropriate number of clusters, all final two to eight cluster solutions were examined: since silhouette coefficients [57] and the total within cluster sum of squares did not give a clear indication for an appropriate number of clusters, the interpretability of the clusters was used as the decision criterion. The three-cluster solution was favored. To evaluate the reproducibility of the cluster solutions, we conducted a cluster analysis in a randomly chosen subsample containing 85% of subjects [58]. This was repeated 10 times for children and adults separately. Compared to the whole sample solutions, the percentage of agreement and the adjusted Rand Index (ARI) [59] were calculated for the three-cluster solutions, leading to a mean agreement of 97% (95%) and a mean ARI of 0.92 (0.87) for adults (children).

Since the dietary patterns of children and parents were very similar, the same cluster names were used. The Euclidian distances between cluster centroids among children and adults were calculated (Table A1), showing that the distances between same labeled clusters were lowest. Two examples illustrating the Euclidean distances between children's and parents' DP are given: a constant difference of 0.1 between children's and parents' *z*-scores leads to a distance of 0.39; a constant difference of 0.6 leads to a distance of 2.32.

Table A1. Cross-tabulation of Euclidean distances between the cluster means of children and parents.

Parents	Children, Adolescents Sweet & Fat	Ref. Cereals	Animal Products
Sweet & Fat	0.45	2.54	2.45
Ref. Cereals	2.7	0.77	2.51
Animal Products	2.48	2.25	0.49

References

1. Patrick, H.; Nicklas, T.A. A review of family and social determinants of children's eating patterns and diet quality. *J. Am. Coll. Nutr.* **2005**, *24*, 83–92. [CrossRef] [PubMed]
2. Campbell, K.J.; Crawford, D.A.; Ball, K. Family food environment and dietary behaviors likely to promote fatness in 5–6 year-old children. *Int. J. Obes. (Lond.)* **2006**, *30*, 1272–1280. [CrossRef] [PubMed]

3. Draxten, M.; Fulkerson, J.A.; Friend, S.; Flattum, C.F.; Schow, R. Parental role modeling of fruits and vegetables at meals and snacks is associated with children's adequate consumption. *Appetite* **2014**, *78*, 1–7. [CrossRef] [PubMed]
4. Brown, R.; Ogden, J. Children's eating attitudes and behaviour: A study of the modelling and control theories of parental influence. *Health Educ. Res.* **2004**, *19*, 261–271. [CrossRef] [PubMed]
5. Johnson, L.; van Jaarsveld, C.H.; Wardle, J. Individual and family environment correlates differ for consumption of core and non-core foods in children. *Br. J. Nutr.* **2011**, *105*, 950–959. [CrossRef] [PubMed]
6. Freeman, E.; Fletcher, R.; Collins, C.E.; Morgan, P.J.; Burrows, T.; Callister, R. Preventing and treating childhood obesity: Time to target fathers. *Int. J. Obes. (Lond.)* **2012**, *36*, 12–15. [CrossRef] [PubMed]
7. Robinson, L.N.; Rollo, M.E.; Watson, J.; Burrows, T.L.; Collins, C.E. Relationships between dietary intakes of children and their parents: A cross-sectional, secondary analysis of families participating in the family diet quality study. *J. Hum. Nutr. Diet.* **2014**, *28*, 443–451. [CrossRef] [PubMed]
8. Raynor, H.A.; Van Walleghen, E.L.; Osterholt, K.M.; Hart, C.N.; Jelalian, E.; Wing, R.R.; Goldfield, G.S. The relationship between child and parent food hedonics and parent and child food group intake in children with overweight/obesity. *J. Am. Diet. Assoc.* **2011**, *111*, 425–430. [CrossRef] [PubMed]
9. Hall, L.; Collins, C.E.; Morgan, P.J.; Burrows, T.L.; Lubans, D.R.; Callister, R. Children's intake of fruit and selected energy-dense nutrient-poor foods is associated with fathers' intake. *J. Am. Diet. Assoc.* **2011**, *111*, 1039–1044. [CrossRef] [PubMed]
10. Wang, Y.; Beydoun, M.A.; Li, J.; Liu, Y.; Moreno, L.A. Do children and their parents eat a similar diet? Resemblance in child and parental dietary intake: Systematic review and meta-analysis. *J. Epidemiol. Community Health* **2011**, *65*, 177–189. [CrossRef] [PubMed]
11. Fisher, J.O.; Mitchell, D.C.; Smiciklas-Wright, H.; Birch, L.L. Parental influences on young girls' fruit and vegetable, micronutrient, and fat intakes. *J. Am. Diet. Assoc.* **2002**, *102*, 58–64. [CrossRef]
12. Grimm, G.C.; Harnack, L.; Story, M. Factors associated with soft drink consumption in school-aged children. *J. Am. Diet. Assoc.* **2004**, *104*, 1244–1249. [CrossRef] [PubMed]
13. Hanson, N.I.; Neumark-Sztainer, D.; Eisenberg, M.E.; Story, M.; Wall, M. Associations between parental report of the home food environment and adolescent intakes of fruits, vegetables and dairy foods. *Public Health Nutr.* **2005**, *8*, 77–85. [CrossRef] [PubMed]
14. Martens, M.K.; van Assema, P.; Brug, J. Why do adolescents eat what they eat? Personal and social environmental predictors of fruit, snack and breakfast consumption among 12–14-year-old dutch students. *Public Health Nutr.* **2005**, *8*, 1258–1265. [CrossRef] [PubMed]
15. Ray, C.; Roos, E.; Brug, J.; Behrendt, I.; Ehrenblad, B.; Yngve, A.; Te Velde, S.J. Role of free school lunch in the associations between family-environmental factors and children's fruit and vegetable intake in four european countries. *Public Health Nutr.* **2013**, *16*, 1109–1117. [CrossRef] [PubMed]
16. Pearson, N.; Biddle, S.J.; Gorely, T. Family correlates of breakfast consumption among children and adolescents. A systematic review. *Appetite* **2009**, *52*, 1–7. [CrossRef] [PubMed]
17. Hannon, P.A.; Bowen, D.J.; Moinpour, C.M.; McLerran, D.F. Correlations in perceived food use between the family food preparer and their spouses and children. *Appetite* **2003**, *40*, 77–83. [CrossRef]
18. Oliveria, S.A.; Ellison, R.C.; Moore, L.L.; Gillman, M.W.; Garrahie, E.J.; Singer, M.R. Parent-child relationships in nutrient intake: The framingham children's study. *Am. J. Clin. Nutr.* **1992**, *56*, 593–598. [PubMed]
19. Neumark-Sztainer, D.; Story, M.; Resnick, M.D.; Blum, R.W. Correlates of inadequate fruit and vegetable consumption among adolescents. *Prev. Med.* **1996**, *25*, 497–505. [CrossRef] [PubMed]
20. Fiese, B.H.; Hammons, A.; Grigsby-Toussaint, D. Family mealtimes: A contextual approach to understanding childhood obesity. *Econ. Hum. Biol.* **2012**, *10*, 365–374. [CrossRef] [PubMed]
21. Welsh, E.M.; French, S.A.; Wall, M. Examining the relationship between family meal frequency and individual dietary intake: Does family cohesion play a role? *J. Nutr. Educ. Behav.* **2011**, *43*, 229–235. [CrossRef] [PubMed]
22. Expert Group on Health Information. The European Core Health Indicators Shortlist. Available online: http://ec.europa.eu/health/indicators/docs/echi_shortlist_by_policy_area_en.pdf (accessed on 7 February 2017).
23. Fismen, A.; Smith, O.R.F.; Torsheim, T.; Rasmussen, M.; Pagh, T.P.; Augustine, L.; Ojala, K.; Samdal, O. Trends in food habits and their relation to socioeconomic status among nordic adolescents 2001/2002-2009/2010. *PLoS ONE* **2016**, *11*. [CrossRef] [PubMed]
24. Mathieson, A.; Koller, T. *Addressing the Socioeconomic Determinants of Healthy Eating Habits and Physical Activity Levels among Adolescents*; World Health Organization: Geneva, Switzerland, 2005.

25. Pinard, C.A.; Davy, B.M.; Estabrooks, P.A. Beverage intake in low-income parent-child dyads. *Eat. Behav.* **2011**, *12*, 313–316. [CrossRef] [PubMed]
26. Ahrens, W.; Siani, A.; de Henauw, S.; Eiben, G.; Gwozdz, W.; Hebestreit, A.; Hunsberger, M.; Kaprio, J.; Krogh, V.; Lissner, L.; et al. Cohort profile: The transition from childhood to adolescence in european children-how I.Family extends the IDEFICS cohort. *Int. J. Epidemiol.* **2016**. [CrossRef] [PubMed]
27. UNESCO. International Standard Classification of Education. Available online: http://www.uis.unesco.org/Education/Documents/isced-2011-en.pdf (accessed on 7 February 2017).
28. Stomfai, S.; Ahrens, W.; Bammann, K.; Kovacs, E.; Marild, S.; Michels, N.; Moreno, L.A.; Pohlabeln, H.; Siani, A.; Tornaritis, M.; et al. Intra- and inter-observer reliability in anthropometric measurements in children. *Int. J. Obes. (Lond.)* **2011**, *35* (Suppl. S1), S45–S51. [CrossRef] [PubMed]
29. Suling, M.; Hebestreit, A.; Peplies, J.; Bammann, K.; Nappo, A.; Eiben, G.; Alvira, J.M.; Verbestel, V.; Kovacs, E.; Pitsiladis, Y.P.; et al. Design and results of the pretest of the IDEFICS study. *Int. J. Obes. (Lond.)* **2011**, *35* (Suppl. S1), S30–S44. [CrossRef] [PubMed]
30. Cole, T.J.; Freeman, J.V.; Preece, M.A. British 1990 growth reference centiles for weight, height, body mass index and head circumference fitted by maximum penalized likelihood. *Stat. Med.* **1998**, *17*, 407–429. [CrossRef]
31. Cole, T.J.; Lobstein, T. Extended international (IOTF) body mass index cut-offs for thinness, overweight and obesity. *Pediatr. Obes.* **2012**, *7*, 284–294. [CrossRef] [PubMed]
32. World Health Organization. The International Classification of Adult Underweight, Overweight and Obesity according to BMI. Available online: http://apps.who.int/bmi/index.jsp?introPage=intro_3.html (accessed on 7 February 2017).
33. Hebestreit, A.; Börnhorst, C.; Barba, G.; Siani, A.; Huybrechts, I.; Tognon, G.; Eiben, G.; Moreno, L.A.; Fernandez Alvira, J.M.; Loit, H.M.; et al. Associations between energy intake, daily food intake and energy density of foods and BMI *z*-score in 2–9-year-old european children. *Eur. J. Nutr.* **2014**, *53*, 673–681. [CrossRef] [PubMed]
34. Livingstone, M.B.; Robson, P.J. Measurement of dietary intake in children. *Proc. Nutr. Soc.* **2000**, *59*, 279–293. [CrossRef] [PubMed]
35. Hebestreit, A.; Barba, G.; De Henauw, S.; Eiben, G.; Hadjigeorgiou, C.; Kovacs, E.; Krogh, V.; Moreno, L.A.; Pala, V.; Veidebaum, T.; et al. Cross-sectional and longitudinal associations between energy intake and BMI z-score in european children. *Int. J. Behav. Nutr. Phys. Act.* **2016**, *13*, 23. [CrossRef] [PubMed]
36. Börnhorst, C.; Huybrechts, I.; Ahrens, W.; Eiben, G.; Michels, N.; Pala, V.; Molnar, D.; Russo, P.; Barba, G.; Bel-Serrat, S.; et al. Prevalence and determinants of misreporting among european children in proxy-reported 24 h dietary recalls. *Br. J. Nutr.* **2012**, *109*, 1257–1265. [CrossRef] [PubMed]
37. Tooze, J.A.; Midthune, D.; Dodd, K.W.; Freedman, L.S.; Krebs-Smith, S.M.; Subar, A.F.; Guenther, P.M.; Carroll, R.J.; Kipnis, V. A new statistical method for estimating the usual intake of episodically consumed foods with application to their distribution. *J. Am. Diet. Assoc.* **2006**, *106*, 1575–1587. [CrossRef] [PubMed]
38. Kipnis, V.; Midthune, D.; Buckman, D.W.; Dodd, K.W.; Guenther, P.M.; Krebs-Smith, S.M.; Subar, A.F.; Tooze, J.A.; Carroll, R.J.; Freedman, L.S. Modeling data with excess zeros and measurement error: Application to evaluating relationships between episodically consumed foods and health outcomes. *Biometrics* **2009**, *65*, 1003–1010. [CrossRef] [PubMed]
39. Lanfer, A.; Hebestreit, A.; Ahrens, W.; Krogh, V.; Sieri, S.; Lissner, L.; Eiben, G.; Siani, A.; Huybrechts, I.; Loit, H.M.; et al. Reproducibility of food consumption frequencies derived from the children's eating habits questionnaire used in the IDEFICS study. *Int. J. Obes. (Lond.)* **2011**, *35* (Suppl. S1), S61–S68. [CrossRef] [PubMed]
40. Bel-Serrat, S.; Mouratidou, T.; Pala, V.; Huybrechts, I.; Bornhorst, C.; Fernandez-Alvira, J.M.; Hadjigeorgiou, C.; Eiben, G.; Hebestreit, A.; Lissner, L.; et al. Relative validity of the children's eating habits questionnaire-food frequency section among young european children: The IDEFICS study. *Public Health Nutr.* **2014**, *17*, 266–276. [CrossRef] [PubMed]
41. Huybrechts, I.; Bornhorst, C.; Pala, V.; Moreno, L.A.; Barba, G.; Lissner, L.; Fraterman, A.; Veidebaum, T.; Hebestreit, A.; Sieri, S.; et al. Evaluation of the children's eating habits questionnaire used in the IDEFICS study by relating urinary calcium and potassium to milk consumption frequencies among european children. *Int. J. Obes. (Lond.)* **2011**, *35* (Suppl. S1), S69–S78. [CrossRef] [PubMed]

42. Drucker, R.R.; Hammer, L.D.; Agras, W.S.; Bryson, S. Can mothers influence their child's eating behavior? *J. Dev. Behav. Pediatr.* **1999**, *20*, 88–92. [CrossRef] [PubMed]
43. Turrell, G. Compliance with the australian dietary guidelines in the early 1990's: Have population-based health promotion programs been effective? *Nutr. Health* **1997**, *11*, 271–288. [CrossRef] [PubMed]
44. Orrell-Valente, J.K.; Hill, L.G.; Brechwald, W.A.; Dodge, K.A.; Pettit, G.S.; Bates, J.E. "Just three more bites": An observational analysis of parents' socialization of children's eating at mealtime. *Appetite* **2007**, *48*, 37–45. [CrossRef] [PubMed]
45. Hammons, A.J.; Fiese, B.H. Is frequency of shared family meals related to the nutritional health of children and adolescents? *Pediatrics* **2011**, *127*, e1565–e1574. [CrossRef] [PubMed]
46. Gillman, M.W.; Rifas-Shiman, S.L.; Frazier, A.L.; Rockett, H.R.; Camargo, C.A., Jr.; Field, A.E.; Berkey, C.S.; Colditz, G.A. Family dinner and diet quality among older children and adolescents. *Arch. Fam. Med.* **2000**, *9*, 235–240. [CrossRef] [PubMed]
47. Cullen, K.W.; Baranowski, T.; Rittenberry, L.; Olvera, N. Social-environmental influences on children's diets: Results from focus groups with african-, euro- and mexican-american children and their parents. *Health Educ. Res.* **2000**, *15*, 581–590. [CrossRef] [PubMed]
48. Birch, L.L. Children's preferences for high-fat foods. *Nutr. Rev.* **1992**, *50*, 249–255. [CrossRef] [PubMed]
49. Boutelle, K.N.; Fulkerson, J.A.; Neumark-Sztainer, D.; Story, M.; French, S.A. Fast food for family meals: Relationships with parent and adolescent food intake, home food availability and weight status. *Public Health Nutr.* **2007**, *10*, 16–23. [CrossRef] [PubMed]
50. Trofholz, A.C.; Tate, A.D.; Draxten, M.L.; Neumark-Sztainer, D.; Berge, J.M. Home food environment factors associated with the presence of fruit and vegetables at dinner: A direct observational study. *Appetite* **2016**, *96*, 526–532. [CrossRef] [PubMed]
51. Hebestreit, A.; Keimer, K.M.; Hassel, H.; Nappo, A.; Eiben, G.; Fernandez, J.M.; Kovacs, E.; Lasn, H.; Shiakou, M.; Ahrens, W. What do children understand? Communicating health behavior in a european multicenter study. *J. Public Health* **2010**, *18*, 391–400. [CrossRef]
52. Subar, A.F.; Freedman, L.S.; Tooze, J.A.; Kirkpatrick, S.I.; Boushey, C.; Neuhouser, M.L.; Thompson, F.E.; Potischman, N.; Guenther, P.M.; Tarasuk, V.; et al. Addressing current criticism regarding the value of self-report dietary data. *J. Nutr.* **2015**, *145*, 2639–2645. [CrossRef] [PubMed]
53. Greenland, P.; Robins, J.M. Confounding and misclassification. *Am. J. Epidemiol.* **1985**, *122*, 495–506. [PubMed]
54. R Core Team. *R: A Language and Environment for Statistical Computing*; R Foundation for Statistical Computing: Vienna, Austria, 2014.
55. Stasinopoulos, D.M.; Rigby, R.A. Generalized additive models for location scale and shape (GAMLSS) in R. *J. Stat. Softw.* **2007**, *23*, 1–46. [CrossRef]
56. Hartigan, J.A.; Wong, M.A. Algorithm AS 136: A k-means clustering algorithm. *Appl. Stat.* **1979**, *28*, 100–108. [CrossRef]
57. Rousseeuw, P.J. Silhouettes: A graphical aid to the interpretation and validation of cluster analysis. *J. Compl. Appl. Math.* **2015**, *20*, 53–65. [CrossRef]
58. Lo, S.G.; Yasui, Y.; Csizmadi, I.; McGregor, S.E.; Robson, P.J. Exploring statistical approaches to diminish subjectivity of cluster analysis to derive dietary patterns: The Tomorrow Project. *Am. J. Epidemiol.* **2011**, *173*, 956–967.
59. Hubert, L.; Arabie, P. Comparing partitions. *J. Classif.* **1985**, *2*, 193–218. [CrossRef]

7

Food Sources of Energy and Nutrients in Infants, Toddlers and Young Children from the Mexican National Health and Nutrition Survey 2012

Liya Denney [1,*], Myriam C. Afeiche [1], Alison L. Eldridge [1] and Salvador Villalpando-Carrión [2,3]

1 Nestlé Research Center, Lausanne 1000, Switzerland; myriam.afeichezehil@rdls.nestle.com (M.C.A.); alison.eldridge@rdls.nestle.com (A.L.E.)

2 Children's Hospital of Mexico Federico Gómez, National Institute of Health, Mexico City 06720, Mexico; salvador.villalpando@MX.nestle.com

3 Nestlé Infant Nutrition, Mexico City 11520, Mexico

* Correspondence: liya.denney@rdls.nestle.com

Abstract: Food sources of nutrients in Mexican children are not well known. To fill the knowledge gap, dietary intake was assessed in 2057 children using a 24-h dietary recall. All reported foods and beverages were assigned to one of 76 food groups. Percent contribution of each food group to nutrient intake was estimated for four age groups: 0–5.9, 6–11.9, 12–23.9, and 24–47.9 months. Breast milk, infant formula, and cow's milk were the top sources of energy and nutrients, especially in younger groups. Among infants aged 6–11.9 months, the top food sources of energy included soups and stews, cookies, fruit, tortillas, eggs and egg dishes, and traditional beverages. The same foods plus sweetened breads, dried beans, and sandwiches and tortas were consumed as the top sources of energy among toddlers and young children. Milk, soups, and stews were the top contributors for all nutrients and tortillas, eggs, and egg dishes were among the top contributors for iron and zinc. This study showed that low nutrient-dense cookies, sweetened breads, and traditional beverages were among the core foods consumed early in life in Mexico. This compromises the intake of more nutritious foods such as vegetables and fortified cereals and increases the risk of obesity.

Keywords: ENSANUT 2012; infants; toddlers; young children; food sources; energy; nutrients

---

1. Introduction

Proper nutrition throughout infancy and early childhood is not only vital for optimal growth and development but also helps to lay the foundation for a child's future health [1,2]. The diet in infancy and early childhood is marked by high nutrient needs [3], a transition from an all-milk diet to family foods in the first year of life [4], and the development of food preferences that may affect long-term food choices later in life [5].

The quality of a child's nutrition is shaped by decisions made by parents and caregivers as well as the social and economic environment. At present, Mexico is facing malnutrition characterized by stunting and micronutrient deficiencies in young children from low-income families, iron deficiency anemia in young children, widespread obesity in all age groups, and a high prevalence of non-communicable chronic diseases [6–10]. As for young children, recent studies from the 2012 Mexican National Health and Nutrition Survey (Encuesta Nacional de Salud y Nutrición; ENSANUT 2012) have observed shortcomings in infant and child feeding practices [11]. Examples include a low prevalence of breastfeeding, low consumption of iron-rich foods, and high consumption of sugar-sweetened beverages and sweet foods [12,13]. These shortcomings very likely contribute to the imbalanced nutrient intakes reported in recent dietary surveys, including inadequate intakes of iron, calcium, vitamin D, vitamin E, folate, and fiber and excessive intakes of energy, added sugars, saturated fat, and sodium [14–18].

Quantitative assessment of food sources of energy and nutrients can show what foods are important contributors of nutrients in the population's diet. This knowledge can assist healthcare professionals to form targeted measures to correct shortcomings. Up to now, detailed quantitative analyses on the dietary sources of nutrients in Mexico have been lacking. One recent study conducted in Mexican children under two years of age reported food sources of energy but not nutrients [12]. To fill the knowledge gap, the aim of this study was to describe and identify the principal sources of energy and nutrients in the diets of infants, toddlers, and young children from the ENSANUT 2012.

2. Materials and Methods

2.1. Study Population

ENSANUT is a cross-sectional, population-based survey that characterizes the health and nutritional status of the Mexican population [19]. The survey used a multi-stage, stratified, and clustered sampling system drawn to represent all states, four geographic regions, and socioeconomic strata in Mexico. The data were collected from 50,528 Mexican households, with a response rate of 87% [19]. A total of 2057 children from birth to four years of age were used in the current analysis. The data are presented for four age groups: infants 0–5.9 months (n = 182), infants 6–11.9 months (n = 229), toddlers 12–23.9 months (n = 538), and young children 24–47.9 months (n = 1108). The survey protocol and data collection instruments were approved by the Ethics Committee of the Mexican National Institute of Public Health (Instituto Nacional de Salud Pública). Written informed consent was obtained from each eligible person 18 years and older or from the parent or caregiver of participants under 18 years. The characteristics of the study population have been described previously [13]. Briefly, the majority of children (70%) lived in urban areas. Of the primary caregivers, most often the mother (85%) had an elementary and/or secondary education; 70% were unemployed and 47% were married.

2.2. Dietary Data Collection

One 24-h dietary recall was collected for each child through a face-to-face interview by trained interviewers with the parent or caregiver. The interviewers asked about all foods and beverages and the amount consumed of each item for the previous 24-h period. Custom recipes or standard recipes developed by the National Institute of Public Health were used to estimate the ingredients in mixed food items. The amount of each food item or ingredient consumed was estimated using common household measurement aids (including spoons, cups, slices, handfuls, etc.) and the information was then converted to grams and milliliters depending on the type of food or beverage consumed. To improve dietary recall data, the ENSANUT 2012 implemented an automated five-step multiple-pass method and collected data on both weekdays and weekend days [16].

Quality control of the dietary intake data was conducted in two stages, as reported previously by Lopez-Olmedo and colleagues [16]. Briefly, in the first stage, the foods reported by a participant were reviewed and information including coding, quantity reported, recipe ingredients, and the context in which the meal or feeding episode took place was scrutinized. In the second stage, energy and nutrient intakes were reviewed to identify implausible values. The ratio of daily energy intake to estimated energy requirement was calculated for each person and each day and transformed to a logarithmic scale to remove outliers below −3 SDs and above +3 SDs. Excessive micronutrient intakes were defined as those that exceeded 1.5 times of the 99th percentile of the observed intake distribution of the nutrient in the corresponding sex and age group [16].

Breast milk consumption was estimated based on the child's age in months and the total amount of other milk (infant formula and cow's milk) reported over the course of the recall day [20,21]. For exclusively breastfed infants aged birth to 5.9 months, an average intake of 780 mL/day of human milk was assumed; for partially breastfed infants, the amount of human milk was computed as 780 mL/day minus the amount of infant formula/other milks consumed. For infants aged six to 11 months fed human milk as the sole milk source, the amount of human milk was assumed to be 600 mL/day. For partially breastfed infants, the amount of human milk was computed as 600 mL/day minus the amount of infant formula/other milks consumed. For breastfed young children aged 12 to 17 months, the amount of human milk was computed as 89 mL per feeding occasion. For breastfed young children aged 18 to 23 months, the amount of human milk was computed as 59 mL per feeding occasion [20,21].

2.3. Analytic Methods

Energy and nutrient intakes were estimated based on the food composition database from the National Institute of Public Health in Mexico (67% foods) [22] and the food composition tables from the United States Department of Agriculture's Nutrient Database for Dietary Studies (33% of foods). [23]. To calculate added sugars, the intake of each food was linked at the ingredient level (single foods, standardized recipes) or dish level (custom recipes) to the U.S. Department of Agriculture's National Nutrient Database for Standard Reference [23] and then further linked to the MyPyramid Equivalents Database [24]. Teaspoon equivalents in the Food Patterns Equivalents Database were converted to grams with the use of the ratio 4.2 g/teaspoon. Vitamin A was estimated in retinol activity equivalents using the following formula [25]: Retinol activity = μg retinol + $\frac{1}{2}$ (μg beta-carotene equivalents/6).

To investigate food sources of energy and nutrients, a list of 76 food groups was formed based on previous dietary intake studies in young children in the USA (Table 1) [26–28]. Two trained Mexican dietary research specialists and a nutrition scientist at Nestlé adjusted food groups to incorporate local food culture and reflect the relative role of specific types of foods and beverages in the diets of infants, toddlers, and young children living in Mexico [13]. Some common food mixtures were estimated "as consumed", such as soups, stews, and mixed dishes, and considered a single food item. All foods, beverages, and nutrient supplements were assigned to one of the 76 food groups (Table 1).

Table 1. Food group classifications *.

Milk and Milk Products	***Vegetables***	Pasta mixed dishes
Breast milk	Baby food (vegetables)	***Sweets***
Infant formula (iron fortified powder or fluid)	Dark green/dark green mixtures	Cookies
Cow's milk (fluid, powdered, flavored, whole or reduced-fat)	White potatoes or starchy/starchy mixtures	Cakes
Cheese	Deep yellow/deep yellow mixtures	Pies & pastries
Yogurt (baby food yogurt or yogurt)	Vegetables (all other/other mixtures)	Sweetened breads (sweet rolls, doughnuts, muffins)
Meat/Poultry/Fish/Meat Alternates	100% vegetable juice	Candy
Baby food (meat)	***Fruit***	Mexican desserts
Meats (chicken, turkey or beef)	Baby food (fruit) (apples and apple mixture, bananas and banana mixtures, pear and pear mixtures, other fruit/fruit mixtures)	Ice cream/frozen yogurt/puddings
Fish/shellfish	Canned fruit	Sugars
Game	Fresh or frozen fruit (bananas, berries, nectarines & peaches, pears, melons, guava, other fruit)	Syrups
Hot dogs/cold cuts/bacon/sausage	100% baby fruit juice	Preserves/jelly
Organ meats	100% fruit juice	Fruit-flavored drinks
Pork/ham	***Mixed Dishes***	Carbonated sodas
Dried beans	Beans & rice, chili, bean mixtures with or without meat	Sweetened tea and coffee
Eggs & egg dishes	Beef or pork with vegetables and /or rice/pasta/potatoes	Artificially sweetened powdered beverages
Peanut/nuts/seeds	Chicken or turkey with vegetables and /or rice/pasta/potatoes	Yakult (skimmed milk fermented with *Lactobacillus casei*)
Vegetarian meat substitutes	Fish or shellfish with vegetables and/or rice/pasta/potatoes	Traditional beverages (*atoles*, *licuados* or *aguas frescas*)
Grains and Grain Products	Soups & stews	***Other***
Infant cereal	Meat tacos	Butter
Breakfast cereals (plain cereal, cereal flakes, corn flakes or oatmeal)	Vegetable & cheese tacos	Sour cream (whole or reduced fat)
Bread/rolls/biscuits/bagels	Enchiladas	Salty snacks (grain snacks and those made from starchy vegetables)
Tortillas (plain)	Tortillas with fillings/toppings	Condiments, herbs and seasonings
Bars/cereal/granola	Tamales	Salad dressing
Crackers/pretzels/rice cakes	Sandwiches & tortas	Water
Pancakes/waffles/French toast	Wheat-based pasta mixed dishes	Mineral water
Pasta	Pizza	Salsas, *moles*, *adobo*
Rice	Rice-based mixed dishes	Supplements (fortified or vitamins)

* The food classification scheme was adapted from the one developed by for the Feeding Infants and Toddlers Study [26] and modified to include commonly consumed foods among Mexican children. All foods and beverages were classified into these 76 mutually exclusive categories.

2.4. Statistical Analysis

Stata (StataCorp. 2015 Stata Statistical Software: Release 14. College Station, TX, USA: StataCorp LP) was used to create data files, assign individual foods and beverages to food groups, and calculate the contribution of each food group to the overall intake of energy and nutrients. The weighted percentage contribution of each food group for all infants, toddlers, and young children was calculated by adding the amount of a given nutrient provided by each food group for all individuals and dividing by the total intake of that nutrient consumed by all individuals from all foods and beverages. All estimates incorporated appropriate sample weights to reflect nationally representative results. Only food groups that contributed over 1% of the nutrient intake are presented in this study. Sources of energy and nutrients were assessed separately and are presented for the four age groups mentioned above.

3. Results

Food sources of energy and 14 nutrients in the diets of infants, toddlers, and young children are presented in Table 2 through 16. In each table, the food groups listed present at least 80% of the total energy or nutrient intake.

3.1. Energy, Macronutrients, and Fiber

Different types of milk were the top sources of energy across all age groups but the relative contribution reduced markedly with age. Breast milk, infant formula, and cow's milk were the first, second, and third sources of energy, collectively contributing 89% of total energy among infants 0–5.9 months (Table 2). These milk sources were still the top three sources of energy among infants 6–11.9 months but the total contribution was lower (53%) as more non-milk foods were consumed. Among toddlers 12–23.9 months, cow's milk was the first source of energy, infant formula was the third, and breast milk dropped to tenth. Among young children 24–47.9 months, cow's milk was still the first source of energy but other milk sources were no longer on the list (Table 2).

Foods and other beverages consumed as the top 10 sources of energy among infants aged 6–11 months included soups and stews, cookies, yogurt, fruit, tortillas, eggs and egg dishes, and traditional beverages (Table 2). Food diversity increased with age, but these top sources of energy for 6–11.9-month-old remained in the top 10 sources of energy among toddlers and young children, except for yogurt (Table 2). Other foods added to the top 10 sources of energy in the two older groups were sweetened breads, which ranked fifth among toddlers and third among young children, dried beans, and sandwiches and tortas (Table 2). Among the top 10 sources of energy, cookies, sweetened breads, and traditional beverages collectively provided 7%, 14%, and 15% of total energy among 6–11.9-month-old infants, toddlers, and young children, respectively. These foods, together with other foods and beverages high in sugar, including sweetened tea and coffee, fruit-flavored drinks, carbonated sodas, and candy, provided 19% and 22% of daily energy intake among toddlers and young children, respectively.

Most of the top 10 milk and food sources of energy were also the top sources of protein and fat (Tables 3 and 4) and saturated fat (Supplementary Table S1) in all age groups. Breast milk, infant formula, and cow's milk were the top three sources of protein and fat among infants of 0–5.9 months and 6–11.9 months; cow's milk, soups and stews, and eggs and egg dishes were the top three sources of protein and fat among toddlers and young children (Table 3, Table 4 and Supplementary Table S1). Meats ranked fifth as a source of protein among both toddlers and young children. Tortillas ranked seventh and fourth as sources of protein among toddlers and young children, respectively. Overall, food sources of total fat and saturated fat were similar, with a slightly varied ranking (Table 4 and Supplementary Table S1).

Table 2. Food sources of energy among Mexican infants, toddlers, and young children aged 0–47.9 months by age group from ENSANUT 2012.

Rank	Age 0–5.9 Months		Age 6–11.9 Months		Age 12–23.9 Months		Age 24–47.9 Months	
	Food Group	% of Total	Food Group	% of Total	Food Group	% of Total	Food Group	% of Total
1	Breast milk	52.6	Breast milk	26.7	Cow's milk	13.2	Cow's milk	10.7
2	Infant formula	34.3	Infant formula	16.5	Soups & stews	7.8	Tortillas (plain)	8.3
3	Cow's milk	1.9	Cow's milk	10.2	Infant formula	6.9	Sweetened breads	7.0
4	Baby food (vegetables)	1.0	Soups & stews	6.5	Tortillas (plain)	5.4	Soups & stews	5.7
5	Infant Cereal	1.0	Cookies	4.3	Sweetened breads	4.9	Eggs & egg dishes	5.3
6			Yogurt	3.6	Traditional beverages	4.7	Cookies	4.2
7			Fresh or frozen fruit	3.2	Eggs & egg dishes	4.3	Dried beans	4.1
8			Tortillas (plain)	3.0	Fresh or frozen fruit	4.1	Sandwiches & tortas	4.1
9			Eggs & egg dishes	2.6	Cookies	3.9	Traditional beverages	3.3
10			Traditional beverages	1.7	Breast milk	3.2	Fresh or frozen fruit	3.2
11			Infant cereal	1.7	Yogurt	3.2	Breakfast cereals	2.9
12			Dried beans	1.4	Dried beans	2.8	Meats	2.9
13			Sweetened breads	1.0	Meats	2.7	Yogurt	2.9
14			100% fruit juice	1.0	Breakfast cereals	2.6	Salty snacks	2.8
15			Salty snacks	1.0	Sweetened tea and coffee	2.6	Sweetened tea and coffee	2.2
16					Salty snacks	2.2	Rice mixed dishes	2.1
17					Pasta mixed dishes	1.9	Carbonated sodas	1.7
18					Sandwiches & tortas	1.7	Candy	1.4
19					Rice mixed dishes	1.5	Vegetable & cheese tacos	1.2
20					100% fruit juice	1.5	Tamales	1.2
21					Fruit-flavored drinks	1.3	Fruit-flavored drinks	1.2
22					Tamales	1.2	Bread/rolls/biscuits/bagels	1.1
23							Beef or pork with vegetables and/or rice/pasta/potatoes	1.1
24							Pasta mixed dishes	1.1
25							100% fruit juice	1.1
26							Meat tacos	1.1
27							Chicken or turkey with vegetables and/or rice/pasta/potatoes	1.0
28							Enchiladas	1.0
29							White potatoes	1.0
All food groups		**90.8**		**84.4**		**83.6**		**86.9**

Table 3. Food sources of protein among Mexican infants, toddlers, and young children aged 0–47.9 months by age group from ENSANUT 2012.

Rank	Age 0–5.9 Months		Age 6–11.9 Months		Age 12–23.9 Months		Age 24–47.9 Months	
	Food Group	% of Total	Food Group	% of Total	Food Group	% of Total	Food Group	% of Total
1	Breast milk	48.0	Breast milk	21.5	Cow's milk	18.2	Cow's milk	14.8
2	Infant formula	40.1	Infant formula	15.9	Soups & stews	9.8	Eggs & egg dishes	10.2
3	Cow's milk	3.3	Cow's milk	13.2	Eggs & egg dishes	8.7	Soups & stews	7.2
4	Yogurt	1.5	Soups & stews	8.9	Infant formula	6.7	Tortillas (plain)	6.4
5	Baby food (vegetables)	1.4	Yogurt	5.3	Meats	6.4	Meats	6.0
6			Eggs & egg dishes	4.7	Dried beans	4.4	Dried beans	5.8
7			Tortillas (plain)	3.0	Tortillas (plain)	4.3	Sweetened breads	5.0
8			Dried beans	2.7	Yogurt	3.5	Sandwiches & tortas	4.9
9			Cookies	2.7	Sweetened breads	3.4	Yogurt	3.1
10			Meats	2.3	Traditional beverages	2.6	Breakfast cereals	2.5
11			Traditional beverages	1.9	Breakfast cereals	2.0	Cookies	2.2
12			Infant cereal	1.7	Cookies	1.9	Beef or pork with vegetables and/or rice/pasta/potatoes	1.7
13			Chicken or turkey with vegetables and/or rice/pasta/potatoes	1.4	Sandwiches & tortas	1.8	Chicken or turkey with vegetables and/or rice/pasta/potatoes	1.6
14					Sweetened tea and coffee	1.8	Traditional beverages	1.6
15					Breast milk	1.8	Sweetened tea and coffee	1.6
16					Chicken or turkey with vegetables and/or rice/pasta/potatoes	1.4	Rice mixed dishes	1.5
17					Pasta mixed dishes	1.1	Meat tacos	1.4
18					Salty snacks	1.1	Salty snacks	1.4
19					Rice mixed dishes	1.1	Fish/shellfish	1.1
20					Tamales	1.0	Bread/rolls/biscuits/bagels	1.1
21							Vegetable & cheese tacos	1.0
22							Tamales	1.0
23							Fresh or frozen fruit	1.0
24							Enchiladas	1.0
All food groups		94.3		85.2		83.0		85.1

Table 4. Food sources of fat among Mexican infants, toddlers, and young children aged 0–47.9 months by age group from ENSANUT 2012.

Rank	Age 0–5.9 Months		Age 6–11.9 Months		Age 12–23.9 Months		Age 24–47.9 Months	
	Food Group	% of Total	Food Group	% of Total	Food Group	% of Total	Food Group	% of Total
1	Breast milk	56.2	Breast milk	33.6	Cow's milk	16.8	Cow's milk	14.2
2	Infant formula	36.2	Infant formula	20.0	Infant formula	9.1	Eggs & egg dishes	9.8
3	Cow's milk	3.4	Cow's milk	13.2	Eggs & egg dishes	7.6	Sweetened breads	9.0
4			Soups & stews	4.8	Soups & stews	7.1	Meats	5.5
5			Cookies	3.7	Sweetened breads	6.1	Soups & stews	5.3
6			Eggs & egg dishes	3.5	Breast milk	4.8	Dried beans	5.1
7			Yogurt	3.2	Cookies	4.0	Sandwiches & tortas	5.0
8			Traditional beverages	1.5	Meats	4.0	Tortillas (plain)	4.2
9			Infant cereal	1.5	Dried beans	4.0	Salty snacks	4.1
10			Salty snacks	1.3	Salty snacks	3.0	Cookies	3.9
11			Dried beans	1.3	Sandwiches & tortas	2.5	Yogurt	2.7
12			Sweetened breads	1.0	Tortillas (plain)	2.4	Breakfast cereals	2.1
13			Tortillas (plain)	1.0	Traditional beverages	2.3	Beef or pork with vegetables and/or rice/pasta/potatoes	1.8
14					Breakfast cereals	2.2	Tamales	1.6
15					Pasta mixed dishes	2.0	Rice mixed dishes	1.6
16					Tamales	1.7	Chicken or turkey with vegetables and/or rice/pasta/potatoes	1.5
17					Yogurt	2.6	Vegetable & cheese tacos	1.4
18					Chicken or turkey with vegetables and/or rice/pasta/potatoes	1.2	Meat tacos	1.4
19					White potatoes	1.1	Pasta mixed dishes	1.3
20							Enchiladas	1.3
21							Traditional beverages	1.2
22							White potatoes	1.0
23							Sweetened tea and coffee	1.0
24							Infant formula	1.0
All food groups		95.8		89.6		84.5		87.0

The top contributors to energy were also the top sources of carbohydrate (Table 5). Tortillas ranked as the seventh source of carbohydrate among infants 6–11.9 months, then became the second and first source of carbohydrates among toddlers and young children, respectively. For added sugar, cookies, yogurt, fruit-flavored drinks, sweetened breads, and traditional beverages were the top sources across the age groups from 6–11.9 months onwards (Table 6). The contribution of carbonated sodas to added sugar was higher with increasing age, ranking fourteenth among infants 6–11.9 months, seventh among toddlers, and second among young children. Overall, the ranking of added sugar from traditional beverages was higher than carbonated sodas.

Fruit was the highest ranked source of dietary fiber among infants in both age categories. Among toddlers and young children, tortillas contributed the most fiber, followed by fruit (Table 7). From six months onwards, soups and stews were also an important source of fiber. Other top sources of fiber were vegetables, dried beans, pasta mixed dishes, and sweetened breads.

3.2. *Vitamins*

Breast milk, infant formula, cow's milk, and soups and stews were the main sources of vitamin A (Table 8), vitamin E (Table 9), folate (Table 10), and other B vitamins (Supplementary Tables 2–5), with a slightly varied order. Among toddlers and young children, in addition to different types of milk and soups and stews, eggs and egg dishes, dried beans, tortillas, breakfast cereals, and sweetened breads were also important sources of vitamin A, vitamin E, and B vitamins. Fruit ranked as the first source of vitamin C among toddlers and young children, followed by cow's milk, soups and stews, infant formula, and traditional beverages (Table 11). For folate, breast milk was the first source among infants; soups and stews were the first and second source among toddlers and young children, respectively, followed by dried beans and eggs and egg dishes (Table 10).

Table 5. Food sources of carbohydrates among Mexican infants, toddlers, and young children aged 0–47.9 months by age group from ENSANUT 2012.

Rank	Age 0–5.9 Months		Age 6–11.9 Months		Age 12–23.9 Months		Age 24–47.9 Months	
	Food Group	**% of Total**	**Food Group**	**% of Total**	**Food Group**	**% of Total**	**Food Group**	**% of Total**
1	Breast milk	50.3	Breast milk	22.5	Cow's milk	9.9	Tortillas (plain)	11.9
2	Infant formula	33.1	Infant formula	13.9	Tortillas (plain)	8.2	Cow's milk	8.2
3	Cow's milk	1.7	Cow's milk	7.2	Soups & stews	7.4	Sweetened breads	6.9
4	Baby food (vegetables)	1.3	Soups & stews	7.0	Fresh or frozen fruit	7.4	Soups & stews	5.5
5	100% fruit juice	1.3	Fresh or frozen fruit	5.5	Traditional beverages	6.4	Cookies	5.1
6	Fresh or frozen fruit	1.2	Cookies	5.3	Infant formula	5.9	Traditional beverages	4.6
7	Baby food (fruit)	1.1	Tortillas (plain)	4.9	Sweetened breads	4.9	Breakfast cereals	3.6
8	Infant cereal	1.1	Yogurt	3.9	Cookies	4.6	Sandwiches & tortas	3.3
9	Sweetened tea and coffee	1.0	Traditional beverages	3.0	Sweetened tea and coffee	3.6	Yogurt	3.3
10			Infant cereal	1.8	Yogurt	3.6	Fresh or frozen fruit	5.5
11			100% fruit juice	1.7	Breakfast cereals	3.0	Dried beans	3.0
12			Fruit-flavored drinks	1.6	100% fruit juice	2.6	Sweetened tea and coffee	2.9
13			Dried beans	1.5	Fruit-flavored drinks	2.6	Carbonated sodas	2.9
14			Infant cereal	1.2	Breast milk	2.6	Salty snacks	2.5
15			Rice mixed dishes	1.0	Pasta mixed dishes	2.2	Rice mixed dishes	2.5
16			Sweetened tea and coffee	1.0	Rice mixed dishes	2.0	Fruit-flavored drinks	2.3
17			Salty snacks	1.0	Dried beans	2.0	Candy	2.0
18			Sweetened breads	1.0	Salty snacks	2.0	100% fruit juice	1.8
19			Eggs & egg dishes	1.0	Tamales	1.1	Bread/rolls/biscuits/bagels	1.6
20			Vegetables	1.0	Sandwiches & tortas	1.1	Vegetable & cheese tacos	1.2
21					Candy	1.0	Pasta mixed dishes	1.2
22					Carbonated sodas	1.0	White potatoes	1.1
23							Tamales	1.1
All food groups		**92.1**		**87.0**		**85.1**		**84.0**

Table 6. Food sources of added sugar among Mexican infants, toddlers, and young children aged 0–47.9 months by age group from ENSANUT 2012.

Rank	Age 0–5.9 Months		Age 6–11.9 Months		Age 12–23.9 Months		Age 24–47.9 Months	
	Food Group	% of Total	Food Group	% of Total	Food Group	% of Total	Food Group	% of Total
1	Yogurt	30.9	Cookies	26.3	Yogurt	14.9	Traditional beverages	12.0
2	Sweetened tea and coffee	14.9	Yogurt	21.6	Cookies	11.8	Carbonated sodas	11.5
3	Traditional beverages	13.1	Fruit-flavored drinks	7.5	Sweetened breads	10.4	Sweetened breads	10.3
4	Bread/rolls/biscuits/bagels	11.6	Sweetened breads	6.4	Traditional beverages	10.3	Yogurt	10.3
5	Mexican desserts	6.0	Ice cream/frozen yogurt/puddings	6.3	Fruit-flavored drinks	8.2	Cookies	7.7
6	Cookies	5.8	Traditional beverages	6.4	Sweetened tea and coffee	7.6	Cow's milk	7.5
7	Fruit-flavored drinks	4.5	Candy	4.8	Carbonated sodas	5.6	Sweetened tea and coffee	6.8
8	Sweet breads	2.6	Bread/rolls/biscuits/bagels	2.3	Breakfast cereals	4.8	Fruit-flavored drinks	6.6
9	Carbonated sodas	2.6	Breakfast cereals	2.0	Candy	4.6	Candy	6.3
10	Canned fruit	1.8	Mexican desserts	1.9	100% fruit juice	3.6	Breakfast cereals	5.1
11	Preserves/jelly	1.8	Salty snacks	1.8	Cow's milk	3.0	Ice cream/frozen yogurt/puddings	2.4
12	Ice cream, frozen yogurt, puddings	1.0	100% fruit juice	1.7	Cakes	2.0	100% fruit juice	1.9
13			Sweetened tea and coffee	1.7	Ice cream/frozen yogurt/puddings	1.8	Bread/rolls/biscuits/bagels	1.6
14			Carbonated sodas	1.5	Mexican desserts	1.7	Cakes	1.5
15			Canned fruit	1.4	Salty snacks	1.6	Yakult	1.5
16			Yakult	1.3	Yakult	1.2	Mexican desserts	1.2
17			Sugars	1.1	Bread/rolls/biscuits/bagels	1.1	Sandwiches & tortas	1.1
18					Artificially sweetened powdered beverage	1.0	Artificially sweetened powdered beverage	1.0
All food groups		**96.6**		**96.0**		**95.2**		**95.3**

Table 7. Food sources of fiber among Mexican infants, toddlers and young children aged 0–47.9 months by age group from ENSANUT 2012.

Rank	Age 0–5.9 Months		Age 6–11.9 Months		Age 12–23.9 Months		Age 24–47.9 Months	
	Food Group	% of Total	Food Group	% of Total	Food Group	% of Total	Food Group	% of Total
1	Baby food (fruit)	22.1	Fresh or frozen fruit	18.8	Tortillas (plain)	17.8	Tortillas (plain)	19.9
2	Fresh or frozen fruit	15.0	Soups & stews	18.0	Fresh or frozen fruit	15.4	Fresh or frozen fruit	11.4
3	Vegetables	9.7	Tortillas (plain)	14.8	Soups & stews	12.5	Soups & stews	8.6
4	Baby food (vegetables)	9.3	Cookies	5.3	Dried beans	5.7	Dried beans	7.0
5	Infant formula	8.1	Vegetables	5.0	Pasta mixed dishes	4.5	Sweetened breads	4.7
6	Infant cereal	7.8	Dried beans	4.3	Sweetened breads	3.4	Sandwiches & tortas	4.3
7	Soups & stews	5.4	Traditional beverages	4.0	Cookies	3.1	Cookies	3.4
8	Pasta mixed dishes	4.3	Infant cereal	2.2	Traditional beverages	5.0	Salty snacks	2.9
9	Sweetened tea and coffee	3.1	Baby food (fruit)	2.1	Breakfast cereals	2.6	Traditional beverages	2.9
10	Tortillas (plain)	2.9	Pasta mixed dishes	2.0	Vegetables	2.4	Breakfast cereals	2.4
11	Yakult	1.6	Eggs & egg dishes	1.6	Salty snacks	2.2	Pasta mixed dishes	2.1
12	Canned fruit	1.5	White potatoes	1.6	Rice mixed dishes	2.1	Vegetables	1.9
13	100% Vegetable juice	1.0	Chicken or turkey with vegetables and/or rice/pasta/potatoes	1.5	Tamales	2.0	Rice mixed dishes	1.8
14	Cookies	1.0	Rice mixed dishes	1.4	Sandwiches & tortas	1.6	Meat tacos	1.8
15			Fruit-flavored drinks	1.3	100% fruit juice	1.4	Vegetable & cheese tacos	1.8
16			Sweetened breads	1.2	Eggs & egg dishes	1.2	Tamales	1.6
17			Salty snacks	1.2	Vegetable & cheese tacos	1.2	Enchiladas	1.6
18			Infant formula	1.0	Fruit-flavored drinks	1.2	Eggs & egg dishes	1.4
19					White potatoes	1.0	Cow's milk	1.3
20							Bread/rolls/biscuits/bagels	1.2
21							White potatoes	1.2
22							Fruit-flavored drinks	1.0
All food groups		**92.8**		**87.3**		**86.3**		**86.2**

Table 8. Food sources of vitamin A among Mexican infants, toddlers, and young children aged 0–47.9 months by age group from ENSANUT 2012.

Rank	Age 0–5.9 Months		Age 6–11.9 Months		Age 12–23.9 Months		Age 24–47.9 Months	
	Food Group	% of Total	Food Group	% of Total	Food Group	% of Total	Food Group	% of Total
1	Breast milk	55.2	Breast milk	34.2	Cow's milk	26.7	Cow's milk	26.3
2	Infant formula	35.3	Infant formula	20.3	Infant formula	10.5	Eggs & egg dishes	12.0
3	Baby food (vegetables)	3.0	Cow's milk	15.6	Soups & stews	9.7	Soups & stews	8.4
4	Cow's milk	1.1	Soups & stews	7.0	Eggs & egg dishes	8.7	Breakfast cereals	6.1
5	Infant cereal	1.0	Eggs & egg dishes	2.9	Breast milk	6.0	Traditional beverages	4.2
6			Infant cereal	1.8	Traditional beverages	4.2	Fresh or frozen fruit	3.5
7			Vegetables	1.5	Breakfast cereals	4.0	Dried beans	3.4
8			Traditional beverages	1.4	Dried beans	2.7	Sandwiches & tortas	3.3
9			Fresh or frozen fruit	1.0	Fresh or frozen fruit	2.7	Sweetened tea and coffee	2.0
10			Breakfast cereals	1.0	100% fruit juice	2.0	Rice mixed dishes	1.9
11					Vegetables	1.8	Infant formula	1.7
12					Rice mixed dishes	1.5	Yogurt	1.6
13					Meats	1.4	Vegetables	1.5
14					Cookies	1.2	100% fruit juice	1.4
15					Sweetened tea and coffee	1.1	Meats	1.2
16					Infant cereal	1.1	Cookies	1.2
17							Tamales	1.1
All food groups		**95.6**		**86.7**		**85.3**		**80.8**

Table 9. Food sources of vitamin E among Mexican infants, toddlers, and young children aged 0–47.9 months by age group from ENSANUT 2012.

Rank	Age 0–5.9 Months		Age 6–11.9 Months		Age 12–23.9 Months		Age 24–47.9 Months	
	Food Group	**% of Total**	**Food Group**	**% of Total**	**Food Group**	**% of Total**	**Food Group**	**% of Total**
1	Infant formula	48.0	Infant formula	24.1	Eggs & egg dishes	11.9	Eggs & egg dishes	14.7
2	Breast milk	41.9	Breast milk	21.2	Infant formula	11.3	Cow's milk	7.9
3	Pasta mixed dishes	1.1	Soups & stews	8.8	Cow's milk	10.1	Soups & stews	6.1
4	Baby food (vegetables)	1.1	Cow's milk	6.9	Soups & stews	9.0	Dried beans	5.5
5	Vegetables	1.0	Eggs & egg dishes	5.3	Fresh or frozen fruit	5.6	Tortillas (plain)	5.0
6			Fresh or frozen fruit	3.6	Pasta mixed dishes	5.0	Salty snacks	5.0
7			Cookies	2.7	Dried beans	4.0	Sandwiches & tortas	4.8
8			Tortillas (plain)	2.4	Salty snacks	3.9	Breakfast cereals	4.8
9			Pasta mixed dishes	1.9	Breakfast cereals	3.3	Fresh or frozen fruit	4.6
10			Infant cereal	1.9	Cookies	3.3	Sweetened breads	3.0
11			Vegetables	1.5	Tortillas (plain)	3.2	Pasta mixed dishes	2.6
12			Breakfast cereals	1.4	Meats	2.2	Cookies	2.3
13			Salty snacks	1.3	Sandwiches & tortas	2.1	Meat tacos	2.2
14			Dried beans	1.1	Traditional beverages	1.9	White potatoes	2.0
15			Traditional beverages	1.1	Sweetened breads	1.8	Rice mixed dishes	1.8
16			Baby food (fruit)	1.1	Breast milk	1.8	Beef or pork with vegetables and/or rice/pasta/potatoes	1.7
17					White potatoes	1.5	Infant formula	1.7
18					Chicken or turkey with vegetables and/or rice/pasta rice/potatoes	1.4	Chicken or turkey with vegetables and/or rice/pasta/potatoes	1.6
19					Tamales	1.3	Vegetable & cheese tacos	1.6
20					Rice mixed dishes	1.2	Enchiladas	1.6
21					100% fruit juice	1.1	Meats	1.5
22							Tamales	1.0
All food groups		**93.1**		**86.3**		**86.9**		**83.0**

Table 10. Food sources of folate among Mexican infants, toddlers, and young children aged 0–47.9 months by age group from ENSANUT 2012.

Rank	Age 0–5.9 Months		Age 6–11.9 Months		Age 12–23.9 Months		Age 24–47.9 Months	
	Food Group	% of Total	Food Group	% of Total	Food Group	% of Total	Food Group	% of Total
1	Breast milk	48.1	Breast milk	20.3	Soups & stews	14.4	Sweetened breads	10.9
2	Infant formula	39.0	Soups & stews	15.3	Dried beans	8.3	Soups & stews	10.7
3	Baby food (vegetables)	2.8	Infant formula	15.2	Fresh or frozen fruit	8.0	Dried beans	10.2
4	Vegetables	2.1	Dried beans	6.3	Eggs & egg dishes	7.5	Eggs & egg dishes	8.8
5	Soups & stews	1.3	Fresh or frozen fruit	5.6	Sweetened breads	7.0	Breakfast cereals	7.0
6	Fresh or frozen fruit	1.0	Vegetables	4.8	Cow's milk	6.8	Fresh or frozen fruit	6.4
7			Cow's milk	3.8	Infant formula	6.7	Cow's milk	4.7
8			Eggs & egg dishes	3.8	Breakfast cereals	5.6	Cookies	3.7
9			Cookies	3.4	Cookies	3.5	Sandwiches & tortas	3.2
10			Sweetened breads	1.6	Rice mixed dishes	2.6	Rice mixed dishes	3.2
11			Breakfast cereals	1.5	Vegetables	2.1	Tortillas (plain)	3.0
12			Rice mixed dishes	1.4	Tortillas (plain)	2.0	Salty snacks	1.6
13			Salty snacks	1.3	Breast milk	1.9	Vegetables	1.6
14			Infant cereal	1.3	100% fruit juice	1.8	100% fruit juice	1.5
15			Yogurt	1.0	Pasta mixed dishes	1.6	Traditional beverages	1.1
16					Salty snacks	1.5	Bread/rolls/biscuits/bagels	1.0
17					Traditional beverages	2.5	Enchiladas	1.0
18					Tamales	1.3	Pasta mixed dishes	1.0
19					Sandwiches & tortas	1.1	Infant formula	1.0
20							Yogurt	1.0
All food groups		**94.3**		**86.6**		**86.2**		**82.6**

Table 11. Food sources of vitamin C among Mexican infants, toddlers, and young children aged 0–47.9 months by age group from ENSANUT 2012.

Rank	Age 0–5.9 Months		Age 6–11.9 Months		Age 12–23.9 Months		Age 24–47.9 Months	
	Food Group	**% of Total**	**Food Group**	**% of Total**	**Food Group**	**% of Total**	**Food Group**	**% of Total**
1	Breast milk	50.5	Breast milk	28.7	Fresh or frozen fruit	17.8	Fresh or frozen fruit	15.1
2	Infant formula	36.5	Infant formula	16.5	Cow's milk	10.8	Cow's milk	11.7
3	100% fruit juice	2.3	Soups & stews	8.8	Soups & stews	9.9	Soups & stews	9.2
4	Vegetables	2.2	Fresh or frozen fruit	8.5	Infant formula	8.9	Traditional beverages	8.0
5	Baby food (vegetables)	1.6	Cow's milk	7.4	Fruit-flavored drinks	7.1	Fruit-flavored drinks	7.3
6	Baby food (fruit)	1.1	Fruit-flavored drinks	3.3	Traditional beverages	6.6	Dried beans	6.2
7			Infant cereal	3.3	100% fruit juice	5.8	Breakfast cereals	4.9
8			Vegetables	3.2	Dried beans	4.5	100% fruit juice	4.5
9			100% fruit juice	2.2	Breast milk	4.3	Rice mixed dishes	2.6
10			Dried beans	1.9	Breakfast cereals	2.9	White potatoes	1.8
11			Traditional beverages	1.6	Rice mixed dishes	2.2	Eggs & egg dishes	1.8
12			White potatoes	1.1	Vegetables	2.0	Sweetened breads	1.6
13			Baby food (fruit)	1.0	Eggs & egg dishes	1.5	Cookies	1.5
14					Pasta mixed dishes	1.4	Pasta mixed dishes	1.4
15					Cookies	1.2	Vegetables	1.4
16							Infant formula	1.3
17							Vegetable & cheese tacos	1.3
18							Beef or pork with vegetables and/or rice/pasta/potatoes	1.2
19							Enchiladas	1.1
20							Tamales	1.0
21							Sandwiches & tortas	1.0
All food groups		94.2		87.5		86.9		85.9

3.3. Minerals and Electrolytes

Among infants, in general, breast milk and infant formula were the top two sources of calcium (Table 12), iron (Table 13), zinc (Table 14), and potassium (Table 15). Among toddlers and young children, in addition to cow's milk, infant formula, yogurt, soups and stews, tortillas, eggs and egg dishes, and dried beans were also important sources of the above minerals.

Except for young children, infant formula ranked as the first source of iron among both infants 0–5.9 months and 6–11.9 months and toddlers, followed by breast milk, soups and stews, cow's milk, and eggs and egg dishes (Table 13). Tortillas ranked fifth as a source of iron among infant 6–11.9 months and toddlers. Cow's milk was the number one source of iron among young children, followed by eggs and egg dishes, tortillas, and sweetened breads. In addition to different types of milk, yogurt and soups and stews were the top sources of potassium. Fruit was another major source of potassium across all age groups, with the contribution higher with increasing age (Table 15). Soups and stews were the highest contributors of sodium among all age groups except infants 0–5.9 months, followed by cow's milk, eggs and egg dishes, and dried beans (Table 16).

Table 12. Food sources of calcium among Mexican infants, toddlers, and young children aged 0–47.9 months by age group from ENSANUT 2012.

Rank	Age 0–5.9 Months		Age 6–11.9 Months		Age 12–23.9 Months		Age 24–47.9 Months	
	Food Group	% of Total	Food Group	% of Total	Food Group	% of Total	Food Group	% of Total
1	Breast milk	47.2	Breast milk	25.8	Cow's milk	30.1	Cow's milk	28.3
2	Infant formula	40.5	Infant formula	20.1	Yogurt	11.7	Yogurt	9.8
3	Yogurt	2.9	Cow's milk	16.4	Infant formula	10.0	Tortillas (plain)	7.5
4	Cow's milk	2.6	Yogurt	12.2	Traditional beverages	4.9	Traditional beverages	5.6
5	Water	1.1	Soups & stews	3.3	Tortillas (plain)	4.3	Sandwiches & tortas	4.8
6			Infant cereal	3.0	Soups & stews	3.7	Breakfast cereals	4.5
7			Tortillas (plain)	2.2	Breast milk	3.5	Eggs & egg dishes	3.8
8			Traditional beverages	2.0	Eggs & egg dishes	3.1	Sweetened tea and coffee	3.3
9			Eggs & egg dishes	1.2	Breakfast cereals	3.0	Sweetened breads	3.3
10					Sweetened tea and coffee	2.8	Dried beans	3.2
11					Dried beans	1.9	Soups & stews	2.1
12					Sweetened breads	1.9	Fresh or frozen fruit	1.5
13					Sandwiches & tortas	1.9	Infant formula	1.4
14					Fresh or frozen fruit	1.7	Salty snacks	1.3
15					Infant cereal	1.3	Candy	1.0
16					Salty snacks	1.0	Vegetable & cheese tacos	1.0
17							Enchiladas	1.0
All food groups		**94.3**		**86.2**		**86.8**		**83.4**

Table 13. Food sources of iron among Mexican infants, toddlers, and young children aged 0–47.9 months by age group from ENSANUT 2012.

Rank	Age 0–5.9 Months		Age 6–11.9 Months		Age 12–23.9 Months		Age 24–47.9 Months	
	Food Group	% of Total	Food Group	% of Total	Food Group	% of Total	Food Group	% of Total
1	Infant formula	47.7	Infant formula	22.7	Infant formula	10.1	Cow's milk	9.8
2	Breast milk	34.1	Soups & stews	11.3	Soups & stews	9.7	Eggs & egg dishes	8.4
3	Cow's milk	2.1	Breast milk	7.1	Cow's milk	9.1	Tortillas (plain)	8.3
4	Soups & stews	1.8	Cow's milk	6.7	Eggs & egg dishes	7.0	Sweetened breads	7.8
5	Water	1.6	Tortillas (plain)	4.9	Tortillas (plain)	5.9	Soups & stews	6.7
6	Baby food (vegetables)	1.6	Cookies	4.9	Sweetened breads	5.8	Breakfast cereals	6.6
7	Vegetables	1.5	Infant cereal	4.4	Dried beans	5.3	Dried beans	5.9
8	Fresh or frozen fruit	1.2	Dried beans	4.3	Breakfast cereals	5.1	Cookies	4.6
9	Baby food (fruit)	1.1	Eggs & egg dishes	3.5	Cookies	4.1	Sandwiches & tortas	3.6
10			Baby food (fruit)	2.5	Traditional beverages	3.7	Meats	2.9
11			Traditional beverages	2.4	Meats	2.7	Traditional beverages	2.7
12			Salty snacks	1.9	Fresh or frozen fruit	2.6	Salty snacks	2.4
13			Rice mixed dishes	1.9	Sweetened tea and coffee	2.3	Rice mixed dishes	2.1
14			Vegetables	1.8	Salty snacks	2.0	Infant formula	1.7
15			Sweetened breads	1.6	100% fruit juice	1.7	Sweetened tea and coffee	1.6
16			Breakfast cereals	1.5	Tamales	1.7	100% fruit juice	1.2
17			Fresh or frozen fruit	1.4	Rice mixed dishes	1.7	Meat tacos	1.1
18			100% fruit juice	1.3	Sandwiches & tortas	1.3	Tamales	1.1
19			Sweetened tea and coffee	1.3	Pasta mixed dishes	1.3	Enchiladas	1.0
20					Infant cereal	1.2	Bread/rolls/biscuits/bagels	1.0
21							Fresh or frozen fruit	1.0
22							Beef or pork with vegetables and/or rice/pasta/potatoes	1.0
All food groups		**92.7**		**87.4**		**84.3**		**82.5**

Table 14. Food sources of zinc among Mexican infants, toddlers, and young children aged 0–47.9 months by age group from ENSANUT 2012.

Rank	Age 0–5.9 Months		Age 6–11.9 Months		Age 12–23.9 Months		Age 24–47.9 Months	
	Food Group	% of Total	Food Group	% of Total	Food Group	% of Total	Food Group	% of Total
1	Breast milk	44.3	Breast milk	21.1	Cow's milk	18.9	Cow's milk	16.0
2	Infant formula	43.3	Infant formula	19.6	Infant formula	9.4	Tortillas (plain)	8.8
3	Yogurt	2.2	Cow's milk	12.6	Soups & stews	7.7	Eggs & egg dishes	7.6
4	Cow's milk	1.9	Yogurt	7.0	Eggs & egg dishes	6.2	Soups & stews	5.9
5	Baby food (vegetables)	1.3	Soups & stews	6.8	Yogurt	6.1	Dried beans	5.7
6			Tortillas (plain)	3.8	Tortillas (plain)	5.8	Yogurt	5.0
7			Infant cereal	3.8	Dried beans	4.2	Breakfast cereals	4.8
8			Dried beans	2.9	Breakfast cereals	4.0	Sandwiches & tortas	4.6
9			Eggs & egg dishes	2.8	Meats	3.8	Meats	4.3
10			Traditional beverages	2.2	Traditional beverages	3.0	Sweetened breads	3.7
11			Vegetables	1.4	Sweetened breads	2.2	Salty snacks	1.8
12			Cookies	1.3	Breast milk	2.0	Cookies	1.7
13			Meats	1.1	Cookies	1.7	Beef or pork with vegetables and/or rice/pasta/potatoes	1.7
14			Breakfast cereals	1.0	Sandwiches & tortas	1.7	Traditional beverages	1.6
15					Pasta mixed dishes	1.4	Rice mixed dishes	1.5
16					Salty snacks	1.4	Meat tacos	1.4
17					Infant cereal	1.3	Sweetened tea and coffee	1.4
18					Sweetened tea and coffee	1.1	Infant formula	1.4
19					Rice mixed dishes	1.0	Vegetable & cheese tacos	1.2
20					Tamales	1.0	Enchiladas	1.1
21							Tamales	1.1
22							Chicken or turkey with vegetables and/or rice/pasta	1.0
All food groups		93.0		87.4		83.9		83.3

Table 15. Food sources of potassium among Mexican infants, toddlers, and young children aged 0–47.9 months by age group from ENSANUT 2012.

Rank	Age 0–5.9 Months		Age 6–11.9 Months		Age 12–23.9 Months		Age 24–47.9 Months	
	Food Group	% of Total	Food Group	% of Total	Food Group	% of Total	Food Group	% of Total
1	Breast milk	48.4	Breast milk	20.8	Cow's milk	15.1	Cow's milk	14.7
2	Infant formula	35.0	Infant formula	14.0	Soups & stews	10.9	Soups & stews	8.6
3	Baby food (vegetables)	2.2	Cow's milk	10.9	Fresh or frozen fruit	8.9	Fresh or frozen fruit	7.2
4	Cow's milk	1.9	Soups & stews	9.9	Infant formula	5.8	Dried beans	6.7
5	Vegetables	1.6	Fresh or frozen fruit	6.8	Dried beans	4.8	Tortillas (plain)	5.3
6	Fresh or frozen fruit	1.5	Eggs & egg dishes	3.6	Sweetened tea and coffee	4.2	Eggs & egg dishes	4.7
7	100% fruit juice	1.5	Yogurt	3.4	Traditional beverages	4.2	Sweetened tea and coffee	4.0
8	Sweetened tea and coffee	1.2	Dried beans	2.9	Tortillas (plain)	3.5	Yogurt	3.8
9	Baby food (fruit)	1.0	100% fruit juice	2.3	Eggs & egg dishes	3.4	Meats	3.1
10			Tortillas (plain)	2.2	100% fruit juice	3.4	Sandwiches & tortas	3.0
11			Vegetables	2.0	Yogurt	3.3	Traditional beverages	2.5
12			Traditional beverages	1.6	Meats	2.7	Breakfast cereals	2.3
13			Infant cereal	1.5	Breast milk	2.3	100% fruit juice	2.3
14			Sweetened tea and coffee	1.5	Fruit-flavored drinks	2.3	Salty snacks	2.0
15			Fruit-flavored drinks	1.3	Vegetables	1.8	Fruit-flavored drinks	1.9
16			Chicken or turkey with vegetables and/or rice/pasta/potatoes	1.2	Breakfast cereals	1.7	Sweetened breads	1.9
17					Pasta mixed dishes	1.4	Rice mixed dishes	1.6
18					Rice mixed dishes	1.4	White potatoes	1.6
19					White potatoes	1.2	Vegetables	1.4
20					Salty snacks	1.2	Beef or pork with vegetables and/or rice/pasta/potatoes	1.3
21					Sandwiches & tortas	1.2	Chicken or turkey with vegetables and/or rice/pasta/potatoes	1.2
22					Sweetened breads	1.0	Vegetable & cheese tacos	1.1
23							Meat tacos	1.1
24							Enchiladas	1.0
25							Tamales	1.0
All food groups		**94.3**		**85.9**		**85.7**		**85.3**

Table 16. Food sources of sodium among Mexican infants, toddlers, and young children aged 0–47.9 months by age group from ENSANUT 2012.

Rank	Age 0–5.9 Months		Age 6–11.9 Months		Age 12–23.9 Months		Age 24–47.9 Months	
	Food Group	% of Total	Food Group	% of Total	Food Group	% of Total	Food Group	% of Total
1	Breast milk	44.6	Soups & stews	16.8	Soups & stews	17.6	Soups & stews	12.2
2	Infant formula	37.4	Breast milk	15.9	Cow's milk	9.9	Eggs & egg dishes	10.6
3	Soups & stews	3.0	Infant formula	12.6	Eggs & egg dishes	8.4	Dried beans	7.3
4	Baby food (vegetables)	2.5	Cow's milk	8.7	Dried beans	7.2	Cow's milk	6.9
5	Vegetables	1.7	Eggs & egg dishes	6.0	Meats	4.2	Sandwiches & tortas	5.8
6	Cow's milk	2.6	Cookies	5.0	Infant formula	4.1	Meats	5.1
7	Water	1.3	Dried beans	3.6	Sweetened breads	3.4	Sweetened breads	4.6
8	Infant cereal	1.0	Yogurt	2.3	Cookies	3.2	Salty snacks	3.9
9			Salty snacks	1.9	Salty snacks	3.2	Rice mixed dishes	3.3
10			Chicken or turkey with vegetables and/or rice/pasta/potatoes	1.9	Traditional beverages	3.2	Tortillas (plain)	3.3
11			Infant cereal	1.7	Rice mixed dishes	2.9	Cookies	3.2
12			Traditional beverages	1.6	Pasta mixed dishes	2.8	Breakfast cereals	2.5
13			Meats	1.4	Breakfast cereals	2.7	Beef or pork with vegetables and/or rice/pasta/potatoes	2.1
14			Rice mixed dishes	1.4	Tortillas (plain)	2.1	White potatoes	1.6
15			Tortillas (plain)	1.1	Sandwiches & tortas	2.0	Bread/rolls/biscuits/bagels	1.6
16			Vegetables	1.1	White potatoes	1.6	Vegetable & cheese tacos	1.5
17			Pasta mixed dishes	1.1	Beef or pork with vegetables and/or rice/pasta/potatoes	1.5	Pasta mixed dishes	1.5
18					Breast milk	1.2	Tamales	1.4
19					Chicken or turkey with vegetables and/or rice/pasta/potatoes	1.1	Enchiladas	1.3
20					Sweetened tea and coffee	1.0	Chicken or turkey with vegetables and/or rice/pasta/potatoes	1.3
21					Bread/rolls/biscuits/bagels	1.0	Carbonated sodas	1.1
22							Meat tacos	1.0
All food groups		**94.1**		**84.1**		**84.3**		**83.1**

4. Discussion

The results of this study provide a comprehensive picture of food sources of energy and nutrients and show the shifts with age among Mexican children aged 0–47.9 months. Previous studies on nutrient intake in this population reported inadequate intakes of iron, calcium, vitamin D, vitamin E, folate, and fiber and excessive intakes of energy, added sugars, saturated fat, and sodium [14–18]. Our data have provided important insights on those findings.

4.1. Milk Sources

Overall, breast milk, infant formula, and cow's milk were the top sources of energy, protein, fat, carbohydrates, vitamins (vitamin A, vitamin E, vitamin C, and B vitamins), and minerals (calcium, iron, zinc, and potassium), especially in younger groups. This is similar to what we observed in studies in the USA [26,29] and in China [30]. However, one difference in this study is that cow's milk was one of the major sources of energy among infants 6–11.9 months. This is a concern because cow's milk is considered to be an inappropriate milk for children under the age of one year as early feeding of cow's milk is associated with an increased risk of developing iron-deficiency anemia [31]. The reasons include its low iron content, poor iron availability, and associated occult intestinal blood loss [32].

4.2. Low Nutrient-Dense Foods and Beverages

As infants and toddlers have a small stomach capacity but high nutrient needs to support their rapid growth, complementary foods should be nutrient-dense, i.e., relatively low in calories and high in vitamins and minerals [3]. However, low nutrient-dense and energy-rich cookies, sweetened breads, and traditional beverages were consumed as core foods in the diet of Mexican children.

These observations are very much aligned with previous findings that showed a high proportion of energy was provided by caloric beverages [12,33] and that added sugar consumption was high among Mexican children aged 1–4 years [16,18]. Our study provided further details as to what foods and beverages contributed to the high added sugar consumption and the relative role of each food. In addition, we found that consumption of sweetened foods and beverages started as early as the second six months of life and some food items shifted with increasing age. For example, the contribution of carbonated sodas to added sugar doubled in young children compared to toddlers. It is important that energy-rich foods, which provide little nutritional benefit, are limited [34]. Reduced consumption of cookies, sweetened breads, sugar sweetened beverages along with lower sugar content of traditional beverages would markedly decrease the total intake of added sugar in Mexican children.

4.3. Food Sources of Iron

Iron-rich foods are lacking in young Mexican children. Iron is of particular importance after six months of age as the infant's iron stores, which are laid down during gestation, are declining [35]. Thus, complementary foods need to provide iron, either from animal-source foods or from fortification, as recommended in the official Mexican guidelines on nutrition [36] and a recent Mexican complementary feeding consensus paper [37]. Given the detrimental consequences of iron deficiency disorders on cognitive and neurological development [38], a recent position paper on complementary feeding stressed the recommendation of iron-rich food consumption [34]. Previous studies in Mexico have shown that iron intake of infants did not meet recommendations [14], heme-iron intake was low [17], and iron-deficiency anemia was prevalent (23%) [10]. It has already been reported that complementary feeding practices in Mexico lack animal foods [39,40]. In our study, we found that meats provided less than 1% of energy among infants 6–11.9 month olds and were not among the top 10 food sources of energy in toddlers and young children. As a result, meats did not markedly contribute to the intake of iron or vitamins. Also of note, iron-fortified infant cereal made a minimal contribution to nutrient intake in this population. However, it is important to note that Mexican tortilla flour is fortified with iron [41], which might explain why tortillas appears as the third to fifth sources of iron after 12 months of age.

Surprisingly, cow's milk was found to be a top source of iron (ranked first among young children). This may be caused by two reasons. One is that a proportion of fortified cow's milk (19.6%) was grouped into cow's milk in this study and hence increased the iron contribution from the cow's milk category. The other reason might be that even though cow's milk is not high in iron, it is frequently consumed, making it a significant iron source.

4.4. Role of Local Foods

The ranking of a food as a source of energy or a nutrient reflects not only the concentration of a nutrient in a food but also the frequency of consumption of the food. Soups and stews were found to be top contributors to energy and almost all nutrients after milk including total fat, saturated fat, and sodium. Soups and stews are frequently consumed in this population [12,13]. Since soups and stews in Mexico typically contain meat (usually chicken), vegetables, and tortillas, it is understandable that these food mixtures can provide a wide range of nutrients.

Tortillas were a top source of energy, protein, carbohydrates, a number of B vitamins, calcium, iron, and zinc, and were the number one source of dietary fiber among toddlers and young children. Again, as a staple food in Mexico, high consumption of tortillas makes them a major contributor to macro- and micronutrients. On the contrary, although the contribution of vegetables (consumed as discrete items rather than as food mixtures) to nutrient intake was minimal, indicating low vegetable consumption, vegetables appeared to be in the top three or top five sources of fiber among infants. This is due to the high content of fiber in vegetables, even though they are infrequently consumed. On the other hand, the fact that tortillas were the number one source of fiber among toddlers and young children suggests that good food sources of fiber are really lacking and explains why fiber intake was low in 87% of children aged 1–4 years in Mexico [16]. In addition to the above, we also found that eggs and egg dishes and dried beans (both among the top 10 sources of energy), were top contributors to a number of key nutrients including protein, vitamin A, folate, iron, zinc, potassium, and fiber (dried beans only) in the diet of this population.

4.5. Limitations

This study was cross-sectional in design, so it is not possible to evaluate changes in food sources among the same children as they grow. We used a single day 24-h dietary recall, which may not reflect usual intake. The grouping of food items was designed to reflect local food culture and to help us understand the relative role of specific types of foods and beverages, but the choice of food groups could have had an influence on the rankings. If no detailed information was available, standard recipes were used for foods prepared at home, which could have led to either underestimation or overestimation of certain nutrients. Nevertheless, a major strength of this study is the use of small age categories and food groups to describe, in detail, the food sources of energy and nutrients and shifts with age in children aged 0–47.9 months using a nationally representative sample of Mexico.

5. Conclusions

This study provides important insights on food sources of energy and nutrients among Mexican children aged 0–47.9 months. The results show that, in addition to milk sources, other types of foods and beverages commonly consumed in Mexico had major contributions to the intakes of energy and nutrients. Foods and beverages high in sugar such as cookies, sweetened breads, and traditional beverages were among the food items commonly consumed from a very young age and contributed increasingly with age to the intake of energy and added sugar. Milk and soups and stews were top contributors to all nutrients. Tortillas and eggs and egg dishes were among the top contributors to iron and zinc. High-fiber foods like vegetables or dried beans were not the top sources of fiber in the diets of children in Mexico. The intake of more nutrient-dense foods such as vegetables, beans, lean meats, and fortified cereals should be encouraged to help address shortfalls in nutrients. Core foods like soups and stews and eggs and egg dishes were the top contributors to sodium, suggesting that they may be suitable targets for sodium reduction. The findings from this study can assist healthcare professionals to develop food-based recommendations to correct the inadequate or excessive intake of certain nutrients in the diets of infants and young children in Mexico.

Acknowledgments: We acknowledge the help of Barry Popkin in accessing and analyzing the ENSANUT data. We thank Phil Bardsley for his work in managing data and programming. Special thanks to Denise Deming, who wrote an initial version of the abstract for the 2016 Experimental Biology Conference and conducted preliminary analyses. We would like to thank the field workers who assisted with the data collection and also the mothers/infants who participated in the study.

Author Contributions: L.D. contributed to data analysis and was responsible for interpreting the data and writing the manuscript, and had final responsibility for this manuscript. M.C.A. contributed to formulating the research question and data analysis, and interpreted the data. A.L.E. and S.V.-C. contributed to data interpretation and the critical review and editing of the manuscript. All authors read and approved the final manuscript.

References

1. Weng, S.F.; Redsell, S.A.; Swift, J.A.; Yang, M.; Glazebrook, C.P. Systematic review and meta-analyses of risk factors for childhood overweight identifiable during infancy. *Arch. Dis. Child.* **2012**, *97*, 1019–1026. [CrossRef] [PubMed]
2. Dyer, J.S.; Rosenfeld, C.R. Metabolic imprinting by prenatal, perinatal, and postnatal overnutrition: A review. *Semin. Reprod. Med.* **2011**, *29*, 266–276. [CrossRef] [PubMed]
3. Dewey, K.G. The challenge of meeting nutrient needs of infants and young children during the period of complementary feeding: An evolutionary perspective. *J. Nutr.* **2013**, *143*, 2050–2054. [CrossRef] [PubMed]
4. Word Health Organization. *Guiding Principles for Complementary Feeding of the Breastfed Child*; Pan American Health Organization: Washington, DC, USA, 2002.
5. Schwartz, C.; Scholtens, P.A.; Lalanne, A.; Weenen, H.; Nicklaus, S. Development of healthy eating habits early in life. Review of recent evidence and selected guidelines. *Appetite* **2011**, *57*, 796–807. [CrossRef] [PubMed]
6. Barquera, S.; Nonato, I.C.; Barrera, L.H.; Pedroza, A.; Rivera, J.Á. Prevalence of obesity in Mexican adults 2000–2012. *Salud Pública Mex.* **2013**, *55*, S151–S160. [PubMed]
7. Rivera, J.Á.; de Cosío, T.G.; Pedraza, L.S.; Aburto, T.C.; Sánchez, T.G.; Martorell, R. Childhood and adolescent overweight and obesity in Latin America: A systematic review. *Lancet Diabetes Endocrinol.* **2014**, *2*, 321–332. [CrossRef]
8. Rivera-Dommarco, J.Á.; Cuevas-Nasu, L.; González de Cosío, T.; Shamah-Levy, T.; García-Feregrino, R. Stunting in Mexico in the last quarter century: Analysis of four national surveys. *Salud Pública Mex.* **2013**, *55*, S161–S169. [PubMed]
9. Villalpando, S.; de la Cruz, V.; Levy, T.S.; Rebollar, R.; Contreras-Manzano, A. Nutritional status of iron, vitamin B12, folate, retinol and anemia in children 1 to 11 years old: Results of the ENSANUT 2012. *Salud Pública Mex.* **2015**, *57*, 372–384. [CrossRef] [PubMed]
10. De la Cruz-Góngora, V.; Villalpando, S.; Mundo-Rosas, V.; Shamah-Levy, T. Prevalence of anemia in Mexican children and adolescents: Results from three national surveys. *Salud Pública Mex.* **2013**, *55*, S180–S189. [PubMed]
11. Rivera, J.Á.; Pedraza, L.S.; Aburto, T.C.; Batis, C.; Sánchez-Pimienta, T.G.; González de Cosío, T.; López-Olmedo, N.; Pedroza-Tobías, A. Overview of the dietary intakes of the Mexican population: Results from the National Health and Nutrition Survey 2012. *J. Nutr.* **2016**, *146*, 1851S–1855S. [CrossRef] [PubMed]
12. Rodríguez-Ramírez, S.; Muñoz-Espinosa, A.; Rivera, J.Á.; González-Castell, D.; González de Cosío, T. Mexican children under 2 years of age consume food groups high in energy and low in micronutrients.

J. Nutr. **2016**, *146*, 1916S–1923S. [CrossRef] [PubMed]
13. Deming, D.M.; Afeiche, M.C.; Reidy, K.C.; Eldridge, A.L.; Villalpando-Carrión, S. Early feeding patterns among Mexican babies: Findings from the 2012 National Health and Nutrition Survey and implications for health and obesity prevention. *BMC Nutr.* **2015**. [CrossRef]
14. Piernas, C.; Miles, D.R.; Deming, D.M.; Reidy, K.C.; Popkin, B.M. Estimating usual intakes mainly affects the micronutrient distribution among infants, toddlers and pre-schoolers from the 2012 Mexican National Health and Nutrition Survey. *Public Health Nutr.* **2016**, *19*, 1017–1026. [CrossRef] [PubMed]
15. Pedroza-Tobías, A.; Hernández-Barrera, L.; López-Olmedo, N.; García-Guerra, A.; Rodríguez-Ramírez, S.; Ramírez-Silva, I.; Villalpando, S.; Carriquiry, A.; Rivera, J.Á. Usual vitamin intakes by Mexican populations. *J. Nutr.* **2016**, *146*, 1866S–1873S. [CrossRef] [PubMed]
16. López-Olmedo, N.; Carriquiry, A.L.; Rodríguez-Ramírez, S.; Ramírez-Silva, I.; Espinosa-Montero, J.; Hernández-Barrera, L.; Campirano, F.; Martínez-Tapia, B.; Rivera, J.Á. Usual intake of added sugars and saturated fats is high while dietary fiber is low in the Mexican population. *J. Nutr.* **2016**, *146*, 1856S–1865S. [CrossRef] [PubMed]
17. Sánchez-Pimienta, T.G.; López-Olmedo, N.; Rodríguez-Ramírez, S.; García-Guerra, A.; Rivera, J.Á.; Carriquiry, A.L.; Villalpando, S. High prevalence of inadequate calcium and iron intakes by Mexican population groups as assessed by 24-hour recalls. *J. Nutr.* **2016**, *146*, 1874S–1880S. [CrossRef] [PubMed]
18. Sánchez-Pimienta, T.G.; Batis, C.; Lutter, C.K.; Rivera, J.A. Sugar-sweetened beverages are the main sources of added sugar intake in the Mexican population. *J. Nutr.* **2016**, *146*, 1888S–1896S. [CrossRef] [PubMed]
19. Romero-Martínez, M.; Shamah-Levy, T.; Franco-Núñez, A.; Villalpando, S.; Cuevas-Nasu, L.; Gutiérrez, J.P.; Rivera-Dommarco, J.Á. National Health and Nutrition Survey 2012: Design and coverage. *Salud Pública Mex.* **2013**, *55*, S332–S340.
20. Devaney, B.; Ziegler, P.; Pac, S.; Karwe, V.; Barr, S.I. Nutrient intakes of infants and toddlers. *J. Am. Diet. Assoc.* **2004**, *104*, S14–S21. [CrossRef] [PubMed]
21. Butte, N.F.; Fox, M.K.; Briefel, R.R.; Siega-Riz, A.M.; Dwyer, J.T.; Deming, D.M.; Reidy, K.C. Nutrient intakes of US infants, toddlers, and preschoolers meet or exceed dietary reference intakes. *J. Am. Diet. Assoc.* **2010**, *110*, S27–S37. [CrossRef] [PubMed]
22. Instituto Nacional de Salud Pública. *Bases de Datos de Valor Nutritivo de los Alimentos (National Institute of Public Health. Food Composition Table)*; National Institute of Public Health: Cuernavaca, Mexico, 2012.
23. United States Department of Agriculture, Agricultural Research Service. SR-27 Home Page. Available online: https://www.ars.usda.gov/northeast-area/beltsville-md/beltsville-human-nutrition-research-center/nutrient-data-laboratory/docs/sr27-home-page/ (accessed on 1 April 2015).
24. Brownman, S.A.; Friday, J.E.; Moshfegh, A.J. MyPyramid Equivalents Database, 2.0 for USDA Survey Foods, 2003–2004. Available online: https://www.ars.usda.gov/ARSUserFiles/80400530/pdf/mped/mped2_doc.pdf (accessed on 16 March 2017).
25. University of Minnesota. Nutrition Coordinating Center—NDSR 2016 User Manual. Appendix 11—Nutrient Information, page A11.5. Available online: http://www.ncc.umn.edu/products/ndsr-user-manual/ (accessed on 12 May 2017).
26. Fox, M.K.; Reidy, K.; Novak, T.; Ziegler, P. Sources of energy and nutrients in the diets of infants and toddlers. *J. Am. Diet. Assoc.* **2006**, *106*, S28–S42. [CrossRef] [PubMed]
27. Fox, M.K.; Condon, E.; Briefel, R.R.; Reidy, K.C.; Deming, D.M. Food consumption patterns of young preschoolers: Are they starting off on the right path? *J. Am. Diet. Assoc.* **2010**, *110*, S52–S59. [CrossRef] [PubMed]
28. Siega-Riz, A.M.; Deming, D.M.; Reidy, K.C.; Fox, M.K.; Condon, E.; Briefel, R.R. Food consumption patterns of infants and toddlers: Where are we now? *J. Am. Diet. Assoc.* **2010**, *110*, S38–S51. [CrossRef] [PubMed]
29. Grimes, C.A.; Szymlek-Gay, E.A.; Campbell, K.J.; Nicklas, T.A. Food sources of total energy and nutrients among U.S. Infants and toddlers: National Health and Nutrition Examination Survey 2005–2012. *Nutrients* **2015**, *7*, 6797–6836. [CrossRef] [PubMed]
30. Wang, H.; Denney, L.; Zheng, Y.; Vinyes Pares, G.; Reidy, K.; Wang, P.; Zhang, Y. Food sources of energy and nutrients in the diets of infants and toddlers in urban areas of China, based on one 24-hour dietary recall. *BMC Nutr.* **2015**. [CrossRef]

31. Griebler, U.; Bruckmuller, M.U.; Kien, C.; Dieminger, B.; Meidlinger, B.; Seper, K.; Hitthaller, A.; Emprechtinger, R.; Wolf, A.; Gartlehner, G. Health effects of cow's milk consumption in infants up to 3 years of age: A systematic review and meta-analysis. *Public Health Nutr.* **2016**, *19*, 293–307. [CrossRef] [PubMed]
32. Borgna-Pignatti, C.; Marsella, M. Iron deficiency in infancy and childhood. *Pediatr Ann.* **2008**, *37*, 329–337. [PubMed]
33. Barquera, S.; Campirano, F.; Bonvecchio, A.; Hernandez-Barrera, L.; Rivera, J.A.; Popkin, B.M. Caloric beverage consumption patterns in Mexican children. *Nutr. J.* **2010**, *9*, 47. [CrossRef] [PubMed]
34. Fewtrell, M.; Bronsky, J.; Campoy, C.; Domellof, M.; Embleton, N.; Fidler Mis, N.; Hojsak, I.; Hulst, J.M.; Indrio, F.; Lapillonne, A.; et al. Complementary feeding: A position paper by the European Society for Paediatric Gastroenterology, Hepatology, and Nutrition (ESPGHAN) committee on nutrition. *J. Pediatr. Gastroenterol. Nutr.* **2017**, *64*, 119–132. [CrossRef] [PubMed]
35. Baker, R.D.; Greer, F.R. Diagnosis and prevention of iron deficiency and iron-deficiency anemia in infants and young children (0–3 years of age). *Pediatrics* **2010**, *126*, 1040–1050. [CrossRef] [PubMed]
36. NORMA Oficial Mexicana NOM-043-SSA2–2012 Basic Health Services. Promotion and Health Education to Food. Criteria to Provide Guidance. Available online: http://dof.gob.mx/nota_detalle_popup.php?codigo=5285372 (accessed on 16 March 2017).
37. Romero-Velarde, E.; Villalpando-Carrión, S.; Pérez-Lizaur, A.B.; Iracheta-Gerez, M.; Alonso-Rivera, C.G.; López-Navarrete, G.E.; García-Contreras, A.; Ochoa-Ortiz, E.; Zarate-Mondragón, F.; López-Pérez, G.T.; et al. Consenso para las prácticas de alimentación complementaria en lactantes sanos. *Bol. Med. Hosp. Infant. Mex.* **2016**, *73*, 338–356.
38. Lozoff, B.; Beard, J.; Connor, J.; Barbara, F.; Georgieff, M.; Schallert, T. Long-lasting neural and behavioral effects of iron deficiency in infancy. *Nutr. Rev.* **2006**, *64*, S34–S43. [CrossRef] [PubMed]
39. González-Cosío, T.; Rivera-Dommarco, J.; Moreno-Macias, H.; Monterrubio, E.; Sepulveda, J. Poor compliance with appropriate feeding practices in children under 2 y in Mexico. *J. Nutr.* **2006**, *136*, 2928–2933.
40. Denney, L.; Reidy, C.K.; Eldridge, A.L. Differences in complementary feeding of 6 to 23 month olds in china, us and Mexico. *J. Nutr. Health Food Sci.* **2016**, *4*, 1–8.
41. Tovar, L.R.; Larios-Saldaña, A. Iron and zinc fortification of corn tortilla made either at the household or at industrial scale. *Int. J. Vitam. Nutr. Res.* **2005**, *75*, 142–148. [CrossRef] [PubMed]

8

Preschool and School Meal Policies: An Overview of What we Know about Regulation, Implementation and Impact on Diet in the UK, Sweden and Australia

Patricia Jane Lucas [1,*] , Emma Patterson [2,3] , Gary Sacks [4], Natassja Billich [4] and Charlotte Elizabeth Louise Evans [5]

1 School for Policy Studies, University of Bristol, Bristol BS8 1TZ, UK
2 Department of Public Health Sciences, Karolinska Institutet, SE-171 77 Stockholm, Sweden; Emma.Patterson@ki.se
3 Centre for Epidemiology and Community Medicine, Stockholm County Council, SE-113 65 Stockholm, Sweden
4 Global Obesity Centre, School of Health and Social Development, Deakin University, Geelong VIC 3220, Australia; gary.sacks@deakin.edu.au (G.S.); natassja.billich@deakin.edu.au (N.B.)
5 Nutritional Epidemiology Group, School of Food Science and Nutrition, University of Leeds, Leeds LS2 9JT, UK; C.E.L.Evans@leeds.ac.uk
* Correspondence: patricia.lucas@bristol.ac.uk

Abstract: School meals make significant contributions to healthy dietary behaviour, at a time when eating habits and food preferences are being formed. We provide an overview of the approaches to the provision, regulation, and improvement of preschool and primary school meals in the UK, Sweden, and Australia, three countries which vary in their degree of centralisation and regulation of school meals. Sweden has a centralised approach; all children receive free meals, and a pedagogical approach to meals is encouraged. Legislation demands that meals are nutritious. The UK system is varied and decentralised. Meals in most primary schools are regulated by food-based standards, but preschool-specific meal standards only exist in Scotland. The UK uses food groups (starchy foods, fruit and vegetables, proteins and dairy) in a healthy plate approach. Australian States and Territories all employ guidelines for school canteen food, predominantly using a "traffic light" approach outlining recommended and discouraged foods; however, most children bring food from home and are not covered by this guidance. The preschool standards state that food provided should be nutritious. We find that action is often lacking in the preschool years, and suggest that consistent policies, strong incentives for compliance, systematic monitoring, and an acknowledgement of the broader school eating environment (including home provided food) would be beneficial.

Keywords: school; preshool; children; school meals; nutrition intake; policy

---

1. Introduction

1.1. Background and Aims

There is increasing interest in policies aimed at establishing schools and Early Education and Care (EEC) as health promoting environments [1], including health education within the school curriculum, and schools as a site for healthy eating [2]. Food eaten in education and care settings makes a significant contribution to children's total diet. Some have even suggested that a failure to provide healthy foods in schools is a breach of children's human rights [3]. Policy, guidance, and regulation in this field has considerable potential to impact on the dietary intake of young children [4].

This paper aims to compare the school meal policies in preschool and primary educational settings in three high-income country contexts: UK, Australia, and Sweden. These were selected to illustrate the variation in OECD countries in approaches to regulation and standard setting at the regional and national level, from entirely centralised (Sweden) to entirely federal (Australia), and from highly standardised (Sweden) to highly varied (UK). We provide an overview [5] of policy and research in the field. Policy documents and regulatory tools do not lend themselves to systematic approaches, and require expert knowledge to locate the associated (grey) literature. We used our local policy knowledge to locate much of the literature included here. In addition, we searched Medline for studies published within the last 10 years in each of our target countries, with search terms for school food/meals and evaluations (the search terms are available from the corresponding author on request). The UK government is unusual in providing a searchable database of policy and government publications, and we reviewed the latest relevant policy documents using the search terms "school meals" and "school food".

We asked: what is the current policy in each country, how many children does it reach, what do we know about how it is implemented, and what evidence exists for the impact of this approach on children's health? We focus here on policy interventions at the national or regional level, not on research or pilot programmes.

1.2. School Food as a Public Health Nutrition Intervention

The diet of preschool and primary children in all three countries leaves room for improvement, with higher than recommended intakes of sugar and saturated fats [6,7], and lower intakes of fruits and vegetables [8]. Moreover, there are stark inequalities with respect to dietary quality, with lower income families reporting poorer diets [6,9–12].

The provision of meals during school hours has a long history as a public health measure [2,13]. Patterns of school food consumption mirror total diet, suggesting both that dietary choices are consistent and that school is an important eating occasion in terms of total intake [14,15]. The contribution of weekday meals for school children is approximately 30% of daily intake in both the UK [16] and Sweden [17]. There is very limited data to comment on the total contribution to diet from meals consumed in preschool [13,18].

Good quality school meals have the potential to improve children's diets and health. The availability of healthy nutritious choices influences diet positively in school children [19]. The provision of fruit and vegetables to children in schools increases their fruit and vegetable consumption [20], and has been shown to level family differences in fruit and vegetable intakes among 11-year-old children [21]. Changes to school cafeteria environments can improve food choices at school [22]. In the earliest years, the behaviour of childcare workers themselves has a positive impact on preschool children's intake of fruit and vegetables [23].

Health promoting schools successfully provide health education and a healthier environment for school aged children across the world [1,24,25]. Health education is an important part of the curriculum in both the primary and preschool years, and in both the UK and Sweden EEC settings are tasked to help children understand their own health choices [26,27].

1.3. Country Contexts

The UK has a total population of 64 million, of whom 18% are aged less than 15; 19% of Australia's population of 24 million are children, and 17% of the 10 million people in Sweden are children [28].

Sweden is a Nordic European nation with a well-developed welfare system and relatively high taxes. Legislation is made centrally, but the 290 local authorities are responsible for the delivery of many services, including education. Preschool care/education for 1–5 year-olds is heavily subsidized (free for many or capped at ~€150 per child per month, even when privately run), and over 90% of children attend, often from 18 months of age. Primary school education covers the ages six to fifteen, is free (even when privately run), and parents incur no charges for education-related expenses, including meals.

The UK is a Western European nation. It has three devolved regions: Scotland, Wales, and Northern Ireland. National policy always applies to England, but applies to different degrees in each devolved region. Children aged 3–4 years in all regions are entitled to 15 h/week in EEC (due to rise to 30 h/week in England in September 2017); parents decide where to spend this provision from within public, private, or voluntary sector settings [29]. In England, Northern Ireland, and Scotland 2 years old in the greatest need (including those living in poverty and those with disabilities) receive the same allocation [29–31]. The government pays a flat rate of £55/week, which is not intended to cover food or other additional costs. Primary education is compulsory for 5–11 years old, but most children begin school aged 4 years. Primary schools may be state funded and maintained, state funded but independently run (academies, free, and church schools), or privately funded and run.

Australia is a Federation of States and Territories (New South Wales, Victoria, South Australia, Western Australia, Queensland, Tasmania, Australian Capital Territory, and Northern Territory). Education in Australia is primarily the responsibility of the states and territories. Early childhood education in Australia is not compulsory and is delivered to children through a range of settings, including childcare centres, kindergartens, and preschools in the year before full-time schooling (age 5 or 6). The Australian Government pays part of the cost of some childcare through the social security system. Compulsory education in Australia starts at around the age of five or six years. Government schools educate approximately 60% of Australian primary school students, with approximately 40% in either private or independent (including Catholic) schools.

Since policy follows organisational structures, not chronological age, we adopt the educational stage cut offs of preschool and primary school in this paper. Thus, for example, 5-year-olds attend school in England but preschool in Sweden. It is important to remember these age differences when comparing between countries. Countries apply adequacy requirements (Table 1) and limits (Table 2), which vary in their regulation, reach, cost to families, and systems of monitoring (Table 3).

Table 1. School food adequacy standards in the UK, Australia, and Sweden.

Food	Standard or Guidance	Level, Country (Jurisdiction)
Fruit and vegetables	Minimum number portions per day/meal	School and Preschool, UK (England, Scotland)
Meat, fish, eggs, and non-dairy protein		
Starchy foods	Recommended number of portions per day	School and Preschool, UK (England, Scotland)
Milk and dairy		
Drinks	Fresh water to be freely available	School and Preschool, UK (England, Scotland)
	Diluted fruit juice or fresh cows' milks	Preschool, UK (England, Scotland)
Traffic Light: "Green" foods	Minimum of 60% of food and snacks sold should be "Green"	School, Australia (WA *)
	Should be available every day the canteen is open	School, Australia (NT, SA, Q, V *)
Every-day (Core) foods	Recommended to make up 75% of food and drinks sold	School, Australia (NSW *)
"Nutritious" meals	Meals must be "nutritious". Preschool meals must also be "varied", and "evenly distributed over the day"	School and Preschool, Sweden
"Good meals in preschool"	Suggestions provided for meal components and nutritional content (e.g., serve fatty fish twice within 4 weeks, serve only milk and water to drink, provide a wide selection of salads, include wholegrain versions of products etc.)	School and Preschool, Sweden
"Good school meals"		

* Northern Territory (NT); South Australia (SA); Queensland (Q); Victoria (V); New South Wales (NSW); Western Australia (WA).

Table 2. School food limiting standards in the UK, Australia, and Sweden.

Food	Standard or Guidance	Level, Country (Jurisdiction)
Meat, fish, eggs, and non-dairy protein	Maximum number portions	School, UK (England), Preschool UK (Scotland)
Starchy foods	Maximum number of occasions higher fat versions offered (fried starchy foods and cheese as protein)	School, UK (England)
Milk and dairy food		
Traffic Light: "Amber" foods	Maximum of 40% of foods and drinks sold should be "Amber"	School, Australia (WA *)
	"Amber" foods should be limited and sold in smaller serve sizes	School, Australia (NT, SA, Q, V *)
Desserts & Puddings	To be served only once per day with main meal	School and Preschool, UK (England, Scotland)
Occasional (non-core) foods	Maximum of 25% of food and drinks sold should be "occasional" and least healthy not sold	School, Australia (NSW *)

Table 2. *Cont.*

Food	Standard or Guidance	Level, Country (Jurisdiction)
Foods high in fat, salt, and sugar	Avoided or limited	School and Preschool, UK (England, Scotland)
Traffic Light: "Red" foods	"Red" foods prohibited or limited to special occasions (no more than twice per term)	School, Australia (NT, SA, Q, V *)
	"Red" foods prohibited	School, Australia (NT, SA, Q, V *)
Salt and condiments	Reduced or not salt in cooking, No salt available to add. Condiments avoided or size limited.	School and Preschool, UK (England, Scotland)
	Should not be available to students	School and Preschool, Sweden
Drinks	All those not specified to be excluded	School and Preschool, UK (England, Scotland)
	"Amber" drinks should be avoided and sold in smaller serve sizes	School, Australia (NT, SA, Q, V *)
	"Red" drinks (sugary) not to be sold and not permitted	School, Australia (all states and territories)
	No sweet drinks containing sugar or sweetener	School and Preschool, Sweden
Confectionary	Not permitted	School and Preschool, UK (England, Scotland)
	Not permitted	School, Australia (all states and territories)
	Should not be provided	School and Preschool, Sweden

* Northern Territory (NT); South Australia (SA); Queensland (Q); Victoria (V); New South Wales (NSW); Western Australia (WA).

Table 3. School food policy regulation and monitoring in the UK, Sweden, and Australia. Abbreviation: EEC, early education and care.

Policy	Country (Jurisdiction)	Level	Reach	Cost to Families	System of Monitoring
Food Based Standards for Schools in England	UK (England)	School	Mandatory for local government controlled schools and schools that became academies before 2010 and after June 2014. Recommended for remaining academies and private schools.	Free for 4–7 years Paid for other years	Included in the Office of Standards in Education (OFSTED) inspection report on healthy eating.
Voluntary Guidance	UK (England)	Preschool	Voluntary	Paid	Not monitored in OFSTED inspections, although the Early Years Foundation Stage (EYFS) requires that provided food must be "healthy balanced and nutritious" (EYFS 2017).
Preschool standards	UK (Scotland)	Preschool	Mandatory for all settings registered with the Care Inspectorate.	Paid	Inspected by the Care Inspectorate. EEC must show they provide opportunities for children to learn about diet and health. EEC must show children have access to a well-balanced and healthy diet. For example, through use of a food policy.

Table 3. *Cont.*

Policy	Country (Jurisdiction)	Level	Reach	Cost to Families	System of Monitoring
Traffic light food groups	Australia (Australia Capital Territory)	School	Policy applies to all food services activities within a school setting. Mandatory for government schools. In independent and Catholic schools, it is not mandatory but highly recommended.	Paid	Independent compliance monitoring. Free assessment, resources and training available for canteens. Facilitate government license agreements with school canteens.
	Australia (Northern Territory)	School	Policy applies to all food services activities within a school setting. Mandatory for government schools	Paid	Independent compliance monitoring, schools responsible for oversight.
	Australia (South Australia)	School	Policy applies to all food services activities within a school setting. Mandatory for government schools. Catholic and independent school sectors support implementation of the policy.	Paid	Independent compliance monitoring, schools responsible for oversight. Resources provided to canteens.
	Australia (Queensland)	School	Policy applies to all food services activities within a school setting. Mandatory for government schools.	Paid	Independent compliance monitoring, schools responsible for oversight. Training and resources provided to canteens.
	Australia (Tasmania)	School	Schools are recommended (not mandatory) to apply to have their canteen accredited.	Paid	Training, resources and monitoring available to canteens.
	Australia (Victoria)	School	Policy applies to all food services activities within a school setting. Mandatory for government schools.	Paid	Independent compliance monitoring, schools responsible for oversight. Optional monitoring and assessment of canteens available. Training and resources provided to canteens.
Every-day vs. occasional foods	Australia (New South Wales)	School	Policy applies to all food services activities within a school setting. Mandatory for government schools. Catholic and independent schools are also encouraged to participate.	Paid	Independent compliance monitoring, schools responsible for oversight. Resources provided to canteens.
Traffic light and core vs. non-core foods	Australia (Western Australia)	School	Policy applies to all food services activities within a school setting. Mandatory for government schools. Catholic schools have a similar mandatory policy.	Paid	Principals are required to develop and implement a whole school-based policy on the provision of healthy food and drinks and ensure that the school canteen/food service menu complies with the requirements of the policy.
Nutritious preschool meals	Sweden	Preschool	Legislation. Mandatory for all (whether local authority or privately run).	Free or subsidized *	Monitoring of provision and cost is not required. Monitoring of nutritional quality falls to the management (i.e., the local authority or owner).
Nutritious school meals	Sweden	School	Legislation. Mandatory for all (whether local authority or privately run).	Free	Monitoring of provision and cost is not required. Monitoring of nutritional quality falls under the School Inspectorate, but is delagated to the school management (i.e., the local authority or owner).
"Good meals in preschool", "Good school meals"	Sweden	Preschool, School	Guidelines. Voluntary for all.	Free or subsidized *	Not applicable, but for schools, compliance with several of the guidelines can be demonstrated using "School Food Sweden" tool.

* Some parents pay a capped low fee for preschool; meals are provided for all.

2. UK National Preschool and Primary Food Policy

In the UK, the provision of a nutritious meal at lunch time in schools dates back over 150 years [32]. Three national school food policies apply UK-wide, while the remainder have some regional variation. Firstly, under the Nursery Milk Scheme, all children under 5 years attending EEC in all UK regions are entitled to 189 mL/day (1/3 pint) of fresh cows' milk for free. Secondly, the Free School Fruit and Vegetable Scheme provides fruit and vegetables (3 times per week) to all state funded schools for 4–6 years old. Thirdly, Free School Meals (FSM) are provided to all children living in low income households, and since 2014, to all 4–7 year-olds in England and all 4–8 year-olds in Scotland.

2.1. UK Regional Preschool Food Policies

In Northern Ireland and Wales, state registered EEC settings must follow the nutritional standards set out for under 12 s (see schools below). England and Scotland have preschool-specific guidance, but while these link to compulsory standards in Scotland, in England they are voluntary.

In England, national voluntary guidelines based on four food groups (starchy foods, fruit and vegetables, non-dairy sources of protein, and dairy) apply [33] (see Tables 1–3, and Table S1). The guidance focuses on balancing intake across the day, suggesting, for instance, that lunch should contribute 30% of energy needs. Nutrient based standards are also provided [34]. For children aged 1–4 years attending full daycare, the food served should provide approximately 116 kcals, 45 g fat, and 155 g carbohydrates; no more than 34.2 Non Milk Extrinsic Sugar (NMES), 810 mg Sodium, and 2.1 g Salt; at least 14 g protein, 7.2 mg Iron, 5.7 mg Zinc, 330 mg Calcium, 390 µg Vit A, and 27 mg Vit C. The guidance makes some provision for foods brought from home (packed meals), including for meal composition, food safety guidance, and the consideration of common allergens.

The Scottish Standards follow the same nutritional guidance as the English model, and include the same food groups (see Tables 1 and 2, and Table S1) [35]. The standards require that the provided food is "well-balanced and healthy" (p. 7) [35], and set out required portions, where a portion is "what a young child can hold in their hand" (p. 50). The standards do not cover home provided food, although additional guidance suggests food items for healthy packed lunches [35].

2.2. UK Regional School Food Policies

The School Food Plan introduced updated food-based standards in England in January 2014. These standards stipulate that a school meal should include an adequate provision of fruit and vegetables, dairy food, low fat proteins, and low fat starchy food (see Table 1, and Table S1). Fried foods, foods high in fats and sugars, and sweetened beverages are restricted (see Table 2). The School Food Plan applies to all state-run schools, and to those state funded but independently run Academies and Free schools created since 2015. Independent schools, along with Academies and Free schools created prior to 2015, are not covered by this policy.

There are no national policies for packed lunches, although some local government and individual schools do recommend foods to include or restrict in packed lunches, such as drinks, fruit and vegetables, and sweet and savoury snacks [36].

2.3. UK Reach and Implementation of Preschool and Primary Food Policy

Policy reach, cost, and monitoring is summarized in Table 3. The majority of English children now attend an EEC setting (93% 3–4 years old in 2012) [37], but we know little about how many are covered by this policy. Given part-time attendance, we do not know how many meals are eaten in EEC. Furthermore, many of these meals may be home-provided. The use of packed meals is under-recognised in preschool children, but estimates in studies have found that between 39% and 49% of Early Years Settings use only packed lunches [38,39]. We do not know whether the guidelines are adhered to in either case.

The school population is very nearly the entire child population [40], so nearly all children eat meals at school. The most recent data on the take up of school meals in England predates the introduction of universal FSM for the youngest children. At that time, 42.6% of children in primary schools ate provided meals, although it was much higher for those eligible for FSM on the basis of household income (75.1%). The average lunch cost was £2.04, and price was predictive of take up, reducing by 1.9% for every 10p more charged for the school meal [41]. The extension of FSM has high take up in Scotland (76% of children) [42].

Both primary and preschools are monitored by the Office for Standards in Education (OFSTED). Inspections should ensure standards are met where they are statutory, but not where voluntary.

2.4. UK Impact of Policy on Diet Quality

There is limited evidence on the quality of food provision in UK EEC, and almost none on consumption [38]. Most nurseries in England are providing meals that contain too much salt and insufficient energy [43]. There is no independent evaluation of the use of the guidelines in England nor the standards in Scotland. A before and after study conducted in England suggests that the guidelines improve staff knowledge and confidence of healthy eating guidelines, and EECs self-report a greater diversity of food and a reduced use of high sugar and salt foods [44]. However, we cannot say whether children's diets have improved as a result of the policy in either region.

The evidence of the use of packed lunches in preschools is worrying, and probably undermines gains in provided meal quality. In one study of preschool packed lunches in the UK, 42% included crisps, 24% confectionary, and most provided a sugar-sweetened drink [38]. In the USA, preschool packed lunches are high in salt, and low in minerals, vegetables, fruit, and dietary fibre [45,46].

A number of evaluations of the primary school meal standards in the UK have demonstrated that lunchtime and whole day intake have improved with the introduction of a high quality school meal. The research mainly includes cross-sectional studies of food intake carried out after the introduction of standards and compared with intakes before the introduction of the standards [47–50]. These suggest that there may have been improvements in food provision, including increases in fruit and vegetables and reductions in non-permitted foods [51–53], but mixed evidence on portion size [54]. Children in schools included in Jamie Oliver's "feed me better campaign" achieved better in standard testing relative to neighbouring schools, and authorised absences (usually for illness or planned appointments) fell [55]. A pilot trial was carried out in two areas of England looking at free meals for infants, which reported better behaviour in pupils in the classroom and healthier food at lunchtime [56].

Packed lunches in primary schools are known to be of poor quality [57], and cross-sectional studies of children across England reported that diet quality over the whole day is higher for children having a school meal compared to a packed lunch [58,59]. To the extent that meal standards and FSM extension increase school meal uptake relative to packed lunches, they therefore probably improve diet.

3. Swedish Preschool and Primary Meals Provision

To our knowledge, Sweden and Finland are the only countries that currently provide free school meals to all children in all years of primary school, regardless of parental income or school form. School meals are regulated by the Education Act, which states that all children attending primary school (age 6–16 years) are entitled to free and nutritious school meals [60], and by extension preschools [61]. All children are offered a prepared warm dish, salad buffet, bread, and a drink at no cost, which should be nutritionally adequate (Table 1); soft drinks are not provided (Table 2), and desserts and fried foods are rare; there are few if any vending machines, and where tuck shops exist these are often closed during lunch. Variation exists in implementation; food can be prepared on site or in an external kitchen, from scratch or from semi-processed components, and local authority or privately run.

Although not an official policy, the concept of "the pedagogic lunch" is well-established in Sweden and Finland. Teachers eat together with the children, and ideally use this opportunity to teach about food and health [62]. Preschools serve food "family style" in communal dishes to tables of approximately 10 children.

3.1. Swedish Preschool and Primary School Meals Guidelines

The provision of free school meals has been required by law since 1997 (Table 3), although most have done so since the 1970s, and charging for meals has not been permitted since 1946. The requirement that meals be "nutritious" (Table 1) was added in 2011, but school meals are not inspected (Table 3). The National Food Agency issues non-binding national guidelines and advice [63,64]. The guidelines focus on the whole meal experience, including quality, timing, composition, and environment. Meals are considered as more than a source of nutrition; and should be tasty, nutritious, safe, pleasant, sustainable, and integrated within the preschool/school day.

In 2010, an audit-and-feedback tool was developed by researchers and stakeholders (SkolmatSverige: School Food Sweden) to assess all of the elements of the meal experience (Figure 1) [65]. The tool aims to aid the evaluation of the impact of the 2011 law, create a nationally representative database of school meal quality, and support schools to undertake their own monitoring and evaluation and thereby improve their own school meal quality. It is web-based, free to use, and requires no training. Feedback is tailored and fully automatic.

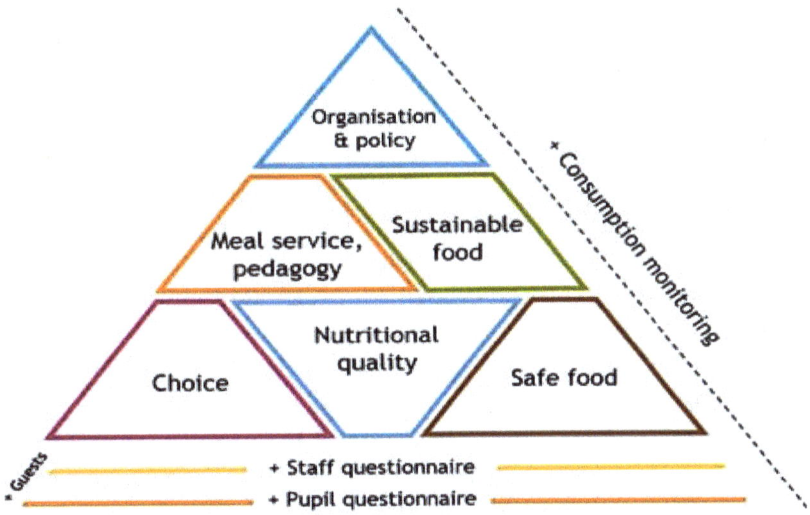

Figure 1. Components of SkolmatSverige instrument.

3.2. Sweden: Reach, Implementation and Impact of Preschool and Primary School Meals Policy

Since policy and provision in Sweden is universal, all children in preschool/school are reached. However, there is some evidence that older children may eat lunch outside of school premises or choose to skip lunch [17]. The very fact of free provision means there are no data available to record uptake (i.e., no till or reimbursement receipts), much less to track the composition of the school meals that students choose. The nature of the traditional Swedish school lunch means that many unhealthy foods (e.g., fried foods) will simply not appear, although the implementation of the newest requirements for nutritious meals is not complete. Sociable, educational interactions modelling good eating habits have been observed in the pedagogic meal, but not among all teachers [62].

The SkolmatSverige instrument is the only current source of national data. To date, 40% of primary schools use it, but the figure is increasing [66]. In a small, but nationally representative, study of schools using the tool before and after the introduction of the law requiring "nutritious" school meals, nutritional quality increased significantly, but remained low [67]. Over a 4-week period in 2014/2015, most schools provided meals that fulfilled iron and fibre requirements (86% and 96%, respectively), but less often met requirements for vitamin D and fat (51% and 41%, respectively). Most schools (71%) offered a choice of warm meals daily, and a salad buffet with at least five components (93%) [68]. Improvements in other aspects of meal quality have not been as marked [68]. These are encouraging signs, although from a self-selecting sample.

The universal nature of Sweden's school meal policy makes evaluation challenging because comparisons can only be historical. While the law may have had some effect, the new national guidelines, national concern about the issue, and related educational activities probably have a role too. Knowledge of the national guidelines for school meals is high [69], and three-quarters of local authorities have developed meal policies. The preliminary results from the first few years of data gathered by SkolmatSverige suggest that the repeated use of the tool results in improvements. As new data becomes available, it will be possible to validate this finding. The tool has also recently been expanded (November 2016) to include a module that helps schools measure uptake and the average amount of food that students actually consume, taking into account plate waste.

No national data on current preschool meal quality are available, and the instrument School Food Sweden was only developed for primary schools [66].

4. Australian Preschool and Primary School Meals

4.1. Australian Preschool Meal Policies

In Australia, EEC services are offered by government, community, and private providers, and are the responsibility of the states and territories (the Federal Government contributes funding to Indigenous preschool services). A National Quality Framework was agreed on by the Council of Australian Governments (COAG), and includes a National Law and Regulations that apply in all States and Territories [70]. National Quality Standards are a key element of the regulations, and apply to most forms of day care and EEC. The standards are overseen by the Australian Children's Education and Care Quality Authority (ACEQUA), and each State and Territory is a regulatory authority with monitoring, compliance, and quality assessment roles.

Food and drink provided in EEC must comply with the legislation, regulations, and standards within the National Quality Framework. Specifically, standard 2.2 states that "healthy eating is embedded in the program for children", and "food and drinks provided by the service are nutritious and appropriate for each child". The meaning of "nutritious and appropriate" is not further stipulated. Each State/Territory provides guidance (see Table 1) and training to support these services to adopt nutrition and healthy eating policies. For example, the Victorian government provides a Healthy Eating Advisory Service [71], the NSW government runs the Munch & Move program [72], and the ACT has a Nutrition Support Service [73]. None of the State/Territory guidelines are mandated (Table 3).

4.2. Australian Primary and Secondary School Meal Policies

In Australia, most school-aged children bring their lunch from home [74,75], but the canteen or "tuckshop" plays an integral role in educating and modelling a healthy food environment [76]. The canteen in Australian schools serves as a small shop where students can purchase lunch, snacks, and drinks, and operate anywhere from one to five days per week [77]. They are operated either by canteen managers, volunteer parents, or are outsourced to external food manufacturing and supply companies.

National voluntary guidelines (based on the Australian Dietary Guidelines [78]) have been published to guide States and Territories in developing healthy school food provision policies. From these, each State/Territory has developed a set of independent healthy canteen guidelines [79–86]. Seven States and Territories have implemented mandatory standards based on their guidelines (Tables 1 and 2).

In the majority of States/Territories, the traffic light system is used in the canteen guidelines to categorise foods into "Green", healthy foods which are encouraged (see Table 1), "Amber" (less healthy), and "Red" (least healthy) items which are discouraged (see Table 2) based on their nutritional quality. The traffic light system is relatively consistent across all States/Territories, and follows the principles outlined in the National Healthy School Canteens Traffic Light criteria (Figure 2). This system enables schools to assess their canteen menu and any other school food provision, and align food and drinks provision to these guidelines. New South Wales (NSW) has recently updated their policy in a move away from the traffic light system, to classify foods as "everyday" or "occasional". The NSW policy mandates that even "occasional" foods are required to maintain a certain degree of healthiness (based on the government-endorsed Health Star Rating system for food labelling).

All of the other States and Territories identify "red category" foods, which are either completely banned in schools or heavily restricted (see Table 2). Guidelines are generally mandatory for government schools in each State/Territory, and are highly encouraged for Independent/Catholic schools (see Table 3).

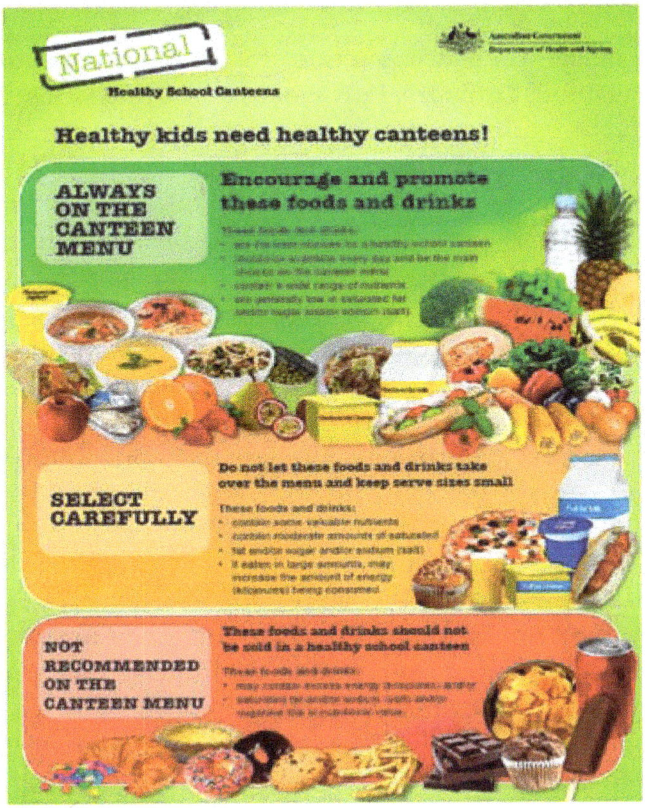
National
Healthy School Canteens
Healthy kids need healthy canteens!
ALWAYS ON THE CANTEEN MENU
Encourage and promote these foods and drinks
SELECT CAREFULLY
Do not let these foods and drinks take over the menu and keep serve sizes small
NOT RECOMMENDED ON THE CANTEEN MENU
These foods and drinks should not be sold in a healthy school canteen

Figure 2. National healthy school canteens traffic light labelling guidelines. © Commonwealth of Australia 2017.

4.3. Australian Reach, Implementation, and Impact of Preschool and School Meals Policies

The monitoring and compliance of policy guidelines in schools varies by State/Territory. In general, the policies are not actively enforced or routinely monitored by government. There is variable implementation across the different jurisdictions, and poor rates of adherence.

A cross-sectional study conducted by Woods et al. collected data in 2012 to assess whether schools were adhering to healthy canteen guidelines. The study explored the compliance of a convenience sample of government schools to healthy canteen guidelines, the proportion of "Green", "Amber", and "Red" on each menu, and the presence of discretionary items [87]. Woods et al. found low to moderate levels of adherence to state canteen guidelines, with the highest rate of compliance in Western Australia (62% of primary and secondary schools) [87]. Four studies report low to moderate rates of compliance with government healthy canteen policies [88–91]. The self-reported implementation of guidelines was demonstrated to be high in one Queensland study [92]. However, Principal and canteen manager self-reporting has been demonstrated to be in poor agreement with the gold standard of compliance assessment [93]. A recently published randomised controlled trial further found that a menu audit and feedback system made only moderate impacts on compliance, although some improvements were seen [94].

Since most school children bring lunch from home, evidence about the content of these and any spillover effect for the canteen guidelines is needed.

Similarly, there is very limited evidence about food provided or eaten in preschool settings. Since the standard is simply that food is "nutritious", monitoring compliance is not particularly meaningful. One qualitative study suggests that the guidelines are not used [95]. Furthermore, due to the highly disparate nature and uptake of EEC services in Australia, it is difficult to know how many children are using preschool provision and how many meals are eaten there.

5. Discussion

Quite different approaches to ensuring school meal quality are taken in the three countries reviewed here. Sweden has almost universal provision and uptake of school meals from preschool through primary years, and a requirement for nutritious meals, but this requirement is not strictly monitored and the guidelines issued for the meals are non-binding. In contrast, Australia largely relies on home-provided meals in the primary years supplemented by in-school canteens. National "traffic light" guidance for canteen food in primary schools exists, but implementation is at a state level and adherence is poor. Preschools in Australia have state-specific support for the provision of healthy food, but national standards simply stipulate food and drinks provided must be "nutritious and appropriate", which makes this standard too vague to be enforceable. The UK uses food-based standards in both the primary and preschool years, but these are only statutory in some contexts. Free school meal uptake is high, but where meals are paid for (including in preschools), the use of home provided meals is common, undermining the positive contribution of food standards to diet. In none of the three countries are the mechanisms for the monitoring of these food standards clearly enforced, limiting our knowledge and potentially limiting impact on diet and health. In both the UK and Australia, there is little regulation and provision for the youngest children.

In the UK, researchers have been active in using opportunistic research designs to estimate the impact of policy changes in the primary years. The introduction of food-based standards for primary school meals combined with an increased uptake following the introduction of universal free meals in the infant years appears to have had positive impacts on children's diet.

The range and breadth of additional guidance and supporting materials available are a strength of the current policy approaches [26,33,71–73]. The wealth of information supplied particularly to preschools is valued by some providers and parents [44], and has the potential to influence diet outside of school too. The ambition to integrate food into the pedagogic environment in Sweden, and to a lesser extent in the UK's preschools, is also a strength. Evidence suggests that embedding discussions about healthy eating and exposing children to healthy food choices is likely to be useful in shaping their long term eating preferences [13,96].

Two core weakness emerge, however. The first is that provided school meals are only part of the picture of food consumed during school hours. Packed lunches commonly provide alternate meals in both Australia and the UK, but additional food sources in all countries include vending machines, tuck shops, bake sales, other foods brought from home, and food provided in care before and after school. As children age, they may also be leaving school premises to purchase food from local food retailers. The nutritional advantages of high quality meal provision are undermined where few children take up this offer and/or where food from other sources is not included in healthy eating plans.

Secondly, all three countries appear to have weak mechanisms for monitoring compliance with healthy eating policies, and lack provisions for monitoring children's actual intake. This means that they are unable to comment with certainty on the extent to which schools provide food as envisaged in the policy, and are unable to assess whether policy changes have resulted in improved nutritional intake. Importantly, we also cannot comment on whether these initiatives counteract health inequalities. The voluntary self-monitoring system in Sweden could enable a comparison of school meal quality between catchment areas of differing socio-economic position in the future, but its use is not widespread enough for this to be the case yet. Where free meals are provided for the most disadvantaged (as is the case among older primary aged children in the UK), nutritionally sound meals have the potential to decrease inequalities, but policy complexity makes this difficult to assess. In England, a particular oddity of the policy evolution is that the youngest children are not included in free meal provision, so although the most disadvantaged children are preferentially provided with free preschool places, their meals are neither free nor covered by school food standards. Anecdotally, we note that some nurseries are providing free meals to the most deprived 2 years old from within their own budget, but this micro-level solution is neither testable nor scalable.

5.1. Implications for Policy

The improvement of school food through national or state nutritional guidelines or standards is ongoing in many countries [2,13,97]. We believe that these policies are likely to be important for the long-term health of our populations through their influence on dietary intake and food habits. Two systematic reviews of methods to increase fruit and vegetable intake in children [20,98] suggest the best evidence for success is for provision through schools.

The implications for school meal policies are that: (a) enforcement of policy is necessary to see improvements; (b) uptake of provided food is crucial to deliver benefits; and (c) monitoring of uptake, nutritional intake, and differential intake by social groups is needed to demonstrate whether provided school food is, in fact, a public health success. Others have reached similar conclusions [4], particularly considering the value of monitoring and evaluation for policy success [99]. Overly burdensome data collection can interfere with policy implementation [51], but light touch regulation, using existing education inspection mechanisms, that requires schools to report on their compliance with guidelines and their uptake of provided food could achieve much with little additional effort. In addition, mechanisms to provide clear accountability for compliance with standards, and strong incentives for compliance (e.g., tied to budget mechanisms, or individual Principal performance assessments) need to be explored. The Swedish self-monitoring tool is working well to encourage quality improvements, and it provides a model for efficient audit.

We also need whole-school approaches to healthy eating which are broader than school meals. This should include the consideration of meals and snacks brought from home, but also wider actions to address attitudes towards healthy foods. Banning adults (staff and visitors) from smoking or using tobacco products on the premises or at any school-related activities is a key feature of tobacco free schools [100]. Adopting similar "whole school" approaches to junk-food free schools may be appropriate.

Population-level improvements in health need population-level responses, and political and policy actions addressing the food environment are needed [101]. Reductions in the extensive marketing of unhealthy food in children's immediate environment (fast food outlets and convenience stores) [102], and increases in the relative price of unhealthy compared to healthy food are needed [103], and would support schools in their efforts.

5.2. Implications for Practice

Canteen-style provision now dominates in primary schools in all three countries, but the pedagogic model used in Sweden deserves greater attention [62]. The use of school meal times as an opportunity to talk about food and food choices may be valuable [104], but only if used by teachers [62]. Although further research is needed, we would consider this to be areas of promising practice.

Similarly, involving parents and carers in changes in school food may promote the generalisability of change [20,105]. Food policies that focus only on safety aspects and the avoidance of allergens are unlikely to engage parents as partners in improving diet. Top down policy has little effect if it is not coupled with, and sensitive to, local implementation [106].

5.3. Implications for Research

We know of few published high quality longitudinal studies or randomised controlled trials evaluating the impact of school meal policies on nutrition behaviour, diet quality, and health [107–111], although some are currently underway [112–114]. A more rigorous evaluation of the benefits of school meals on diet quality and health outcomes (such as obesity), including longitudinal studies or randomised controlled trials, are needed to assess the impact of policies, particularly on reducing inequalities in diet and health.

Much of the practice outlined in this paper has not been monitored or evaluated. While guidelines themselves are often based on extensive and expert review of nutritional needs in children, the evidence to support the implementation of such guidelines is regrettably lacking. The research needs are many in this field, but we propose the most urgent ones here: (a) the exploitation of routinely collected data to comment on the impact of policy roll-out when innovation occurs; (b) research on the implementation of nutritional and food-based guidelines; (c) research into the contribution of foods consumed during school hours to total diet across the preschool and primary years; and (d) research into the long term effects of healthy school meal provision on diet and educational achievement. Core to this would be (e) the introduction of standard measures and indicators to assess food intake [97].

6. Conclusions

There is good evidence to suggest that meals eaten in the preschool and primary years should be a target for improving children's dietary habits and preferences. In the three countries reviewed, action in the preschool years generally lags behind schools, and policies tend to lack enforceability. Policies are needed which have clear standards, systems for monitoring compliance and reach, and which acknowledge the whole school eating environment including home provided meals. While important, school food policies will have limited impact in the absence of broader public health and political action to improve our food environment.

Acknowledgments: G.S. is the recipient of an Australian Research Council Discovery Early Career Researcher Award (project number DE160100307). No other funds supported the preparation of this manuscript.

Author Contributions: P.J.L. and C.E.L.E. conceived of the paper. P.J.L. and C.E.L.E. wrote the UK sections, E.P. the Swedish and G.S. and N.B. the Australian. All authors contributed to the introduction and discussion sections. All authors reviewed and agreed on the final version.

References

1. WHO. What Is a Health Promoting School? Available online: http://www.who.int/school_youth_health/gshi/hps/en/ (accessed on 12 April 2017).
2. McKenna, M.L. Policy options to support healthy eating in schools. *Can. J. Public Health* **2010**, *101*, S14–S17. [PubMed]
3. Mikkelsen, B.E.; Engesveen, K.; Afflerbach, T.; Barnekow, V. The human rights framework, the school and healthier eating among young people: A European perspective. *Public Health Nutr.* **2016**, *19*, 15–25. [CrossRef] [PubMed]
4. Nelson, M.; Breda, J. School food research: Building the evidence base for policy. *Public Health Nutr.* **2013**, *16*, 958–967. [CrossRef] [PubMed]
5. Grant, M.J.; Booth, A. A typology of reviews: An analysis of 14 review types and associated methodologies. *Health Inf. Libr. J.* **2009**, *26*, 91–108. [CrossRef] [PubMed]
6. Public Health England. *National Diet And Nutrition Survey Results from Years 5 and 6 Combined of the Rolling Programme for 2012 and 2013 to 2013 and 2014: Report*; Public Health England: London, UK, 2016.
7. Barbieri, H.E.; Pearson, M.; Becker, W. *Riksmaten—Barn 2003. Livsmedels-och Näringsintag Bland Barn i Sverige [Food and Nutrient Intake of Children in Sweden]*; Livsmedelsverket: Uppsala, Sweden, 2006. (In Swedish)

8. Australian Bureau of Statistics. *Australian Health Survey: Nutrition First Results—Food and Nutrients, 2011–2012*; Australian Bureau of Statistics: Canberra, Australia, 2014.
9. Public Health England. *National Diet And Nutrition Survey: Results from Years 1 to 4 (Combined) of the Rolling Programme (2008/2009–2011/12): Executive Summary*; Public Health England and Food Standards Agency: London, UK, 2015.
10. Nelson, M.; Erens, B.; Bates, B.; Church, S.; Boshier, T. *Low Income Diet and Nutrition Survey*; The Stationary Office: London, UK, 2007; Volume 3.
11. Rasmussen, M.; Krolner, R.; Klepp, K.; Lytle, L.A.; Brug, J.; Bere, E.; Due, P. Determinants of fruit and vegetable consumption among children and adolescents: A review of the literature. Part I: Quantitative studies. *Int. J. Behav. Nutr. Phys. Act.* **2006**, *3*, 22. [CrossRef] [PubMed]
12. Mattisson, I. *Socioekonomiska Skillnader i Matvanor i Sverige [Socioeconomic Differences in Food Habits in Sweden]*; Livsmedelsverket: Uppsala, Sweden, 2016. (In Swedish)
13. Brambila-Macias, J.; Shankar, B.; Capacci, S.; Mazzocchi, M.; Perez-Cueto, F.J.; Verbeke, W.; Traill, W.B. Policy interventions to promote healthy eating: A review of what works, what does not, and what is promising. *Food Nutr. Bull.* **2011**, *32*, 365–375. [CrossRef] [PubMed]
14. Tilles-Tirkkonen, T.; Pentikainen, S.; Lappi, J.; Karhunen, L.; Poutanen, K.; Mykkanen, H. The quality of school lunch consumed reflects overall eating patterns in 11–16-year-old schoolchildren in Finland. *Public Health Nutr.* **2011**, *14*, 2092–2098. [CrossRef] [PubMed]
15. Raulio, S.; Roos, E.; Prattala, R. School and workplace meals promote healthy food habits. *Public Health Nutr.* **2010**, *13*, 987–992. [CrossRef] [PubMed]
16. Rogers, I.S.; Ness, A.R.; Hebditch, K.; Jones, L.R.; Emmett, P.M. Quality of food eaten in English primary schools: School dinners vs. packed lunches. *Eur. J. Clin. Nutr.* **2007**, *61*, 856–864. [CrossRef] [PubMed]
17. Persson Osowski, C.; Lindroos, A.K.; Enghardt Barbieri, H.; Becker, W. The contribution of school meals to energy and nutrient intake of swedish children in relation to dietary guidelines. *Food Nutr. Res.* **2015**, *59*, 27563. [CrossRef] [PubMed]
18. Syrad, H.; Llewellyn, C.H.; van Jaarsveld, C.H.; Johnson, L.; Jebb, S.A.; Wardle, J. Energy and nutrient intakes of young children in the UK: Findings from the gemini twin cohort. *Br. J. Nutr.* **2016**, *115*, 1843–1850. [CrossRef] [PubMed]
19. Bevans, K.B.; Sanchez, B.; Teneralli, R.; Forrest, C.B. Children's eating behavior: The importance of nutrition standards for foods in schools. *J. Sch. Health* **2011**, *81*, 424–429. [CrossRef] [PubMed]
20. De Costa, P.; Moller, P.; Frost, M.B.; Olsen, A. Changing children's eating behaviour—A review of experimental research. *Appetite* **2017**, *113*, 327–357. [CrossRef] [PubMed]
21. Ray, C.; Roos, E.; Brug, J.; Behrendt, I.; Ehrenblad, B.; Yngve, A.; te Velde, S.J. Role of free school lunch in the associations between family-environmental factors and children's fruit and vegetable intake in four European countries. *Public Health Nutr.* **2013**, *16*, 1109–1117. [CrossRef] [PubMed]
22. Williamson, D.A.; Han, H.; Johnson, W.D.; Martin, C.K.; Newton, R.L., Jr. Modification of the school cafeteria environment can impact childhood nutrition. Results from the wise mind and la health studies. *Appetite* **2013**, *61*, 77–84. [CrossRef] [PubMed]
23. Gubbels, J.S.; Gerards, S.M.; Kremers, S.P. Use of food practices by childcare staff and the association with dietary intake of children at childcare. *Nutrients* **2015**, *7*, 2161–2175. [CrossRef] [PubMed]
24. Mukoma, W.; Flisher, A.J. Evaluations of health promoting schools: A review of nine studies. *Health Promot. Int.* **2004**, *19*, 357–368. [CrossRef] [PubMed]
25. Lister-Sharp, D.; Chapman, S.; Stewart-Brown, S.; Sowden, A. Health promoting schools and health promotion in schools: Two systematic reviews. *Health Technol. Assess.* **1999**, *3*, 1–207. [PubMed]
26. Skolverket [Swedish National Agency for Education]. *Curriculum for the Preschool Lpfö 98 Revised 2010*; Skolverket: Stockholm, Sweden, 2010.
27. Department for Education. *Statutory Framework for the Early Years Foundation Stage. Setting the Standards for Learning, Development and Care for Children from Birth to Five*; Department for Education: London, UK, 2012.
28. The Organisation for Economic Co-operation and Development (OCED). *Country Statistical Profiles: Key Tables from OECD*; The Organisation for Economic Co-operation and Development (OECD): Paris, France, 2017.
29. Gov.Uk. Help Paying for Childcare. Available online: https://www.gov.uk/help-with-childcare-costs/free-childcare-and-education-for-2-to-4-year-olds (accessed on 22 April 2017).

30. Department for Education. Will I Qualify for 30 h Free Childcare? Available online: https://www.gov.uk/government/uploads/system/uploads/attachment_data/file/600592/30_h_free_childcare_eligibility.pdf (accessed on 22 April 2017).
31. Family and Childcare Trust. Help with My Childcare Costs. Available online: https://www.familyandchildcaretrust.org/help-my-childcare-costs (accessed on 10 July 2017).
32. Evans, C.E.; Harper, C.E. A history and review of school meal standards in the UK. *J. Hum. Nutr. Diet.* **2009**, *22*, 89–99. [CrossRef] [PubMed]
33. The Children's Food Trust. *Eat Better Start Better, Voluntary Food and Drink Guidelines for Early Years Settings in England—A Practical Guide*; Children's Food Trust: Sheffield, UK, 2012; p. 80.
34. Advisory Panel on Food and Nutrition in Early Years. *Laying the Table. Recommendations for National Food and Nutrition Guidance for Early Years Settings in England*; Main Report; Schools Food Trust: Sheffield, UK, 2010; Volume 1.
35. NHS Scotland. *Setting the Table. Nutritional Guidance and Food Standards for Early Years Childcare Providers in Scotland*; NHS Scotland: Edinburgh, UK, 2015.
36. Children's Food Trust. Available online: http://www.childrensfoodtrust.org.uk/childrens-food-trust/parents/your-childs-food-at-school/packed-lunches/packed-lunch-information/ (accessed on 10 July 2017).
37. Department for Education. *Provision for Children under Five Years of Age in England*; Statistical First Release; Department for Education: London, UK, 2013.
38. Nicholas, J.; Stevens, L.; Briggs, L.; Wood, L. *Pre-School Food Survey*; Children's Food Trust: Sheffield, UK, 2013.
39. Lucas, P.; Richards, H.; Johnson, L. How common are packed or sack lunches in English early education and care? (Bristol, England). Personal communication, 2017.
40. FOI Directory. Reference from Freedom of Information Directory. Available online: http://www.foi.directory/updates/foi-reveals-rising-numbers-of-pupils-home-educated/ (accessed on 10 July 2017).
41. Wollny, I.; Lord, C.; Tanner, E.; Fry, A.; Tipping, S.; Kitchen, S. *School Lunch Take-Up Survey 2013 to 2014 Research Report*; Department for Education: London, UK, 2015.
42. Chambers, S.; Ford, A.; Boydell, N.; Moore, L.; Stead, M.; Eadie, D. Universal free school meals in Scotland: A process evaluation of implementation and uptake. *Eur. J. Public Health* **2016**, *26*, ckw169. [CrossRef]
43. Parker, M.; Lloyd-Williams, F.; Weston, G.; Macklin, J.; McFadden, K. Nursery nutrition in liverpool: An exploration of practice and nutritional analysis of food provided. *Public Health Nutr.* **2011**, *14*, 1867–1875. [CrossRef] [PubMed]
44. Mucavele, P.; Sharp, L.; Wall, C.; Nicholas, J. Children's food trust 'eat better, start better' programme: Outcomes and recommendations. *Perspect. Public Health* **2014**, *134*, 67–69. [PubMed]
45. Sweitzer, S.J.; Briley, M.E.; Robert-Gray, C. Do sack lunches provided by parents meet the nutritional needs of young children who attend child care? *J. Am. Diet. Assoc.* **2009**, *109*, 141–144. [CrossRef] [PubMed]
46. Romo-Palafox, M.J.; Ranjit, N.; Sweitzer, S.J.; Roberts-Gray, C.; Hoelscher, D.M.; Byrd-Williams, C.E.; Briley, M.E. Dietary quality of preschoolers' sack lunches as measured by the healthy eating index. *J. Acad. Nutr. Diet.* **2015**, *115*, 1779–1788. [CrossRef] [PubMed]
47. Spence, S.; Delve, J.; Stamp, E.; Matthews, J.N.; White, M.; Adamson, A.J. Did school food and nutrient-based standards in England impact on 11–12Y olds nutrient intake at lunchtime and in total diet? Repeat cross-sectional study. *PLoS ONE* **2014**, *9*, e112648. [CrossRef] [PubMed]
48. Spence, S.; Delve, J.; Stamp, E.; Matthews, J.N.; White, M.; Adamson, A.J. The impact of food and nutrient-based standards on primary school children's lunch and total dietary intake: A natural experimental evaluation of government policy in England. *PLoS ONE* **2013**, *8*, e78298. [CrossRef] [PubMed]
49. Golley, R.; Pearce, J.; Nelson, M. Children's lunchtime food choices following the introduction of food-based standards for school meals: Observations from six primary schools in sheffield. *Public Health Nutr.* **2011**, *14*, 271–278. [CrossRef] [PubMed]
50. Adamson, A.; Spence, S.; Reed, L.; Conway, R.; Palmer, A.; Stewart, E.; McBratney, J.; Carter, L.; Beattie, S.; Nelson, M. School food standards in the UK: Implementation and evaluation. *Public Health Nutr.* **2013**, *16*, 968–981. [CrossRef] [PubMed]
51. Moore, L.; Tapper, K. The impact of school fruit tuck shops and school food policies on children's fruit consumption: A cluster randomised trial of schools in deprived areas. *J. Epidemiol. Commun. Health* **2008**, *62*, 926–931. [CrossRef] [PubMed]

52. Haroun, D.; Harper, C.; Wood, L.; Nelson, M. The impact of the food-based and nutrient-based standards on lunchtime food and drink provision and consumption in primary schools in England. *Public Health Nutr.* **2011**, *14*, 209–218. [CrossRef] [PubMed]
53. Nicholas, J.; Wood, L.; Harper, C.; Nelson, M. The impact of the food-based and nutrient-based standards on lunchtime food and drink provision and consumption in secondary schools in England. *Public Health Nutr.* **2013**, *16*, 1052–1065. [CrossRef] [PubMed]
54. Pearce, J.; Wood, L.; Stevens, L. Portion weights of food served in english schools: Have they changed following the introduction of nutrient-based standards? *J. Hum. Nutr. Diet.* **2013**, *26*, 553–562. [CrossRef] [PubMed]
55. Belot, M.; James, J. Healthy school meals and educational outcomes. *J. Health Econom.* **2011**, *30*, 489–504. [CrossRef] [PubMed]
56. Department for Education. Available online: www.gov.uk/government/publications/evaluation-of-the-free-school-meals-pilot-impact-report (accessed on 10 July 2017).
57. Evans, C.E.; Greenwood, D.C.; Thomas, J.D.; Cade, J.E. A cross-sectional survey of children's packed lunches in the UK: Food- and nutrient-based results. *J. Epidemiol. Commun. Health* **2010**, *64*, 977–983. [CrossRef] [PubMed]
58. Evans, C.E.; Mandl, V.; Christian, M.S.; Cade, J.E. Impact of school lunch type on nutritional quality of english children's diets. *Public Health Nutr.* **2016**, *19*, 36–45. [CrossRef] [PubMed]
59. Harrison, F.; Jennings, A.; Jones, A.; Welch, A.; van Sluijs, E.; Griffin, S.; Cassidy, A. Food and drink consumption at school lunchtime: The impact of lunch type and contribution to overall intake in british 9–10-year-old children. *Public Health Nutr.* **2013**, *16*, 1132–1139. [CrossRef] [PubMed]
60. Sveriges Riksdag [The Swedish Parliament]. *Den nya Skollagen—för Kunskap, Valfrihet och Trygghet [The New School Law—For Knowledge, Choice and Security]*; Sveriges Riksdag, Ed.; Sveriges Riksdag: Stockholm, Sweden, 2010. (In Swedish)
61. Skolverket [Swedish National Agency for Education]. *Måluppfyllelse i förskolan [Goal Achievement in Preschool]*; Skolverket: Stockholm, Sweden, 2017. (In Swedish)
62. Persson Osowski, C.; Goranzon, H.; Fjellstrom, C. Teachers' interaction with children in the school meal situation: The example of pedagogic meals in Sweden. *J. Nutr. Educ. Behav.* **2013**, *45*, 420–427. [CrossRef] [PubMed]
63. Swedish National Food Agency. *Good School Meals*; Livsmedelsverket: Uppsala, Sweden, 2014.
64. Livsmedelsverket [Swedish National Food Agency]. *Bra måltider i Förskolan [Good Meals in Preschool]*; Livsmedelsverket: Uppsala, Sweden, 2016. (In Swedish)
65. Patterson, E.; Quetel, A.-K.; Lilja, K.; Simma, M.; Olsson, L.; Schäfer Elinder, L. Design, testing and validation of an innovative web-based instrument to evaluate school meal quality. *Public Health Nutr.* **2013**, *16*, 1028–1036. [CrossRef] [PubMed]
66. SkolmatSverige. What Is Skolmatsverige? Available online: www.skolmatsverige.se/in-english (accessed on 22 June 2017).
67. Patterson, E.; Elinder, L.S. Improvements in school meal quality in Sweden after the introduction of new legislation-a 2-year follow-up. *Eur. J. Public Health* **2015**, *25*, 655–660. [CrossRef] [PubMed]
68. Patterson, E.; Regnander, M.; Elinder, L.S. *SkolmatSveriges Kartläggning av Skolmåltidens Kvalitet—Läsåret 2014/15 [School Food Sweden's Survey of School Meal Quality—For the School Year 2014/15]*; Centrum för Epidemiologi och Samhällsmedicin, Stockholms Läns Landsting: Stockholm, Sweden, 2015. (In Swedish)
69. Skolmatens Vänner; Livsmedelsverket. Kartläggning av Sveriges Kommuner Gällande Skolmaten i Grundskolan [Survey of Sweden's Municpalities Concerning School Food in Primary School]. Available online: https://www.livsmedelsverket.se/globalassets/rapporter/2016/rapport-2016---maltidsverksamheten-i-kommunala-grundskolor.pdf (accessed on 10 July 2017).
70. Australian Children's Education and Care Quality Authority (ACEQUA). The National Quality Framework. Available online: http://www.acecqa.gov.au/national-quality-framework (accessed on 10 July 2017).
71. Nutrition Australia Victoria Division. Healthy Eating Advisory Service. Available online: http://heas.health.vic.gov.au/ (accessed on 10 July 2017).
72. New South Wales Office of Preventative Health. The Munch & Move Program. Available online: http://www.preventivehealth.net.au/munch--move.html (accessed on 10 July 2017).

73. Nutrition Australia ACT Division. Act Nutrition Support Service. Available online: http://www.actnss.org/ (accessed on 10 July 2017).
74. Bell, A.C.; Swinburn, B.A. What are the key food groups to target for preventing obesity and improving nutrition in schools? *Eur. J. Clin. Nutr.* **2004**, *58*, 258–263. [CrossRef] [PubMed]
75. Sanigorski, A.M.; Bell, A.C.; Kremer, P.J.; Swinburn, B.A. Lunchbox contents of Australian school children: Room for improvement. *Eur. J. Clin. Nutr.* **2005**, *59*, 1310–1316. [CrossRef] [PubMed]
76. Department of Health. Role of the School Canteen in Contributing to a Health Promoting School. Available online: http://health.gov.au/internet/publications/publishing.nsf/Content/canteen-mgr-tr1~role-school-canteen (accessed on 10 July 2017).
77. Lawlis, T.; Knox, M.; Jamieson, M. School canteens: A systematic review of the policy, perceptions and use from an Australian perspective. *Nutr. Diet.* **2016**, *73*, 389–398. [CrossRef]
78. NHMRC. *Australian Dietary Guidelines*; NHMRC: Canberra, Australia, 2013.
79. NSW School Canteen Advisory Committee. *Fresh Tastes @ School: NSW Healthy School Canteen Strategy*; NSW School Canteen Advisory Committee: Sydney, Australia, 2006.
80. Department of Education. *Healthy Food And Drink Policy*; Department of Education: Perth, Australia, 2014.
81. Department of Education. *Smart Choices: Healthy Food and Drink Supply Strategy for Queensland Schools*; Department of Education: Brisbane, Australia, 2016.
82. Victorian Government. *Healthy Canteen Kit: School Canteens and Other School Food Services Policy*; Victorian Government: Melbourne, Australia, 2012.
83. Department of Education. *Canteen, Nutrition and Healthy Eating*; Department of Education: Darwin, Australia, 2013.
84. Tasmanian School Canteen Association Inc. *School Canteen Handbook: A Whole School Approach to Healthy Eating*; Tasmanian School Canteen Association Inc.: Hobart, Australia, 2014.
85. Department of Health. *National Healthy School Canteens: Guidelines for Healthy Foods and Drinks Supplied in School Canteens*; Department of Health: Canberra, Australia, 2014.
86. Department for Education and Child Development. *Right Bite, Easy Guide to Healthy Food and Drink Supply for South Australian Schools and Preschools*; Department for Education and Child Development: Adelaide, Australia, 2008.
87. Woods, J.; Bressan, A.; Langelaan, C.; Mallon, A.; Palermo, C. Australian school canteens: Menu guideline adherence or avoidance? *Health Promot. J. Aust.* **2014**, *25*, 110–115. [CrossRef] [PubMed]
88. Ardzejewska, K.; Tadros, R.; Baxter, D. A descriptive study on the barriers and facilitators to implementation of the NSW (Australia) healthy school canteen strategy. *Health Educ. J.* **2012**, *72*, 136–145. [CrossRef]
89. De Silva-Sanigorski, A.; Breheny, T.; Jones, L.; Lacy, K.; Kremer, P.; Carpenter, L.; Bolton, K.; Prosser, L.; Gibbs, L.; Waters, E.; et al. Government food service policies and guidelines do not create healthy school canteens. *Aust. N. Z. J. Public Health* **2011**, *35*, 117–121. [CrossRef] [PubMed]
90. Pettigrew, S.; Donovan, R.J.; Jalleh, G.; Pescud, M. Predictors of positive outcomes of a school food provision policy in Australia. *Health Promot. Int.* **2014**, *29*, 317–327. [CrossRef] [PubMed]
91. Hills, A.; Nathan, N.; Robinson, K.; Fox, D.; Wollfenden, L. Improvement in primary school adherence to the NSW healthy school canteen strategy in 2007 and 2010. *Health Promot. J. Aust.* **2015**, *26*, 89–92. [CrossRef] [PubMed]
92. Dick, M.; Lee, A.; Bright, M.; Turner, K.; Edwards, R.; Dawson, J.; Miller, J. Evaluation of implementation of a healthy food and drink supply strategy throughout the whole school environment in queensland state schools, Australia. *Eur. J. Clin. Nutr.* **2012**, *66*, 1124–1129. [CrossRef] [PubMed]
93. Reilly, K.; Nathan, N.; Wolfenden, L.; Wiggers, J.; Sutherland, R.; Wyse, R.; Yoong, S.L. Validity of four measures in assessing school canteen menu compliance with state-based healthy canteen policy. *Health Promot. J. Aust.* **2016**, *27*, 215–221. [CrossRef] [PubMed]
94. Yoong, S.L.; Nathan, N.; Wolfenden, L.; Wiggers, J.; Reilly, K.; Oldmeadow, C.; Wyse, R.; Sutherland, R.; Delaney, T.; Butler, P.; et al. Cafe: A multicomponent audit and feedback intervention to improve implementation of healthy food policy in primary school canteens: A randomised controlled trial. *Int. J. Behav. Nutr. Phys. Act.* **2016**, *13*, 126. [CrossRef] [PubMed]

95. Cole, A.; Vidgen, H.; Cleland, P. Food provision in early childhood education and care services: Exploring how staff determine nutritional adequacy. *Nutr. Diet.* **2017**, *74*, 105–110. [CrossRef]
96. Council on School Health; Committee on Nutrition. Snacks, sweetened beverages, added sugars, and schools. *Pediatrics* **2015**, *135*, 575–583.
97. Perez-Cueto, F.J.; Aschemann-Witzel, J.; Shankar, B.; Brambila-Macias, J.; Bech-Larsen, T.; Mazzocchi, M.; Capacci, S.; Saba, A.; Turrini, A.; Niedzwiedzka, B.; et al. Assessment of evaluations made to healthy eating policies in Europe: A review within the eatwell project. *Public Health Nutr.* **2012**, *15*, 1489–1496. [CrossRef] [PubMed]
98. Ganann, R.; Fitzpatrick-Lewis, D.; Ciliska, D.; Peirson, L.J.; Warren, R.L.; Fieldhouse, P.; Delgado-Noguera, M.F.; Tort, S.; Hams, S.P.; Martinez-Zapata, M.J.; et al. Enhancing nutritional environments through access to fruit and vegetables in schools and homes among children and youth: A systematic review. *BMC Res. Notes* **2014**, *7*, 422. [CrossRef] [PubMed]
99. Treasury, H. *The Magenta Book. Guidance for Evaluation*; HM Treasury: London, UK, 2011.
100. Campaign for Tobacco Free Kids. How Schools Can Help Students Stay Tobacco-Free. Available online: http://www.tobaccofreekids.org/research/factsheets/pdf/0153.pdf (accessed on 27 June 2017).
101. Oliver, T.R. The politics of public health policy. *Annu. Rev. Public Health* **2006**, *27*, 195–233. [CrossRef] [PubMed]
102. Centre for Disease Control. Zoning to Encourage Healthy Eating. Available online: https://www.cdc.gov/phlp/winnable/zoning_obesity.html (accessed on 27 June 2017).
103. Parliamentary Office for Science and Technology (POST). *Barriers to Healthy Food*; Parliamentary Office for Science and Technology: London, UK, 2016.
104. Dudley, D.A.; Cotton, W.G.; Peralta, L.R. Teaching approaches and strategies that promote healthy eating in primary school children: A systematic review and meta-analysis. *Int. J. Behav. Nutr. Phys. Act.* **2015**, *12*, 28. [CrossRef] [PubMed]
105. Sansolios, S.; Mikkelsen, B.E. Views of parents, teachers and children on health promotion in kindergarten—First results from formative focus groups and observations. *J. Paediatr. Obes.* **2011**, *6*, 28–32. [CrossRef] [PubMed]
106. Moore, S.; Murphy, S.; Tapper, K.; Moore, L. From policy to plate: Barriers to implementing healthy eating policies in primary schools in Wales. *Health Policy* **2010**, *94*, 239–245. [CrossRef] [PubMed]
107. Evans, C.E.; Greenwood, D.C.; Thomas, J.D.; Cleghorn, C.L.; Kitchen, M.S.; Cade, J.E. Smart lunch box intervention to improve the food and nutrient content of children's packed lunches: UK wide cluster randomised controlled trial. *J. Epidemiol. Commun. Health* **2010**, *64*, 970–976. [CrossRef] [PubMed]
108. Sweitzer, S.J.; Briley, M.E.; Roberts-Gray, C.; Hoelscher, D.M.; Staskel, D.M.; Almansour, F.D. How to help parents pack better preschool sack lunches: Advice from parents for educators. *J. Nutr. Educ. Behav.* **2011**, *43*, 194–198. [CrossRef] [PubMed]
109. Sweitzer, S.J.; Ranjit, N.; Calloway, E.E.; Hoelscher, D.M.; Almansor, F.; Briley, M.E.; Roberts-Gray, C.R. Examining how adding a booster to a behavioral nutrition intervention prompts parents to pack more vegetables and whole gains in their preschool children's sack lunches. *Behav. Med.* **2016**, *42*, 9–17. [CrossRef] [PubMed]
110. Williams, P.A.; Cates, S.C.; Blitstein, J.L.; Hersey, J.; Gabor, V.; Ball, M.; Kosa, K.; Wilson, H.; Olson, S.; Singh, A. Nutrition-education program improves preschoolers' at-home diet: A group randomized trial. *J. Acad. Nutr. Diet.* **2014**, *114*, 1001–1008. [CrossRef] [PubMed]
111. Hutchinson, J.; Christian, M.S.; Evans, C.E.; Nykjaer, C.; Hancock, N.; Cade, J.E. Evaluation of the impact of school gardening interventions on children's knowledge of and attitudes towards fruit and vegetables. A cluster randomised controlled trial. *Appetite* **2015**, *91*, 405–414. [CrossRef] [PubMed]
112. De Silva-Sanigorski, A.; Prosser, L.; Carpenter, L.; Honisett, S.; Gibbs, L.; Moodie, M.; Sheppard, L.; Swinburn, B.; Waters, E. Evaluation of the childhood obesity prevention program Kids—'Go for your life'. *BMC Public Health* **2010**, *10*, 288. [CrossRef] [PubMed]

113. Williams, C.M.; Nathan, N.; Delaney, T.; Yoong, S.L.; Wiggers, J.; Preece, S.; Lubans, N.; Sutherland, R.; Pinfold, J.; Smith, K.; et al. Cafe: A multicomponent audit and feedback intervention to improve implementation of healthy food policy in primary school canteens: Protocol of a randomised controlled trial. *BMJ Open* **2015**, *5*, e006969. [CrossRef] [PubMed]
114. Waling, M.; Olafsdottir, A.S.; Lagstrom, H.; Wergedahl, H.; Jonsson, B.; Olsson, C.; Fossgard, E.; Holthe, A.; Talvia, S.; Gunnarsdottir, I.; et al. School meal provision, health, and cognitive function in a nordic setting—The promeal-study: Description of methodology and the nordic context. *Food Nutr. Res.* **2016**, *60*, 30468. [CrossRef] [PubMed]

9

Dietary Patterns in Primary School are of Prospective Relevance for the Development of Body Composition in Two German Pediatric Populations

Maike Wolters [1,†,*], Gesa Joslowski [2,†], Sandra Plachta-Danielzik [3], Marie Standl [4], Manfred J. Müller [3], Wolfgang Ahrens [1] and Anette E. Buyken [2,5]

1 Leibniz Institute for Prevention Research and Epidemiology—BIPS, Department: Epidemiological Methods and Etiologic Research, Achterstr. 30, 28359 Bremen, Germany; ahrens@leibniz-bips.de

2 IEL—Nutritional Epidemiology, University of Bonn, DONALD Study, Heinstück 11, 44225 Dortmund, Germany; gesa.joslowski@gmx.de (G.J.); anette.buyken@uni-paderborn.de (A.E.B.)

3 Institute of Human Nutrition and Food Science, Christian-Albrechts University, 24118 Kiel, Germany; s.plachta-danielzik@kompetenznetz-ced.de (S.P.-D.); mmueller@nutrfoodsc.uni-kiel.de (M.J.M.)

4 Institute of Epidemiology I, Helmholtz Zentrum München—German Research Center for Environmental Health, D-85764 Neuherberg, Germany; marie.standl@helmholtz-muenchen.de

5 Institute of Nutrition, Consumption and Health, Faculty of Natural Science, University Paderborn, 33098 Paderborn, Germany

* Correspondence: wolters@leibniz-bips.de

† These authors contributed equally to this work.

Abstract: This study performed comparative analyses in two pediatric cohorts to identify dietary patterns during primary school years and examined their relevance to body composition development. Nutritional and anthropometric data at the beginning of primary school and two or four years later were available from 298 and 372 participants of IDEFICS-Germany (Identification and prevention of Dietary-induced and lifestyle-induced health Effects In Children and infants Study) and the KOPS (Kiel Obesity Prevention Study) cohort, respectively. Principal component analyses (PCA) and reduced rank regression (RRR) were used to identify dietary patterns at baseline and patterns of change in food group intake during primary school years. RRR extracted patterns explaining variations in changes in body mass index (BMI), fat mass index (FMI), and waist-to-height-ratio (WtHR). Associations between pattern adherence and excess gain in BMI, FMI, or WtHR (>75th percentile) during primary school years were examined using logistic regression. Among PCA patterns, only a change towards a more Mediterranean food choice during primary school years were associated with a favorable body composition development in IDEFICS-Germany ($p < 0.05$). In KOPS, RRR patterns characterized by a frequent consumption of fast foods or starchy carbohydrate foods were consistently associated with an excess gain in BMI and WtHR (all $p < 0.005$). In IDEFICS-Germany, excess gain in BMI, FMI, and WtHR were predicted by a frequent consumption of nuts, meat, and pizza at baseline and a decrease in the consumption frequency of protein sources and snack carbohydrates during primary school years (all $p < 0.01$). The study confirms an adverse impact of fast food consumption on body composition during primary school years. Combinations of protein and carbohydrate sources deserve further investigation.

Keywords: body composition; primary school; dietary pattern; principal component analysis; reduced rank regression; prevention

1. Introduction

Most Western societies report the highest prevalence of overweight/obesity among children and adolescents at the end of primary school [1,2]. Thus, primary school years are now regarded as a further window of opportunity when interventions targeting development or the reversal of becoming overweight or obese are particularly warranted [3–8].

Upon entry into primary school, many aspects of a child's daily routine change, which may all contribute to the lower remission of overweight during primary school years as compared to pre-school years. Importantly, nutritional behavior may change substantially and these changes may best be captured by dietary pattern analysis, which allows insights into the joint relevance of multiple dietary components for overweight development. Yet, to date, few studies examined the prospective relevance of dietary patterns for the development of body composition [9–15] and most of these were performed among adolescents [10,11,13]. In addition, such analyses should often consider BMI only [10–12], which is, however, only a proxy measure of adiposity. Consideration of more adiposity-specific measures such as fat mass or waist circumference is, therefore, warranted [16–19].

Additionally, patterns of dietary change during primary school years may be of relevance for an unfavorable development of body composition during this period. In a previous analysis, we observed that both the selection of unfavorable carbohydrate sources (more white bread, less pulses, and whole grain bread) at the beginning of primary school and an increased consumption of processed savory food during primary school years were related to adverse changes in BMI and fat mass during primary school years in a sample of German school children participating in the DONALD Study (Dortmund Nutritional and Longitudinally Designed Study) [9]. These patterns were identified by using reduced rank regression (RRR) to identify dietary patterns best explaining variation in changes of body composition during primary school years. Ideally, these dietary patterns should be applied to another cohort so as to confirm their relevance for German pediatric populations in general. In practice, this is, however, not possible because of different dietary assessment methods used in different studies (e.g., German pediatric cohort studies often assess consumption frequency only, i.e., use food propensity questionnaires [20]). Comparative analysis based on a different dietary assessment method but using a similar analytic approach is, therefore, a feasible alternative approach. Similar dietary patterns identified with this analytical approach would be highly informative for the formulation of preventive and interventional strategies targeted at primary school age children.

Therefore, the aims of the present study were to identify and describe dietary patterns at the beginning of the primary school period as well as patterns of dietary changes during the course of primary school in two German pediatric cohort studies known as the Kiel Obesity Prevention Study (KOPS) and the Identification and prevention of Dietary-induced and lifestyle-induced health Effects In Children and infants (IDEFICS)-Germany cohort. In a further step, we illustrated the impact of adherence to the identified dietary patterns on excess gain in the body mass index (BMI), fat mass index (FMI), or waist-to-height ratio (WtHR) (increases >75th percentile) during primary school years.

2. Methods

2.1. Study Populations

The study designs of the KOPS and the IDEFICS-Germany study were described previously [16,21,22]. KOPS is a cohort study to investigate determinants and preventive measures of childhood obesity. It was performed between 1996 and 2001 in the context of a school entry health examination [23,24]. A representative group of 4997 children participated in the study [24,25]. At the end of the primary school period (fourth grade), follow-up information was collected from 1764 children (35% of the original population) during examinations performed in the school setting between 2000 and 2005 [23,24]. For the present analyses, complete information on dietary habits at baseline (age 5 to 7 years) and follow-up (age 9 to 11 years) was available for 415 children. Of these, 372 had complete anthropometric data at both time points as well as information on potential confounding factors.

The IDEFICS-Germany study is a multicenter study designed to investigate and prevent diet-related and lifestyle-related disorders among European children (aged 2–9.9 years at baseline). The present analysis is based on data of the German subsample. In 2007/2008, 2066 children were recruited from kindergartens and schools in Germany. Anthropometric measurements were performed at baseline and at the two-year follow-up and dietary and lifestyle questionnaires were administered. A total of 993 children had complete dietary data at baseline and follow-up. Of these, 312 children provided dietary data at the beginning of primary school (i.e., age 5 to 7 years) and at least two years later. Complete anthropometric measurements at baseline and follow-up and data on potential covariates were available for 298 children included in the analyses.

This study was conducted according to the guidelines laid down in the Declaration of Helsinki and all procedures involving human subjects were approved by the local ethics committee in Kiel and the ethics review board of the University of Bremen written informed consent was obtained from the parents or legal caregivers of all children.

2.2. Nutritional Assessment

In KOPS, dietary intake was assessed using a 24 item food propensity questionnaire (FPQ) based on the WHO MONICA FFQ (food frequency questionnaire) adapted to children [26] (see Table S1). It was completed by the parents or primary caregiver who provided dietary information over the last six months. The FPQ—i.e., an FFQ inquiring consumption frequencies but not the amounts consumed was validated against a seven day diet record in 24 and 61 5–7 and 9–11 year old children, respectively [27]. Consumption frequencies were asked from mutually exclusive alternatives: never or less than once a week, 1 to 2 times per week, and 3 to 6 times per week or daily.

The Children's Eating Habits Questionnaire (CEHQ) was used to assess dietary intake in the IDEFICS-Germany study [28]. This reproducible and validated instrument [28–30] inquiring the consumption frequency of 43 foods and beverages (see Table S2) was completed by parents or other caregivers. Frequencies of consumption during the past month were asked from mutually exclusive alternatives: never or less than once a week, 1 to 3 times per week, 4 to 6 times per week, once per day, twice per day, and three or more times per day.

2.3. Anthropometric Measurements and Calculations

Anthropometric measurements in KOPS were performed by trained nutritionists and physicians [25]. Weight and height were measured to the nearest of 0.1 kg and 0.5 cm with a calibrated electronic scale and a stadiometer (Seca, Hamburg, Germany). Waist circumference was measured midway between the lowest rib and the top of the iliac crest at the end of gentle expiration with an inelastic tape. A bioelectrical impedance analysis (BIA) was performed by using a terapolar bio-impedance analyzer (BIA 2000-C, Data Input, Frankfurt/M, Germany) and fat mass was calculated with an algorithm developed in Kiel using air-displacement plethysmography as the reference method [16,31].

In IDEFICS-Germany, anthropometric measurements included weight, height, BIA, and waist circumference. Children were barefoot and wore only underwear and a T-shirt. Weight measurements to the nearest 0.1 kg and BIA were carried out using an electronic scale (Tanita BC 420 SMA, Tanita Europe GmbH, Sindelfingen, Germany). Height was measured using a telescopic height measuring instrument (Seca 225 stadiometer, Hamburg, Germany) to the nearest 0.1 cm. Fat mass was calculated with an algorithm derived from BIA [32]. Waist circumference was measured using an inelastic Seca 200 tape (Seca, Hamburg, Germany) according to World Health Organization Standards [33].

For both study samples, BMI was calculated from measured height and weight (weight (kg)/height^2 (m^2)). FMI and FFMI were calculated relating fat mass and fat free mass (weight—fat mass) to height^2 (m^2). For WtHR (waist circumference(m)/height(cm), a simple practical non-invasive tool reflecting visceral fat of a value >0.5 was considered to indicate excessive upper body fat accumulation [34]. Since absolute measures are considered a better alternative than *z*-scores when assessing adiposity changes [35], the response variables were the changes in BMI, FMI, and WtHR between the end and the beginning of the primary school period. Being overweight was defined according to the International Obesity Task Force criteria [36].

2.4. Statistical Methods

To facilitate comparison to the findings from the DONALD study, the statistical approach in the present analysis was analogous to that in Diethelm et al. [9]. Dietary patterns at the beginning of the primary school period and patterns of changes during primary school years were derived by two different empirical methods: PCA and RRR. Intake frequencies were standardized by using z-scores (by age group and sex (mean = 0, SD = 1)). Due to the extracted dietary patterns being similar for boys and girls in both cohorts, the data were pooled for the analyses.

2.4.1. PCA

PCA analyses were conducted by using the PROC FACTOR procedure in SAS. The first PCA was conducted to identify dietary patterns at the beginning of the primary school period (PCA baseline pattern) while the second PCA identified patterns of dietary changes between the end and the beginning of the primary school period (PCA change pattern). For this purpose, changes in the intake frequencies of food groups were obtained (standardized intake frequencies at the end of the primary school period minus standardized intake frequencies at the beginning of the primary school period).

To select the baseline and change patterns to be retained in analyses, the following criteria were used: (1) eigenvalues exceeding 1 (based on the rationale that each component should explain more variance than a single variable in the data set), (2) the scree plot (a graphical presentation of the eigenvalues where a break indicates how many factors should be retained), and (3) factor interpretability [37,38]. Two baseline patterns and three change patterns were retained for further analyses. After a varimax rotation, food groups with factor loadings $\geq |0.4|$ were considered as contributing to a pattern. For each pattern, more than three food groups were retained, which is considered an adequate number for good interpretability [38]. According to the approach of simplified pattern variables, the individual PCA factor scores (resembling adherence to the respective pattern) were based solely on the sum of the unweighted standardized frequencies of food groups that were loaded high (i.e., $\geq |0.4|$) at the respective pattern [39].

2.4.2. RRR

RRR analyses were used as a second approach. RRR is commonly applied to a set of intermediary response variables presumed to link diet to the health outcome [40]. Since current scientific evidence does not substantiate strong associations between specific nutrients and body composition development, RRR was used to directly extract dietary patterns best explaining the variation of changes in BMI, FMI, and WtHR during the primary school period; i.e., the method was used in a purely exploratory way.

RRR analyses were conducted via the PROC PLS procedure in SAS (option method = RRR) [40]. The RRR extracts linear combinations (i.e., RRR patterns) of predictor variables that explain as much variation in response variables as possible. For the first RRR, standardized intake frequencies of food groups at the beginning of the primary school period were used as predictor variables. The response variables were the changes in BMI, FMI, and WtHR between the end and the beginning of the primary school period in which each was adjusted for baseline BMI, FMI, and WtHR at the beginning of the primary school period, respectively, by applying the residual method [41] (RRR baseline factors). For the second RRR, changes in standardized intake frequencies of food groups between the end and the beginning of the primary school period were used as predictor variables. Changes in BMI, FMI, and WtHR between the end and the beginning of the primary school period adjusted for the baseline body composition were, again, the response variables (RRR change factors).

The number of factors extracted by RRR from the predictor variables is always equal to the number of response variables, i.e., three factors were identified by each RRR. However, only those patterns explaining the largest amount of response variation (as indicated by a break) were retained for further analyses. As for PCA, the individual RRR factor scores were calculated, according to the simplified pattern approach [39] including all food groups with a factor loading $\geq |0.2|$.

2.4.3. Logistic Regression Analyses

The PCA and RRR factors were used as independent predictors in the logistic regression models (PROC LOGISTIC) by estimating odds ratios (ORs) with 95% confidence intervals (95% CIs) of excess gain in BMI, FMI, or WtHR during primary school years with the lower three quartiles of increases in BMI, FMI, or WtHR serving as the reference category.

By definition, RRR patterns will be predictive of changes in BMI, FMI, and WtHR during primary school years, i.e., the response variables for which they were derived. Thus, our main interest was to (i) illustrate the effect sizes of the predicted OR and (ii) to investigate whether the obtained pattern would still be predictive after adjustment for potentially confounding factors [9]. Adjusted OR for excess gain in BMI, FMI, and WtHR are categorized by tertiles of RRR or PCA factors scores of adherence. The *p*-values for a linear trend refer to logistic regression models with continuous pattern scores of adherence as the independent variable. Potentially confounding variables were initially examined separately and included in the fully adjusted model only if they modified regression coefficients of the pattern scores in the unadjusted models by $\geq$10%. To ensure comparability between the models, we included all variables that met this criterion in any of the models investigating the relationship between a dietary pattern (baseline or change patterns) and the outcomes (excess gain in BMI, FMI, or WtHR).

The following covariates inquired from the parents by self-administered questionnaires were considered as potentially confounding factors: child's birth weight, breast feeding practice, smoking during pregnancy, parental education, parental weight and height, income, the child's physical activity, and the migration background (IDEFICS only).

Differences between baseline and follow-up were tested using the Wilcoxon rank sum test for continuous variables and the Chi-square test for categorical variables. SAS procedures (SAS, version 9.2, SAS Institute Inc., Cary, NC, USA) were used for data analysis. A *p*-value <0.05 was considered statistically significant.

3. Results

The characteristics of both study samples are given in Table 1. The anthropometric characteristics of the participants stratified by the beginning and the end of primary school years are summarized in Table 2. In the KOPS sample, waist circumference, BMI, and FFMI increased during primary school years while WtHR decreased and FMI did not change. Similarly, waist circumference, BMI, FMI, and FFMI increased during primary school years in the IDEFICS-Germany sample while WtHR decreased.

3.1. Dietary Patterns

For the KOPS sample, the dietary pattern obtained by PCA and RRR are presented in Table 3. The PCA baseline pattern 1 is characterized by a frequent consumption of 'fast food' (fish fingers, curry-sausage, or lasagna) while food groups characterizing PCA baseline pattern 2 could be summarized as 'healthy' (wholegrain, vegetables, and fruits). The PCA change pattern 1 reflects an increase in the consumption frequency of fast foods while the PCA change patterns 2 and 3 reflect changes in diet towards a healthier and an unhealthier dietary pattern, i.e., an 'increase in the consumption of vegetables and fruits' and a 'change towards unhealthy carbohydrates' (increase in white bread and savory bakery goods and decrease in whole-grain bread), respectively. The RRR patterns contained more disjoint food groups than the PCA patterns. The RRR baseline pattern was labelled a 'fast food pattern' characterized by a frequent intake of lemonade, children's yogurt, and a seldom intake of whole-grain bread, cheese, curd, and yogurt. The RRR change pattern increase in frequency of fast foods and starchy carbohydrate foods was characterized by an increase in the consumption frequency of carbohydrate sources such as whole-grain bread, potatoes, and pizza as well as fish sticks while the consumption frequency of vegetables decreased.

Table 1. Characteristics of the KOPS and IDEFICS-Germany samples included in the present analyses.

	KOPS		IDEFICS-Germany	
	Median or *n*-Number	**P25, P75 or Percentage**	**Median or *n*-Number**	**P25, P75 or Percentage**
n (% female)	372	49.5	298	47.3
Birth and infancy				
Birth year (min–max)	1991–1996		2000–2003	
Gestational age (weeks)	40	39, 40	n/a	
Birth weight < 3500 g, *n* (%)	184	49.5	113	37.9
Appropriate for gestational age, *n* (%)	276	74.2	n/a	
Fully breast fed, *n* (%) [a]	317	85.2	182	61.1
Smoking during pregnancy, *n* (%)	63	16.9	50	17.2
Family				
Maternal overweight, *n* (%) [b,c]	104	28.0	116	39.2
Paternal overweight, *n* (%) [b,c]	161	44.9	165	61.3
Parental overweight, *n* (%) [b,d]	209	56.2	205	68.8
Parental education, *n* (%) [e]	217	58.3	149	50.0
Single parenting, *n* (%) [c,f]	57	15.5	33	11.1
Low income, *n* (%) [c,g]	10	8.3	47	17.2

Numbers are medians (P25, P75) or *n*-numbers (percentages) unless otherwise indicated. [a] KOPS: defined as full breastfeeding > 0.5 months. IDEFICS-Germany: defined as full breastfeeding > 1 months vs. no breastfeeding/missing. [b] BMI ≥ 25 kg/m^2. [c] Missing data KOPS: paternal overweight: *n* = 13. Single parenting: *n* = 4. Low income: *n* = 251. Missing data IDEFICS-Germany: maternal overweight: *n* = 2, paternal overweight: *n* = 29, and low income: *n* = 24. [d] At least one parent is overweight. [e] At least one parent had ≥12 years of schooling. [f] IDEFICS-Germany: Single parenting defined as living with mother or father or 50% of the time with each mother and father. [g] KOPS: low or low/medium income level, i.e., <1,000 € per months. IDEFICS-Germany: low income level, i.e., <1,100 € per months.

Table 2. Anthropometric characteristics of the KOPS and IDEFICS-Germany samples at the beginning (baseline) and the end (follow-up) of the primary school period.

	Beginning of the Primary School Period		End of the Primary School Period		Mean Difference between End and Beginning of Primary School Period	
	Median or *n*-Number	**P25, P75, or Percentage**	**Median or *n*-Number**	**P25, P75, or Percentage**	**Median or *n*-Number**	**P25, P75, or Percentage**
KOPS						
n (% female)	372	49.5	372	49.5		
Age	6.2	6.0, 6.5	9.8	9.6, 10.1	3.6	3.5, 3.7
Anthropometry						
BMI (kg/m^2)	15.41	14.63, 16.31	16.85	15.55, 18.35	1.32	0.58, 2.55
Overweight, *n* (%)[a]	37	10.0	58	15.6		
FMI (kg/m^2)	3.18	2.59, 3.91	3.17	2.28, 4.31	−0.02	−0.70, 1.00
FFMI (kg/m^2)	12.31	11.68, 12.91	13.67	13.11, 14.40	1.46	0.92, 1.97
Waist circumference (cm)	54.5	52.3, 57.5	62.0	58.0, 66.0	7.0	4.0, 10.5
Waist-to-height ratio	0.46	0.44, 0.48	0.43	0.42, 0.46	−0.02	−0.04, 0.01
WtHR >0.5[b], *n* (%)	46	12.4	36	9.7		
IDEFICS-Germany						
n (% female)	298	47.3	298	47.3		
Age	6.5	5.6, 6.9	8.5	7.7, 9.0	2.0	2.0, 2.1
Anthropometry						
BMI (kg/m^2)	15.50	14.60, 16.60	16.15	14.90, 17.80	0.60	0.10, 1.30
Overweight, *n* (%) [a]	34	11.4	48	16.1		
FMI (kg/m^2)	4.33	3.68, 5.17	4.42	3.40, 5.68	0.07	−0.44, 0.73
FFMI (kg/m^2)	11.23	10.58, 11.79	11.85	11.22, 12.36	0.61	0.39, 0.82
Waist circumference (cm)	51.6	49.5, 54.1	56.5	53.3, 60.1	4.8	2.7, 6.9
Waist-to-height ratio	0.43	0.41, 0.45	0.42	0.40, 0.45	−0.01	−0.02, 0.01
WtHR >0.5 [b], *n* (%)	12	4.0	16	5.4		

The numbers are medians (P25, P75) or *n*-numbers (percentages). Differences between baseline and follow-up were tested using the Wilcoxon rank sum test for continuous variables and a Chi-square test for categorical variables. BMI, body mass index, FMI, fat-mass index, WtHR, waist-to-height ratio, [a] Derived from the age-specific and sex-specific cut-points proposed by the International Obesity Task Force [36]. [b] The cut-off >0.5 was proposed by McCarthy et al. [34] as indicated whether the amount of upper body fat accumulation is excessive and a risk to health.

Table 3. Food groups included in the PCA and RRR patterns—KOPS sample, $n = 372$.

	Included Food Groups	Factor Loading	Explained Variance in the Food Group Intake (%)
PCA pattern [a]			
PCA baseline pattern 1 ('fast food pattern')	+ Fish sticks + Curry-sausage + Lasagna + Pancakes + Potato fritters + Pizza + Meat balls	0.62 0.62 0.57 0.55 0.52 0.51 0.5	12.7
PCA baseline pattern 2 ('wholegrain, vegetables & fruits')	+ Whole-grain bread + Vegetables, salad + Fruits + Cheese, curd, yogurt + Muesli	0.66 0.65 0.56 0.47 0.43	8.1
PCA change pattern 1 ('increase in the consumption of fast food')	+Δ Meat balls +Δ Fish sticks +Δ Lasagna +Δ Pizza +Δ Pancakes +Δ Curry-sausage +Δ Potato fritters	0.61 0.57 0.54 0.52 0.48 0.44 0.43	9.4
PCA change pattern 2 ('increase in the consumption of vegetables and fruits')	+Δ Vegetables, salad +Δ Fruits +Δ Meat +Δ Potatoes	0.61 0.57 0.47 0.44	6.8
PCA change pattern 3 ('change towards unhealthy carbohydrates')	+Δ White bread +Δ Savory bakery goods −Δ Whole-grain bread	0.64 0.49 −0.51	6.4
	Included Food Groups	**Factor Loading**	**Explained Variance in Response Variables [b] (%)**
RRR pattern [a]			
RRR baseline pattern ('fast food pattern')	− Whole-grain bread − Cheese, curd, yogurt + Lemonade + Children's yogurt + Potato fritters + Meat balls + Meat	−0.32 −0.32 0.55 0.41 0.27 0.24 0.21	Changes in BMI: 9.1 Changes in FMI: 5.5 Changes in WtHR: 7.9 Total variance: 7.5
RRR change pattern ('increase in the consumption of fast foods and starchy carbohydrate foods')	+Δ Fish sticks +Δ Whole-grain bread +Δ Pizza +Δ Potatoes −Δ Vegetables −Δ Lemonade −Δ Sweets −Δ Chocolate spread −Δ Meat balls	0.49 0.26 0.21 0.2 −0.44 −0.33 −0.28 −0.21 −0.21	Changes in BMI: 7.7 Changes in FMI: 5.9 Changes in WtHR: 8.6 Total variance: 7.4

+, positive loading, −, negative loading, Δ, change, BMI, body mass index, FMI, fat-mass index, WtHR, waist-to-height ratio. [a] PCA patterns consider food groups with factor loadings ≥ |0.4|, RRR patterns consider food groups with factor loadings ≥ |0.2|. [b] Changes in response variables between the beginning of the primary school period (baseline) and the end of the primary school period adjusted for the baseline.

For the IDEFICS-Germany sample, dietary patterns obtained by PCA and RRR are given in Table 4. The PCA baseline pattern 1 termed 'snack pattern' was characterized by the frequent consumption of snack foods (sweet snacks, fried potatoes, croquettes, ketchup, savory snacks, and sweetened drinks) while frequent consumption of plain unsweetened yogurt or kefir, dishes of milled cereals, nuts, and pizza dominate the PCA baseline pattern 2 ('Mediterranean type pattern'). The PCA change pattern 1 termed 'change towards a Mediterranean type pattern' is dominated by increases in the consumption frequency of nuts, pasta, fresh meat, and pizza. Increases in the consumption frequency of cooked vegetables, potatoes, beans, and legumes but also sweetened drinks, butter/ margarine, and fresh fruits characterize the PCA change pattern 2 ('change towards a traditional type pattern') while the PCA change pattern 3 ('change towards a snack pattern') is dominated by increases in the consumption frequency of sweet snacks such as biscuits or pastries, candies, ice creams, and savory snack foods such as crisps or popcorn. The RRR baseline pattern was labeled 'Nuts, meat, and pizza pattern' because it is characterized by frequent intakes of nuts, fresh meats, pizza but also yogurt, jam, and honey as well as a seldom consumption of cooked vegetables, potatoes, beans, legumes, and sweetened breakfast cereals. The RRR change pattern, 'decrease in the consumption of animal protein sources and snack carbohydrates', was characterized by an increase in the consumption of 'reduced-fat products on bread' and decreases in the consumption frequency of fresh meat, savory pastries, fried or scrambled eggs, sweetened drinks, nuts, seeds, and dried fruits.

Table 4. Food groups included in the PCA and RRR patterns—IDEFICS-Germany sample, n = 298.

	Included Food Groups	Factor Loading	Explained Variance in Food Group Intake (%)
PCA pattern[a]			
PCA baseline pattern 1 ('snack pattern')	+ Sweet snacks (biscuits, packaged cakes, pastries, puddings) + Potatoes (fried, croquettes) + Ketchup and similar + Savory snacks (Crisps, corn crisps, popcorn) + Sweetened drinks + Chocolate, candy bars + Candies, loose candies, marshmallows + Ice cream, milk, or fruit-based bars	0.57 0.52 0.51 0.51 0.45 0.44 0.44 0.43	10.3
PCA baseline pattern 2 ('Mediterranean type pattern')	+ Plain unsweetened yogurt or kefir + Dish of milled cereals + Nuts, seeds, dried fruits + Pizza as main dish + Cheese (sliced and spreadable) + Fresh meat, not fried + Plain unsweetened milk + Fresh fruits with added sugar + Water + Pasta, noodles, rice	0.66 0.57 0.56 0.45 0.44 0.44 0.42 0.41 0.41 0.41	6.5
PCA change pattern 1 ('change towards a Mediterranean type pattern')	+Δ Nuts, seeds, dried fruits +Δ Pasta, noodles, rice +Δ Fresh meat, not fried +Δ Pizza as main dish +Δ Dish of milled cereals +Δ Sweet yogurt, fermented milk beverages +Δ Fried meat	0.6 0.56 0.52 0.49 0.48 0.43 0.41	8.9
PCA change pattern 2 ('change towards a traditional type pattern')	+Δ Cooked vegetables, potatoes, beans, and legumes +Δ Sweetened drinks +Δ Butter, margarine on bread +Δ Fresh fruits without added sugar	0.54 0.49 0.48 0.47	4.8
PCA change pattern 3 ('change towards a snack pattern')	+Δ Sweet snacks (biscuits, packaged cakes, pastries, puddings) +Δ Candies, loose candies, marshmallows +Δ Ice cream, milk, or fruit-based bars +Δ Savory snacks (Crisps, corn crisps, popcorn) +Δ Chocolate, candy bars	0.65 0.58 0.52 0.51 0.46	4.5
	Included Food Groups	**Factor Loading**	**Explained Variance in Response Variables b (%)**
RRR pattern [a]			
RRR baseline pattern ('Nuts, meat, and pizza pattern')	+ Nuts, seeds, dried fruits + Fresh meat, not fried + Pizza as main dish + Plain unsweetened yogurt or kefir + Jam, honey + Savory pastries, fritters + Dish of milled cereals − Cooked vegetables, potatoes, beans, and legumes − Breakfast cereals, muesli, sweetened	0.37 0.36 0.3 0.23 0.22 0.23 0.24 −0.29 −0.23	Changes in BMI: 11.5 Changes in FMI: 11.9 Changes in WtHR: 12.3 Total variance: 11.9
RRR change pattern ('decrease in the consumption of protein sources and snack carbohydrates')	+Δ Reduced-fat products on bread −Δ Fresh meat, not fried −Δ Savory pastries, fritters −Δ Fried or scrambled eggs −Δ Sweetened drinks −Δ Nuts, seeds, dried fruits −Δ Dish of milled cereals	0.24 −0.36 −0.33 −0.29 −0.27 −0.3 −0.24	Changes in BMI: 14.0 Changes in FMI: 14.3 Changes in WtHR: 12.0 Total variance: 13.5

+, positive loading, −, negative loading, Δ, change, BMI, body mass index, FMI, fat-mass index, WtHR, waist-to-height ratio. [a] PCA patterns consider food groups with factor loadings ≥ |0.4|, RRR patterns consider food groups with factor loadings ≥ |0.2|. [b] Changes in response variables between the beginning of the primary school period (baseline) and the end of the primary school period adjusted for baseline.

3.2. Logistic Regression Analyses

In KOPS, no significant association was found between PCA baseline patterns ('fast food pattern' and 'wholegrain, vegetables & fruits') and excess gain in BMI, FMI, or WtHR during the primary school period (Table 5). Among the PCA change patterns, only the adherence to an 'increase in the consumption of fast food' was significantly associated with higher odds for an excess gain in FMI after adjustment for parental overweight, parental education, and physical activity (p_{trend} = 0.0411). However, no similar associations were seen with odds for an excess gain in BMI or WtHR.

Figure 1 shows that a closer adherence to the RRR baseline pattern ('fast food pattern') was independently related to higher odds for an excess gain in BMI (Panel A, p_{trend} = 0.0006) and WtHR (Panel C, p_{trend} = 0.0047) but not in FMI (Panel B, p_{trend} = 0.2465) during primary school in the KOPS sample. Similarly, a closer adherence to the RRR change pattern ('increase in frequency of fast foods and starchy carbohydrate foods') predicted excess gain in BMI, FMI, and WtHR during the primary school period (Panel D–F, all p_{trend} < 0.002). Overall, those in the highest tertile of adherence were at least two times more likely to have excessively gained than their counterparts in the lowest tertile of adherence.

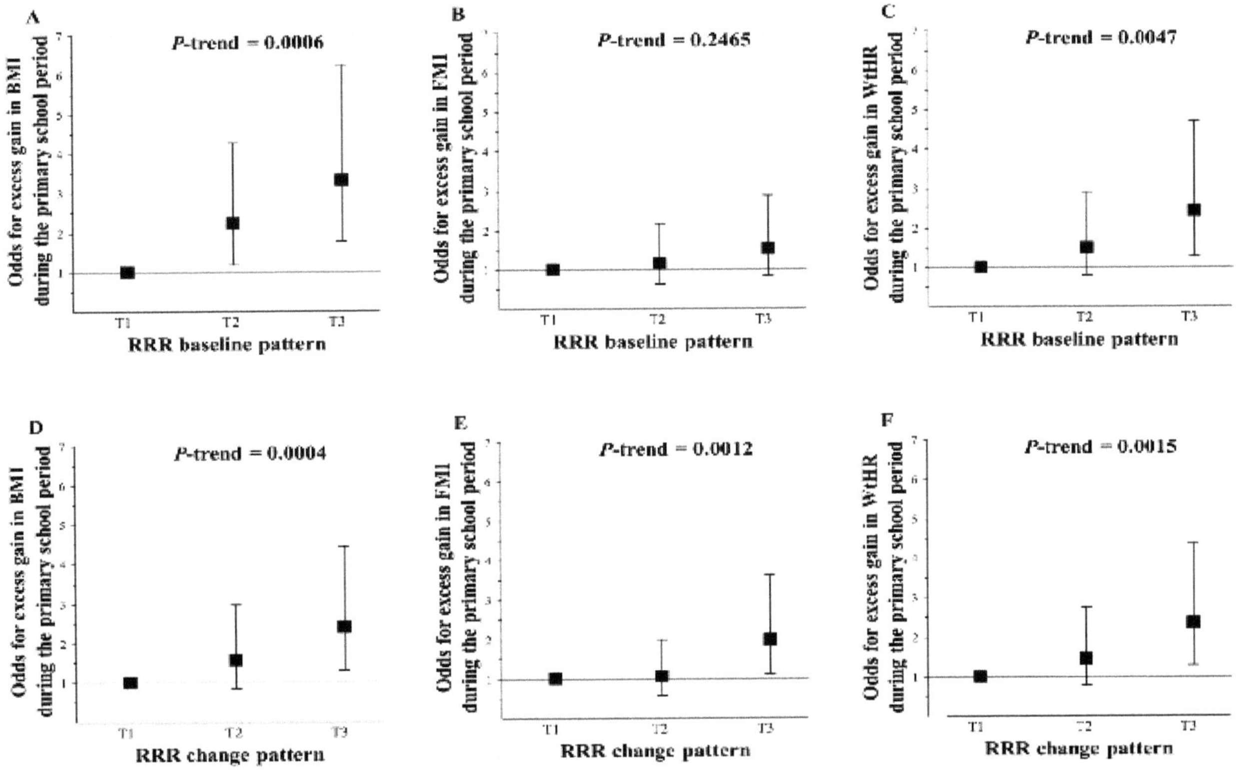

Figure 1. Odds for excess gains in BMI (panel **A** and **D**), fat-mass index (FMI, panel **B** and **E**), and waist-to-height ratio (WtHR, panel **C** and **F** during the primary school period according to tertiles of adherence to RRR baseline and change patterns ('fast food pattern' and 'increase in the consumption of fast foods and starchy carbohydrate foods', respectively)–KOPS sample (n = 372). Values are odd ratios (95% confidence intervals) presented in tertiles of adherence to the respective dietary pattern. Changes in body composition were adjusted for baseline body composition using the residual method. For the logistic regression analyses, the outcomes were excess gains in BMI, FMI, or WtHR defined as gains >75th percentile, adjusted for parental overweight (BMI $\geq$ 25 kg/m^2, yes/no), parental education ($\geq$12 years of schooling, yes/no), and physical activity (very low, low, middle, and high). The p-values are based on logistic regression models with dietary pattern scores as a continuous variable. T, Tertile.

In IDEFICS-Germany, higher adherence to the PCA change pattern ('change towards a Mediterranean type pattern was associated with lower odds for excess gain in FMI, WtHR, and BMI

($p < 0.05$) (Table 6). All other PCA baseline and change patterns were not associated with changes in body composition during primary school years.

Figure 2 illustrates that both the RRR baseline and change patterns remained independently associated with substantially increased odds for excess gains in BMI, FMI, and WtHR during the primary school years in the IDEFICS-Germany sample after an adjustment for potential confounders (all $p_{\text{trend}} < 0.01$).

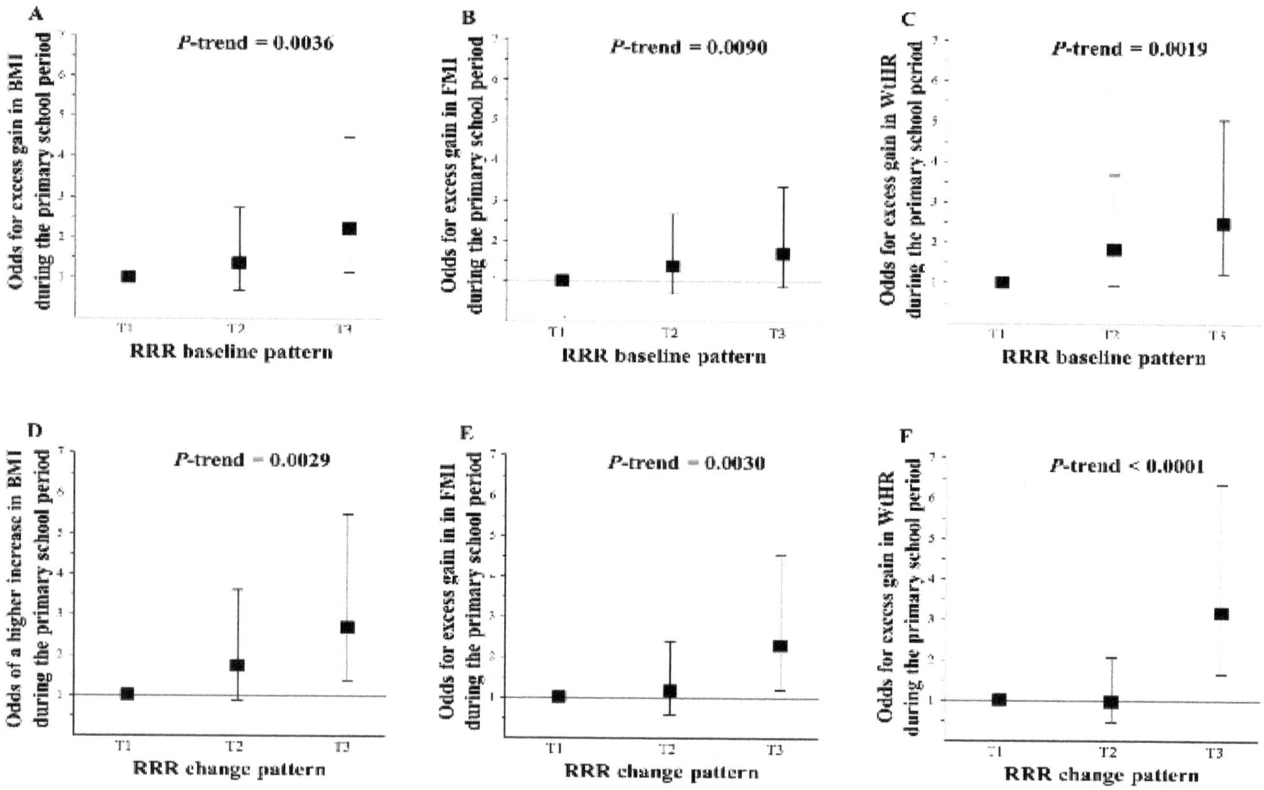

Figure 2. Odds for excess gains in BMI (panel **A** and **D**), fat-mass index (FMI, panel **B** and **E**), and waist-to-height ratio (WtHR, panel **C** and **F** during the primary school period according to tertiles of adherence to the RRR baseline and change patterns ('Nuts, meat, and pizza pattern' and 'decrease in the consumption of protein sources and snack carbohydrates', respectively)—IDEFICS-Germany sample ($n = 298$). Values are odd ratios (95% confidence intervals) presented in tertiles of the respective dietary pattern. Changes in body composition were adjusted for baseline body composition (BMI, FMI, or WtHR, respectively) using the residual method. For the logistic regression analyses, the outcomes were excess gains in BMI, FMI, or WtHR, which were defined as gains >75th percentile, adjusted for parental overweight (BMI $\geq$ 25 kg/m^2; yes/no), smoking during pregnancy (yes/no), and migration background (born in Germany, yes/no). Models for BMI and FMI also adjust for low income (<1.100 € per month, (no/yes/unknown): 8% of values were inputted using the missing indicator method resulting in a coding of 0, 1, and 2, respectively [42]), p-values based on multiple logistic regression models with dietary pattern scores as continuous variables. T, Tertile.

Table 5. Odds for excess gains in BMI, fat-mass index (FMI), or waist-to-height ratio (WtHR) [a] during the primary school period, according to tertiles of adherence to the PCA patterns—KOPS sample (n = 372).

	PCA Baseline Pattern 1 ('Fast Food Pattern')								PCA Change Pattern 1 ('Increase in the Consumption of Fast Food')							
	T1	T2		T3		Continuous [b]		p_{trend} [c]	T1	T2		T3		Continuous [b]		p_{trend} [c]
		OR	95% CI	OR	95% CI	OR	95% CI			OR	95% CI	OR	95% CI	OR	95% CI	
BMI																
Model A	1	0.89	0.50, 1.60	1.26	0.72, 2.21	1.03	0.98, 1.09	0.2768	1	0.91	0.50, 1.65	1.39	0.79, 2.46	1.04	0.99, 1.10	0.1478
Model B		0.81	0.44, 1.49	1.00	0.55, 1.80	1.01	0.95, 1.07	0.8457	1	0.95	0.51, 1.75	1.49	0.83, 2.68	1.05	0.99, 1.10	0.1133
								FMI								
Model A	1	0.79	0.44, 1.40	0.98	0.56, 1.73	1.02	0.97, 1.08	0.4590	1	1.10	0.60, 2.01	1.73	0.97, 3.07	1.05	1.00, 1.11	0.0538
Model B	1	0.67	0.37, 1.24	0.73	0.41, 1.33	0.99	0.94, 1.06	0.8556	1	1.19	0.64, 2.21	1.86	1.03, 3.38	1.06	1.00, 1.12	0.0411
								WtHR								
Model A	1	0.59	0.32, 1.07	1.11	0.64, 1.93	1.03	0.97, 1.09	0.3318	1	0.76	0.42, 1.38	1.28	0.73, 2.23	1.02	0.97, 1.08	0.4498
Model B	1	0.54	0.29, 1.01	0.88	0.49, 1.57	1.00	0.95, 1.06	0.9329	1	0.79	0.43, 1.46	1.35	0.76, 2.40	1.02	0.97, 1.08	0.3665
	PCA Baseline Pattern 2 ('Wholegrain, Vegetables & Fruits')								PCA Change Pattern 2 ('Increase in the Consumption of Vegetables and Fruits')							
	T1	T2		T3		Continuous [b]		p_{trend} [c]	T1	T2		T3		Continuous [b]		p_{trend} [c]
		OR	95% CI	OR	95% CI	OR	95% CI			OR	95% CI	OR	95% CI	OR	95% CI	
BMI																
Model A	1	0.94	0.54, 1.64	0.60	0.33, 1.09	0.95	0.88, 1.03	0.2316	1	1.01	0.57, 1.79	0.87	0.49, 1.55	1.00	0.92, 1.09	0.9687
Model B		1.10	0.62, 1.95	0.77	0.41, 1.43	1.00	0.91, 1.08	0.9079	1	1.03	0.57, 1.86	0.76	0.42, 1.39	0.98	0.90, 1.08	0.7236
FMI																
Model A	1	1.20	0.69, 2.09	0.68	0.37, 1.25	0.96	0.89, 1.04	0.2859	1	0.85	0.47, 1.52	1.03	0.59, 1.82	1.02	0.93, 1.11	0.7210
Model B	1	1.42	0.80, 2.53	0.89	0.47, 1.67	1.00	0.92, 1.09	0.9971	1	0.86	0.47, 1.57	0.92	0.51, 1.65	1.00	0.91, 1.09	0.9852
WtHR																
Model A	1	0.87	0.50, 1.51	0.58	0.32, 1.05	0.96	0.89, 1.04	0.3049	1	0.65	0.36. 1.17	0.91	0.52, 1.59	0.98	0.90, 1.07	0.6387
Model B	1	0.97	0.55, 1.72	0.72	0.39, 1.34	1.00	0.92, 1.09	0.9676	1	0.61	0.33, 1.13	0.80	0.45, 1.43	0.96	0.88, 1.05	0.3628
									PCA Change Pattern 3 ('Change towards Unhealthy Carbohydrates')							
									T1	T2		T3		Continuous [b]		p_{trend} [c]
										OR	95% CI	OR	95% CI	OR	95% CI	
BMI																
Model A									1	0.83	0.47, 1.46	0.80	0.45, 1.42	0.97	0.87, 1.08	0.5265
Model B									1	0.89	0.50, 1.61	0.90	0.50, 1.63	0.99	0.88, 1.10	0.8046
FMI																
Model A									1	0.69	0.39, 1.24	0.84	0.48, 1.47	0.95	0.85, 1.06	0.3516
Model B									1	0.75	0.41, 1.35	0.96	0.53, 1.72	0.97	0.87, 1.09	0.6091
WtHR																
Model A									1	0.87	0.49, 1.52	0.67	0.37, 1.20	0.91	0.81, 1.01	0.0836
Model B									1	0.92	0.52, 1.64	0.71	0.39, 1.30	0.92	0.82, 1.03	0.1262

Values are odds ratios (95% confidence intervals) presented in tertiles of adherence to the respective dietary pattern. [a] Change in body composition was adjusted for the respective baseline value using the residual method. Odds refer to excess gains in BMI, FMI, or WtHR' defined as gains >75th percentile. [b] Continuous, i.e., per unit of pattern score. [c] Based on logistic regression models with dietary pattern scores as a continuous variable. Model A: Unadjusted. Model B: Adjusted for parental overweight (BMI $\geq$ 25 kg/m^2, yes/no), parental education ($\geq$12 years of schooling, yes/no), and physical activity (very low, low, middle, high).

Table 6. Odds for excess gains in BMI, fat-mass index (FMI), or waist-to-height ratio (WtHR) [a] during the primary school period according to tertiles of adherence to the PCA patterns—IDEFICS-Germany sample (n = 298).

	PCA Baseline Pattern 1 ('Snack Pattern')								PCA Change Pattern 1 ('Increase in the Consumption of Fast Food')								
	T1	T2		T3		Continuous [b]		p_{trend} [c]	T1	T2		T3		Continuous [b]		p_{trend} [c]
		OR	95% CI	OR	95% CI	OR	95% CI			OR	95% CI	OR	95% CI	OR	95% CI	
BMI																
Model A	1	0.69	0.37, 1.29	0.52	0.27, 1.00	0.95	0.88, 1.02	0.1537	1	1.15	0.62, 2.15	0.67	0.34, 1.30	0.93	0.87, 1.00	0.0395
Model B		0.67	0.35, 1.26	0.47	0.23, 0.91	0.94	0.87, 1.01	0.0810	1	1.12	0.60, 2.11	0.65	0.33, 1.30	0.93	0.87, 0.99	0.0436
FMI																
Model A	1	1.10	0.58, 2.07	0.85	0.44, 1.63	0.99	0.92, 1.06	0.8102	1	1.21	0.65, 2.27	0.75	0.38, 1.46	0.93	0.87, 0.99	0.0454
Model B	1	1.06	0.55, 2.03	0.78	0.39, 1.52	0.98	0.91, 1.05	0.6013	1	1.05	0.55, 1.99	0.79	0.40, 1.56	0.94	0.87, 0.99	0.0490
WtHR																
Model A	1	1.29	0.68, 2.45	1.00	0.52, 1.94	0.99	0.92, 1.06	0.8259	1	1.04	0.55, 1.95	0.76	0.39, 1.46	0.93	0.87, 0.99	0.0409
Model B	1	1.18	0.62, 2.28	0.95	0.48, 1.87	0.98	0.92, 1.05	0.6481	1	1.04	0.55, 1.99	0.79	0.40, 1.56	0.93	0.87, 0.99	0.0490
	PCA Baseline Pattern 2 ('Mediterranean Type Pattern')								PCA Change Pattern 2 ('Change towards a Traditional Type Pattern')								
	T1	T2		T3		Continuous [b]		p_{trend} [c]	T1	T2		T3		Continuous [b]		p_{trend} [c]
		OR	95% CI	OR	95% CI	OR	95% CI			OR	95% CI	OR	95% CI	OR	95% CI	
BMI																
Model A	1	0.65	0.33, 1.25	0.92	0.49. 1.71	1.04	0.99, 1.09	0.1456	1	1.04	0.55, 1.99	1.06	0.55, 2.02	1.02	0.92, 1.13	0.7179
Model B		0.65	0.33, 1.27	0.92	0.47, 1.79	1.04	0.99, 1.11	0.1403	1	1.02	0.52, 1.98	1.06	0.54, 2.07	1.02	0.92, 1.14	0.6587
FMI																
Model A	1	0.96	0.51, 1.82	0.86	0.45, 1.64	1.03	0.98, 1.09	0.1957	1	1.10	0.58, 2.07	0.85	0.44, 1.63	0.99	0.89, 1.10	0.8205
Model B	1	1.00	0.52, 1.92	0.91	0.46, 1.81	1.05	0.99, 1.12	0.1073	1	1.02	0.53, 1.96	0.83	0.42, 1.63	0.99)	0.89, 1.10	0.8780
WtHR																
Model A	1	0.62	0.32, 1.19	0.83	0.44, 1.55	1.04	0.98, 1.10	0.2349	1	0.75	0.39, 1.44	0.90	0.48, 1.70	0.95	00.86, 1.05	0.3343
Model B	1	0.60	0.31, 1.17	0.86	0.44, 1.67	1.04	0.98, 1.11	0.1764	1	0.63	0.32, 1.24	0.77	0.40, 1.50	0.94	0.85, 1.04	0.2324
									PCA Change Pattern 3 ('Change towards a Snack Pattern')								
									T1	T2		T3		Continuous [b]		p_{trend} [c]
										OR	95% CI	OR	95% CI	OR	95% CI	
BMI																
Model A									1	1.53	0.80, 2.99	1.41	0.73, 2.76	1.01	0.93, 1.10	0.7551
Model B									1	1.60	0.83, 3.15	1.46	0.75, 2.87	1.02	0.94, 1.11	0.6363
FMI																
Model A									1	1.24	0.64, 2.41	1.47	0.77, 2.83	0.98	0.90, 1.06	0.6550
Model B									1	1.27	0.65, 2.50	1.49	0.78, 2.90	0.99	0.91, 1.08	0.8546
WtHR																
Model A									1	1.11	0.57, 2.18	1.62	0.85, 3.11	1.03	0.95, 1.12	0.5336
Model B									1	1.17	0.59, 2.33	1.64	0.86, 3.19	1.03	0.95, 1.12	0.4342

Values are odds ratios (95% confidence intervals) presented in tertiles of adherence to the respective dietary pattern. [a] Change in body composition was adjusted for the respective baseline value using the residual method. Odds refer to excess gains in BMI, FMI, or WtHR defined as gains >75th percentile. [b] Continuous, i.e., per unit of pattern score. [c] Based on logistic regression models with dietary pattern scores as a continuous variable. Model A: Unadjusted. Model B: Adjusted for parental overweight (BMI $\geq$ 25 kg/m^2, yes/no), smoking during pregnancy (yes/no), and migration background (born in Germany, yes/no) in models for BMI and FMI additional adjustment for low income (<1.100 € per months, (no/yes/unknown): 8% of values were imputed using the missing indicator method resulting in a coding of 0, 1, and 2, respectively [42]).

4. Discussion

The present study provides new prospective evidence from two pediatric samples suggesting a relevance of dietary patterns during the primary school period identified by RRR for the development of body composition in primary school years. Our data support a potentially detrimental role of dietary patterns characterized by fast foods for BMI, FMI, and WtHR development during this critical time period. On a more exploratory level, this study also suggests that future research should shed light on the relevance of combinations of protein and carbohydrate sources for body composition development in school children.

Both PCA and RRR identified dietary patterns characterized by a preferred consumption of fast foods, which were associated with excess gains in adiposity measures both prospectively and concurrently in the KOPS cohort. Our findings are broadly in line with the ALSPAC study, which reported that an energy-dense, low-fiber, high-fat RRR dietary pattern at 7 years of age but not at 5 years of age, was predictive of fat mass at 9 years of age among UK children [14]. In addition, the preferred consumption of fast foods itself has repeatedly been related to an unfavorable body composition among children and adolescents [43–46] even though it is possible that associations with measures of obesity risk may partly reflect relations to the associated behaviors rather than the preferred consumption of these foods [47,48]. The fact that no predictive fast food pattern was identified for the IDEFICS-Germany cohort may, in part, result from differences in the focused inquiry of these foods by the employed FPQs: in KOPS, one-third of the inquired food groups (8 out of 22) referred to fast foods while only four out of 43 items in IDEFICS-Germany addressed fast foods.

Our study did also confirm a protective role of a Mediterranean type pattern identified by PCA, which was prospectively related to lower odds for excess gains in BMI, FMI, and WtHR in the German IDEFICS-Germany cohort. Similar associations have previously been reported by some [49–53] but not all [54,55] pediatric studies that were explicitly investigating the relevance of Mediterranean dietary indices or scores for body composition. Recently, a Mediterranean type diet was observed to be associated with a more favorable BMI, glucose, and lipid profile among children and adolescents presenting with components of the metabolic syndrome than a standard diet [56]. Similarly, evidence from both intervention and prospective cohort studies support benefits of Mediterranean type diets for body composition among adults [57–60].

Snacking habits have also been suggested as a potential cause contributing to the development of overweight and obesity among children. Evidence for the prospective role of a 'snacking' pattern among children is available from two prospective observational studies. In a cohort of 5-year-old to 12-year-old Columbian children, the adherence to this PCA-derived 'snacking' pattern was associated with greater increases in BMI, subscapular: triceps skinfold thickness ratio, and waist circumference over a median 2.5 year follow-up [13]. By contrast, a PCA-derived 'snacking' pattern in 2-year-old and 9.9-year-old participants of the IDEFICS-multicenter cohort was not related to a two-year BMI change [12]. In line with this, the PCA 'snack food pattern' and the 'change towards a snack pattern' identified in the IDEFICS-Germany cohort were not related to a higher BMI, FMI, or WtHR. PCA generally yields interpretable patterns, but they may not be relevant for disease outcomes because PCA is purely exploratory, which explains maximal variation in food intake [61]. In addition, PCA patterns generally tend to account for only a small amount of the total variance in food intake in pediatric populations [61–65]. Similarly, in our study, the PCA patterns accounted for only 6.4% to 12.7% and 4.5% to 10.3% of the total variance in food intake in KOPS and IDEFICS-Germany, respectively.

RRR may be more informative since it explicitly derives predictors that explain maximal variation in response variables [40,66]. In the present study, three of the RRR patterns point towards a specific relevance of combinations of unfavorable carbohydrate sources and (animal) protein sources (RRR patterns 'fast food', 'increase in the consumption of fast foods and starchy carbohydrate foods,' and 'decrease in the consumption of protein sources and snack carbohydrates.' The protein leverage hypothesis proposes that a preference for protein in combination with a decrease in the ratio of protein to carbohydrates and fat in the diet is related to excess energy intake and the risk of obesity [67,68]. The two RRR change patterns in the present study are in line with this since they suggest that either increases in (starchy) carbohydrate sources or decreases in the consumption of protein sources during primary school years were associated with an unfavorable development of body composition. Data from a large animal study conducted by the advocates of the protein leverage hypothesis revealed that a high ratio of protein to carbohydrate rather than total caloric intake was related to lower body fat content but may adversely affect cardio-metabolic health [69]. However, in adults, diets with higher plant and animal protein intake were associated with lower central adiposity [70,71] and favorable cardiometabolic markers [71]. Furthermore, in eight-year-old school children, high protein intake was positively associated with a higher fat-free mass index two years later [72]. The relevance of macronutrient ratios or of the combinations of carbohydrate and protein sources for body composition remains to be elucidated.

Despite some similarities in the identified pattern and their association with body composition development in primary school years as outlined above, the patterns differ substantially between both cohorts. Our analyses do, therefore, not confirm our initial hypothesis that similar detrimental or protective dietary patterns may be identified in the three German pediatric cohorts, i.e., DONALD, KOPS, and IDEFICS-Germany. It is likely that this largely reflects the considerable methodological differences, i.e., the different nutrition assessment methods as well as differences in the examined food groups. Comparison with other pediatric studies is further hampered by differences in the method to identify dietary patterns, e.g., the definition of high factor loadings and the fact that the simplified pattern approach is not universally applied.

To overcome some of the issues of comparability, both the criteria for sample selections and the analytical approach of the present study were similar to those previously applied in the DONALD study [9]. Additional strengths of the present study include its prospective nature, which covered the period of two and 3.6 years of primary school for IDEFICS-Germany and KOPS, respectively, with completion of one FPQ at the beginning and one at the end of the observation period as well as anthropometric examination at both points in time, which allows the analysis of changes in diet and growth. In addition, in both cohorts, FMI and WtHR—i.e., more sensitive measurements of obesity and central adiposity, respectively, were examined in addition to BMI. Nonetheless, the fact that fat mass was estimated by two different algorithms derived from the respective BIA may be seen as a limitation. In addition, changes in body composition after puberty onset are known to differ between early-maturing and late-maturing children of the same age [73]. However, puberty onset was not assessed in the studies. KOPS data stem from 2001 and one can assume that dietary behavior and other lifestyle factors may have changed in the meantime. However, results of examinations conducted in a further cohort after 10 years at school entry (2006–2008) and at the end of the primary school period (4th grade, 2010–2012) indicate that these data are still comparable [74,75]. In addition, our study is limited by the comparably small samples from the KOPS and IDEFICS-Germany cohorts. However, it has been suggested that the ratio of the sample size to the number of food groups may be more important than the absolute number of subjects [76]. We performed a number of statistical tests. Therefore, the chance may be an explanation for our findings. However, for the RRR results in particular consistency of findings across the different body composition outcomes argues against chance findings. Another limitation arises from the fact that the FPQ used in KOPS and IDEFICS-Germany did not inquire the consumption frequencies of the same food groups. Therefore, pooled analyses of the KOPS and IDEFICS-Germany samples were not possible. However, as outlined above, comparative analyses using similar analytic approaches based on the food-group specific data available from different assessment methods are desirable and were conducted.

5. Conclusions

The present study confirms an unfavorable impact of fast foods on the development of body composition during primary school years. The role of combinations of unfavorable carbohydrate sources and (animal) protein sources requires further investigation.

Author Contributions: Conceptualization, A.E.B. Data curation, M.W. and S.P.-D. Formal analysis, G.J. Funding acquisition, M.J.M., W.A., and A.E.B. Investigation, M.J.M., W.A., and A.E.B. Methodology, A.E.B and G.J. Writing-original draft, M.W. and G.J. Writing-review & editing, M.W., G.J., S.P.-D., M.S., M.J.M., W.A., and A.E.B.

Acknowledgments: The participation of all children and their families in the KOPS and IDEFICS-Germany cohort is gratefully acknowledged.

References

1. Kurth, B.M.; Schaffrath Rosario, A. [The prevalence of overweight and obese children and adolescents living in germany. Results of the german health interview and examination survey for children and adolescents (kiggs)]. *Bundesgesundheitsblatt Gesundheitsforschung Gesundheitsschutz* **2007**, *50*, 736–743. [CrossRef] [PubMed]
2. Ogden, C.L.; Carroll, M.D.; Kit, B.K.; Flegal, K.M. Prevalence of childhood and adult obesity in the united states, 2011–2012. *JAMA* **2014**, *311*, 806–814. [CrossRef] [PubMed]
3. von Kries, R.; Reulen, H.; Bayer, O.; Riedel, C.; Diethelm, K.; Buyken, A.E. Increase in prevalence of adiposity between the ages of 7 and 11 years reflects lower remission rates during this period. *Pediatr. Obes.* **2013**, *8*, 13–20. [CrossRef] [PubMed]
4. Hughes, A.R.; Sherriff, A.; Lawlor, D.A.; Ness, A.R.; Reilly, J.J. Incidence of obesity during childhood and adolescence in a large contemporary cohort. *Prev. Med.* **2011**, *52*, 300–304. [CrossRef] [PubMed]
5. Plachta-Danielzik, S.; Pust, S.; Asbeck, I.; Czerwinski-Mast, M.; Langnase, K.; Fischer, C.; Bosy-Westphal, A.; Kriwy, P.; Muller, M.J. Four-year follow-up of school-based intervention on overweight children: The kops study. *Obesity (Silver Spring)* **2007**, *15*, 3159–3169. [CrossRef] [PubMed]
6. Datar, A.; Shier, V.; Sturm, R. Changes in body mass during elementary and middle school in a national cohort of kindergarteners. *Pediatrics* **2011**, *128*, e1411–e1417. [CrossRef] [PubMed]
7. Verrotti, A.; Penta, L.; Zenzeri, L.; Agostinelli, S.; De Feo, P. Childhood obesity: Prevention and strategies of intervention. A systematic review of school-based interventions in primary schools. *J. Endocrinol. Invest.* **2014**, *37*, 1155–1164. [CrossRef] [PubMed]
8. Li, X.H.; Lin, S.; Guo, H.; Huang, Y.; Wu, L.; Zhang, Z.; Ma, J.; Wang, H.J. Effectiveness of a school-based physical activity intervention on obesity in school children: A nonrandomized controlled trial. *BMC Public Health* **2014**, *14*, 1282. [CrossRef] [PubMed]
9. Diethelm, K.; Gunther, A.L.; Schulze, M.B.; Standl, M.; Heinrich, J.; Buyken, A.E. Prospective relevance of dietary patterns at the beginning and during the course of primary school to the development of body composition. *Br. J. Nutr.* **2014**, *111*, 1488–1498. [CrossRef] [PubMed]
10. Cutler, G.J.; Flood, A.; Hannan, P.J.; Slavin, J.L.; Neumark-Sztainer, D. Association between major patterns of dietary intake and weight status in adolescents. *Br. J. Nutr.* **2012**, *108*, 349–356. [CrossRef] [PubMed]
11. Oellingrath, I.M.; Svendsen, M.V.; Brantsaeter, A.L. Tracking of eating patterns and overweight—a follow-up study of norwegian schoolchildren from middle childhood to early adolescence. *Nutr. J.* **2011**, *10*, 106. [CrossRef] [PubMed]
12. Pala, V.; Lissner, L.; Hebestreit, A.; Lanfer, A.; Sieri, S.; Siani, A.; Huybrechts, I.; Kambek, L.; Molnar, D.; Tornaritis, M.; et al. Dietary patterns and longitudinal change in body mass in european children: A follow-up study on the idefics multicenter cohort. *Eur. J. Clin. Nutr.* **2013**, *67*, 1042–1049. [CrossRef] [PubMed]

13. Shroff, M.R.; Perng, W.; Baylin, A.; Mora-Plazas, M.; Marin, C.; Villamor, E. Adherence to a snacking dietary pattern and soda intake are related to the development of adiposity: A prospective study in school-age children. *Public Health Nutr.* **2014**, *17*, 1507–1513. [CrossRef] [PubMed]
14. Johnson, L.; Mander, A.P.; Jones, L.R.; Emmett, P.M.; Jebb, S.A. Energy-dense, low-fiber, high-fat dietary pattern is associated with increased fatness in childhood. *Am. J. Clin. Nutr.* **2008**, *87*, 846–854. [CrossRef] [PubMed]
15. Emmett, P.M.; Jones, L.R.; Northstone, K. Dietary patterns in the avon longitudinal study of parents and children. *Nutr. Rev.* **2015**, *73 Suppl 3*, 207–230. [CrossRef]
16. Danielzik, S.; Pust, S.; Landsberg, B.; Muller, M.J. First lessons from the kiel obesity prevention study (KOPS). *Int. J. Obes. (Lond.)* **2005**, *29 Suppl 2*, S78–S83. [CrossRef]
17. Brambilla, P.; Bedogni, G.; Heo, M.; Pietrobelli, A. Waist circumference-to-height ratio predicts adiposity better than body mass index in children and adolescents. *Int. J. Obes. (Lond.)* **2013**, *37*, 943–946. [CrossRef] [PubMed]
18. Nagy, P.; Kovacs, E.; Moreno, L.A.; Veidebaum, T.; Tornaritis, M.; Kourides, Y.; Siani, A.; Lauria, F.; Sioen, I.; Claessens, M.; et al. Percentile reference values for anthropometric body composition indices in european children from the idefics study. *Int. J. Obes. (Lond.)* **2014**, *38 Suppl 2*, S15–S25. [CrossRef]
19. Schroder, H.; Ribas, L.; Koebnick, C.; Funtikova, A.; Gomez, S.F.; Fito, M.; Perez-Rodrigo, C.; Serra-Majem, L. Prevalence of abdominal obesity in spanish children and adolescents. Do we need waist circumference measurements in pediatric practice? *PLoS One* **2014**, *9*. [CrossRef] [PubMed]
20. Subar, A.F.; Dodd, K.W.; Guenther, P.M.; Kipnis, V.; Midthune, D.; McDowell, M.; Tooze, J.A.; Freedman, L.S.; Krebs-Smith, S.M. The food propensity questionnaire: Concept, development, and validation for use as a covariate in a model to estimate usual food intake. *J. Am. Diet. Assoc.* **2006**, *106*, 1556–1563. [CrossRef] [PubMed]
21. Muller, M.J.; Asbeck, I.; Mast, M.; Langnase, K.; Grund, A. Prevention of obesity-more than an intention. Concept and first results of the kiel obesity prevention study (KOPS). *Int. J. Obes. Relat. Metab. Disord.* **2001**, *25* (Suppl 1), S66–S74. [CrossRef] [PubMed]
22. Ahrens, W.; Bammann, K.; Siani, A.; Buchecker, K.; De Henauw, S.; Iacoviello, L.; Hebestreit, A.; Krogh, V.; Lissner, L.; Marild, S.; et al. The idefics cohort: Design, characteristics and participation in the baseline survey. *Int. J. Obes. (Lond.)* **2011**, *35 Suppl 1*, S3–S15. [CrossRef]
23. Von Kries, R.; Beyerlein, A.; Muller, M.J.; Heinrich, J.; Landsberg, B.; Bolte, G.; Chmitorz, A.; Plachta-Danielzik, S. Different age-specific incidence and remission rates in pre-school and primary school suggest need for targeted obesity prevention in childhood. *Int. J. Obes. (Lond.)* **2012**, *36*, 505–510. [CrossRef] [PubMed]
24. Plachta-Danielzik, S.; Landsberg, B.; Seiberl, J.; Gehrke, M.I.; Gose, M.; Kehden, B.; Muller, M.J. Longitudinal data of the kiel obesity prevention study (KOPS). *Bundesgesundheitsblatt Gesundheitsforschung Gesundheitsschutz* **2012**, *55*, 885–891. [CrossRef] [PubMed]
25. Plachta-Danielzik, S.; Landsberg, B.; Lange, D.; Seiberl, J.; Muller, M.J. Eight-year follow-up of school-based intervention on childhood overweight–the kiel obesity prevention study. *Obes Facts* **2011**, *4*, 35–43. [CrossRef] [PubMed]
26. Mast, M.; Kortzinger, I.; Konig, E.; Muller, M.J. Gender differences in fat mass of 5–7-year old children. *Int. J. Obes. Relat. Metab. Disord.* **1998**, *22*, 878–884. [CrossRef] [PubMed]
27. Pust, S. *Evaluation eines Adipositas-Präventionsprogrammes für Kinder. Ergebnisse der Kieler Adipositas-Präventionsstudie (Kops)*; Der Andere Verlag: Tönning, Lübeck, Marburg, Germany, 2006.
28. Lanfer, A.; Hebestreit, A.; Ahrens, W.; Krogh, V.; Sieri, S.; Lissner, L.; Eiben, G.; Siani, A.; Huybrechts, I.; Loit, H.M.; et al. Reproducibility of food consumption frequencies derived from the children's eating habits questionnaire used in the idefics study. *Int. J. Obes. (Lond.)* **2011**, *35* (Suppl 1), S61–S68. [CrossRef] [PubMed]
29. Huybrechts, I.; Bornhorst, C.; Pala, V.; Moreno, L.A.; Barba, G.; Lissner, L.; Fraterman, A.; Veidebaum, T.; Hebestreit, A.; Sieri, S.; et al. Evaluation of the children's eating habits questionnaire used in the idefics study by relating urinary calcium and potassium to milk consumption frequencies among european children. *Int. J. Obes. (Lond.)* **2011**, *35* (Suppl 1), S69–S78. [CrossRef] [PubMed]
30. Bel-Serrat, S.; Mouratidou, T.; Pala, V.; Huybrechts, I.; Bornhorst, C.; Fernandez-Alvira, J.M.; Hadjigeorgiou, C.; Eiben, G.; Hebestreit, A.; Lissner, L.; et al. Relative validity of the children's eating habits questionnaire-food frequency section among young european children: The idefics study. *Public Health Nutr.* **2014**, *17*, 266–276. [CrossRef] [PubMed]

31. Plachta-Danielzik, S.; Gehrke, M.I.; Kehden, B.; Kromeyer-Hauschild, K.; Grillenberger, M.; Willhoft, C.; Bosy-Westphal, A.; Muller, M.J. Body fat percentiles for german children and adolescents. *Obes Facts* **2012**, *5*, 77–90. [CrossRef] [PubMed]
32. Tyrrell, V.J.; Richards, G.; Hofman, P.; Gillies, G.F.; Robinson, E.; Cutfield, W.S. Foot-to-foot bioelectrical impedance analysis: A valuable tool for the measurement of body composition in children. *Int. J. Obes. Relat. Metab. Disord.* **2001**, *25*, 273–278. [CrossRef] [PubMed]
33. World Health Organization. Waist circumference and waist–hip ratio: Report of a who expert consultation, 8–11 December 2008. Available online: http://whqlibdoc.who.int/publications/2011/9789241501491_eng.pdf (accessed on 9 November.2017).
34. McCarthy, H.D.; Ashwell, M. A study of central fatness using waist-to-height ratios in uk children and adolescents over two decades supports the simple message-'keep your waist circumference to less than half your height'. *Int. J. Obes. (Lond.)* **2006**, *30*, 988–992. [CrossRef] [PubMed]
35. Cole, T.J.; Faith, M.S.; Pietrobelli, A.; Heo, M. What is the best measure of adiposity change in growing children: Bmi, bmi %, bmi *z*-score or bmi centile? *Eur. J. Clin. Nutr.* **2005**, *59*, 419–425. [CrossRef] [PubMed]
36. Cole, T.J.; Bellizzi, M.C.; Flegal, K.M.; Dietz, W.H. Establishing a standard definition for child overweight and obesity worldwide: International survey. *BMJ* **2000**, *320*, 1240–1243. [CrossRef] [PubMed]
37. Schulze, M.B.; Hoffmann, K.; Kroke, A.; Boeing, H. Dietary patterns and their association with food and nutrient intake in the european prospective investigation into cancer and nutrition (epic)-potsdam study. *Br. J. Nutr.* **2001**, *85*, 363–373. [CrossRef] [PubMed]
38. Hatcher, L. *A Step-by-Step Approach to Using the SAS System for Factor Analysis and Structural Equation Modeling*; SAS Institute: Cary, NC, USA, 2007; p. 588.
39. Schulze, M.B.; Hoffmann, K.; Kroke, A.; Boeing, H. An approach to construct simplified measures of dietary patterns from exploratory factor analysis. *Br. J. Nutr.* **2003**, *89*, 409–419. [CrossRef] [PubMed]
40. Hoffmann, K.; Schulze, M.B.; Schienkiewitz, A.; Nothlings, U.; Boeing, H. Application of a new statistical method to derive dietary patterns in nutritional epidemiology. *Am. J. Epidemiol.* **2004**, *159*, 935–944. [CrossRef] [PubMed]
41. Willett, W. *Nutritional Epidemiology*, 2nd ed.; Oxford University Press: New York, NY, USA, 1998; p. 514.
42. Haukoos, J.S.; Newgard, C.D. Advanced statistics: Missing data in clinical research-part 1: An introduction and conceptual framework. *Acad. Emerg. Med.* **2007**, *14*, 662–668. [PubMed]
43. Rosenheck, R. Fast food consumption and increased caloric intake: A systematic review of a trajectory towards weight gain and obesity risk. *Obes. Rev.* **2008**, *9*, 535–547. [CrossRef] [PubMed]
44. Braithwaite, I.; Stewart, A.W.; Hancox, R.J.; Beasley, R.; Murphy, R.; Mitchell, E.A. Fast-food consumption and body mass index in children and adolescents: An international cross-sectional study. *BMJ Open* **2014**, *4*. [CrossRef] [PubMed]
45. Whitton, C.; Ma, Y.; Bastian, A.C.; Fen Chan, M.; Chew, L. Fast-food consumers in singapore: Demographic profile, diet quality and weight status. *Public Health Nutr.* **2014**, *17*, 1805–1813. [CrossRef] [PubMed]
46. Shang, L.; O'Loughlin, J.; Tremblay, A.; Gray-Donald, K. The association between food patterns and adiposity among canadian children at risk of overweight. *Appl. Physiol. Nutr. Metab.* **2014**, *39*, 195–201. [CrossRef] [PubMed]
47. Poti, J.M.; Duffey, K.J.; Popkin, B.M. The association of fast food consumption with poor dietary outcomes and obesity among children: Is it the fast food or the remainder of the diet? *Am. J. Clin. Nutr.* **2014**, *99*, 162–171. [CrossRef] [PubMed]
48. Alexy, U.; Libuda, L.; Mersmann, S.; Kersting, M. Convenience foods in children's diet and association with dietary quality and body weight status. *Eur. J. Clin. Nutr.* **2011**, *65*, 160–166. [CrossRef] [PubMed]
49. Tognon, G.; Moreno, L.A.; Mouratidou, T.; Veidebaum, T.; Molnar, D.; Russo, P.; Siani, A.; Akhandaf, Y.; Krogh, V.; Tornaritis, M.; et al. Adherence to a mediterranean-like dietary pattern in children from eight european countries. The idefics study. *Int. J. Obes. (Lond.)* **2014**, *38 Suppl 2*, S108–S114. [CrossRef]
50. Lydakis, C.; Stefanaki, E.; Stefanaki, S.; Thalassinos, E.; Kavousanaki, M.; Lydaki, D. Correlation of blood pressure, obesity, and adherence to the mediterranean diet with indices of arterial stiffness in children. *Eur. J. Pediatr.* **2012**, *171*, 1373–1382. [CrossRef] [PubMed]
51. Schroder, H.; Mendez, M.A.; Ribas-Barba, L.; Covas, M.I.; Serra-Majem, L. Mediterranean diet and waist circumference in a representative national sample of young spaniards. *Int. J. Pediatr. Obes.* **2010**, *5*, 516–519. [CrossRef] [PubMed]

52. Martin-Calvo, N.; Chavarro, J.E.; Falbe, J.; Hu, F.B.; Field, A.E. Adherence to the mediterranean dietary pattern and bmi change among us adolescents. *Int. J. Obes. (Lond.)* **2016**, *40*, 1103–1108. [CrossRef] [PubMed]
53. Tognon, G.; Hebestreit, A.; Lanfer, A.; Moreno, L.A.; Pala, V.; Siani, A.; Tornaritis, M.; De Henauw, S.; Veidebaum, T.; Molnár, D.; et al. Mediterranean diet, overweight and body composition in children from eight european countries: Cross-sectional and prospective results from the idefics study. *Nutr. Metab. Cardiovasc. Dis.* **2014**, *24*, 205–213. [CrossRef] [PubMed]
54. Farajian, P.; Risvas, G.; Karasouli, K.; Pounis, G.D.; Kastorini, C.M.; Panagiotakos, D.B.; Zampelas, A. Very high childhood obesity prevalence and low adherence rates to the mediterranean diet in greek children: The greco study. *Atherosclerosis* **2011**, *217*, 525–530. [CrossRef] [PubMed]
55. Jennings, A.; Welch, A.; van Sluijs, E.M.; Griffin, S.J.; Cassidy, A. Diet quality is independently associated with weight status in children aged 9–10 years. *J. Nutr.* **2011**, *141*, 453–459. [CrossRef] [PubMed]
56. Velazquez-Lopez, L.; Santiago-Diaz, G.; Nava-Hernandez, J.; Munoz-Torres, A.V.; Medina-Bravo, P.; Torres-Tamayo, M. Mediterranean-style diet reduces metabolic syndrome components in obese children and adolescents with obesity. *BMC Pediatr.* **2014**, *14*, 175. [CrossRef] [PubMed]
57. Romaguera, D.; Norat, T.; Vergnaud, A.C.; Mouw, T.; May, A.M.; Agudo, A.; Buckland, G.; Slimani, N.; Rinaldi, S.; Couto, E.; et al. Mediterranean dietary patterns and prospective weight change in participants of the epic-panacea project. *Am. J. Clin. Nutr.* **2010**, *92*, 912–921. [CrossRef] [PubMed]
58. Buckland, G.; Bach, A.; Serra-Majem, L. Obesity and the mediterranean diet: A systematic review of observational and intervention studies. *Obes. Rev.* **2008**, *9*, 582–593. [CrossRef] [PubMed]
59. Shai, I.; Schwarzfuchs, D.; Henkin, Y.; Shahar, D.R.; Witkow, S.; Greenberg, I.; Golan, R.; Fraser, D.; Bolotin, A.; Vardi, H.; et al. Weight loss with a low-carbohydrate, mediterranean, or low-fat diet. *N. Engl. J. Med.* **2008**, *359*, 229–241. [CrossRef] [PubMed]
60. Bonaccio, M.; Di Castelnuovo, A.; Costanzo, S.; De Lucia, F.; Olivieri, M.; Donati, M.B.; de Gaetano, G.; Iacoviello, L.; Bonanni, A. Nutrition knowledge is associated with higher adherence to mediterranean diet and lower prevalence of obesity. Results from the moli-sani study. *Appetite* **2013**, *68*, 139–146. [CrossRef] [PubMed]
61. Michels, K.B.; Schulze, M.B. Can dietary patterns help us detect diet-disease associations? *Nutr. Res. Rev.* **2005**, *18*, 241–248. [CrossRef] [PubMed]
62. McNaughton, S.A.; Ball, K.; Mishra, G.D.; Crawford, D.A. Dietary patterns of adolescents and risk of obesity and hypertension. *J. Nutr.* **2008**, *138*, 364–370. [CrossRef] [PubMed]
63. Northstone, K.; Emmett, P.M. Are dietary patterns stable throughout early and mid-childhood? A birth cohort study. *Br. J. Nutr.* **2008**, *100*, 1069–1076. [CrossRef] [PubMed]
64. Craig, L.C.; McNeill, G.; Macdiarmid, J.I.; Masson, L.F.; Holmes, B.A. Dietary patterns of school-age children in scotland: Association with socio-economic indicators, physical activity and obesity. *Br. J. Nutr.* **2010**, *103*, 319–334. [CrossRef] [PubMed]
65. Richter, A.; Heidemann, C.; Schulze, M.B.; Roosen, J.; Thiele, S.; Mensink, G.B. Dietary patterns of adolescents in Germany—associations with nutrient intake and other health related lifestyle characteristics. *BMC Pediatr.* **2012**, *12*, 35. [CrossRef] [PubMed]
66. Weikert, C.; Schulze, M.B. Evaluating dietary patterns: The role of reduced rank regression. *Curr. Opin. Clin. Nutr. Metab. Care* **2016**, *19*, 341–346. [CrossRef] [PubMed]
67. Simpson, S.J.; Raubenheimer, D. Perspective: Tricks of the trade. *Nature* **2014**, *508*, S66. [CrossRef] [PubMed]
68. Gosby, A.K.; Conigrave, A.D.; Raubenheimer, D.; Simpson, S.J. Protein leverage and energy intake. *Obes. Rev.* **2014**, *15*, 183–191. [CrossRef] [PubMed]
69. Solon-Biet, S.M.; McMahon, A.C.; Ballard, J.W.; Ruohonen, K.; Wu, L.E.; Cogger, V.C.; Warren, A.; Huang, X.; Pichaud, N.; Melvin, R.G.; et al. The ratio of macronutrients, not caloric intake, dictates cardiometabolic health, aging, and longevity in ad libitum-fed mice. *Cell Metab.* **2014**, *19*, 418–430. [CrossRef] [PubMed]
70. Berryman, C.E.; Agarwal, S.; Lieberman, H.R.; Fulgoni, V.L., 3rd; Pasiakos, S.M. Diets higher in animal and plant protein are associated with lower adiposity and do not impair kidney function in us adults. *Am. J. Clin. Nutr.* **2016**, *104*, 743–749. [CrossRef] [PubMed]
71. Pasiakos, S.M.; Lieberman, H.R.; Fulgoni, V.L. , 3rd. Higher-protein diets are associated with higher hdl cholesterol and lower bmi and waist circumference in us adults. *J. Nutr.* **2015**, *145*, 605–614. [CrossRef] [PubMed]

72. Jen, V.; Karagounis, L.G.; Jaddoe, V.W.V.; Franco, O.H.; Voortman, T. Dietary protein intake in school-age children and detailed measures of body composition: The generation r study. *Int. J. Obes. (Lond.)* **2018**. [CrossRef] [PubMed]
73. Buyken, A.E.; Bolzenius, K.; Karaolis-Danckert, N.; Gunther, A.L.; Kroke, A. Body composition trajectories into adolescence according to age at pubertal growth spurt. *Am. J. Hum. Biol.* **2011**, *23*, 216–224. [CrossRef] [PubMed]
74. Johannsen, M. *Übergewicht bei 5–7-jährigen Kindern. Analyse von Trends, Determinanten und gesundheitlichen Auswirkungen*; eine Untersuchung im Rahmen der Kieler Adipositas-Präventionsstudie (KOPS). Der Andere Verlag: Tönning, Lübeck, Marburg, Germany, 2009.
75. Gose, M.; Plachta-Danielzik, S.; Kehden, B.; Johannsen, M.; Landsberg, B.; Müller, M. Trends in incidence and determinants of overweight among 9–11-year-old children–kiel obesity prevention study (KOPS). *Obesity Facts* **2013**, *6*, 202.
76. Costello, A.B.; Osborne, J. Best practices in exploratory factor analysis: Four recommendations for getting the most from your analysis. *Pract. Assess. Res. Eval.* **2005**, *10*, 1–9.

10

International Study of Childhood Obesity, Lifestyle and the Environment (ISCOLE): Contributions to Understanding the Global Obesity Epidemic

Peter T. Katzmarzyk [1,*], Jean-Philippe Chaput [2], Mikael Fogelholm [3], Gang Hu [1], Carol Maher [4], Jose Maia [5], Timothy Olds [4], Olga L. Sarmiento [6], Martyn Standage [7], Mark S. Tremblay [2] and Catrine Tudor-Locke [8]

1 Pennington Biomedical Research Center, 6400 Perkins Road, Baton Rouge, LA 70808, USA; gang.hu@pbrc.edu
2 Children's Hospital of Eastern Ontario Research Institute, Ottawa, ON K1H 8L1, Canada; jpchaput@cheo.on.ca (J.-P.C.); mtremblay@cheo.on.ca (M.S.T.)
3 Department of Food and Environmental Sciences, University of Helsinki, 00014 Helsinki, Finland; mikael.fogelholm@helsinki.fi
4 School of Health Sciences, Sansom Institute, University of South Australia, Adelaide, SA 5001, Australia; Carol.Maher@unisa.edu.au (C.M.); timothy.olds@unisa.edu.au (T.O.)
5 Faculdade de Desporto, University of Porto, Rua Dr. Plácido Costa, 91, 4200-450 Porto, Portugal; jmaia@fade.up.pt
6 School of Medicine, Universidad de los Andes, Bogota 11001000, Colombia; osarmien@uniandes.edu.co
7 Department for Health, University of Bath, Bath BA2 7AY, UK; m.standage@bath.ac.uk
8 Department of Kinesiology, University of Massachusetts, Amherst, MA 01003, USA; ctudorlocke@umass.edu
* Correspondence: peter.katzmarzyk@pbrc.edu

Abstract: The purpose of this review is to summarize the scientific contributions of the International Study of Childhood Obesity, Lifestyle and the Environment (ISCOLE) in extending our understanding about obesity in children from around the world. ISCOLE was a multi-national study of 9 to 11 year-old children from sites in 12 countries from all inhabited continents. The primary purpose was to investigate relationships between lifestyle behaviors and obesity, and the influence of higher-order characteristics such as behavioral settings, and physical, social and policy environments. ISCOLE has made several advances in scientific methodology related to the assessment of physical activity, dietary behavior, sleep and the neighborhood and school environments. Furthermore, ISCOLE has provided important evidence on (1) epidemiological transitions in obesity and related behaviors, (2) correlates of obesity and lifestyle behaviors at the individual, neighborhood and school levels, and (3) 24-h movement behaviors in relation to novel analytical techniques. A key feature of ISCOLE was the development of a platform for international training, data entry, and data quality for multi-country studies. Finally, ISCOLE represents a transparent model for future public-private research partnerships across low, middle and high-income countries.

Keywords: pediatric; overweight; epidemiological transition; collaboration

---

1. Introduction

The prevalence of childhood obesity has increased significantly in recent years and remains high in many countries [1]. Given the global nature of the problem, a greater understanding of context-specific correlates of obesity is required in order to develop effective interventions that can be translated from one setting to another. To date, there have been only limited attempts to understand the correlates of adiposity or obesity in specific world regions using standardized methods. Large multi-country studies of childhood obesity and/or related behavioral risk factors (physical activity, diet, etc.) have been largely limited to the European region [2–6]. Therefore, the primary aim of the International Study of Childhood Obesity, Lifestyle and the Environment (ISCOLE) was to investigate relationships between lifestyle behaviors and obesity, and the influence of higher-order characteristics such as behavioral settings, and the physical, social and policy environments, on the observed relationships within and between countries that vary widely in levels of human development [7]. ISCOLE was a multi-national study of 9–11 year-old children from research sites in 12 countries from all inhabited continents ranging widely in environmental and socio-cultural contexts.

The purpose of this paper is to summarize the scientific contributions of ISCOLE in extending our understanding about obesity in children from around the world. The focus is primarily on the results from analyses that utilized the 12-country dataset; nevertheless, a large number of papers have also been generated using country-specific datasets or data from small clusters of countries. A complete list of scientific peer-reviewed papers to date from ISCOLE can be found in the online Supplementary Materials (Supplementary File S1).

2. Study Design

A detailed description of the ISCOLE design and methods has been published elsewhere [7]. Briefly, ISCOLE was a multi-national, cross-sectional study conducted in 12 countries (Australia, Brazil, Canada, China, Colombia, Finland, India, Kenya, Portugal, South Africa, United Kingdom, United States) from all inhabited continents. A total of 7372 9–11 year old children participated in ISCOLE [8]. In addition to including sites from countries across a wide range of human development, children were sampled across a range of family socio-economic status within each country. By design, the ISCOLE samples are not representative of the populations from which the participants were drawn. However, an analysis of ISCOLE data compared to other available studies across many world regions suggests that there is no evidence that the ISCOLE samples are systematically biased [9]. These results suggest that ISCOLE data could be used cautiously to inform the development of country-level interventions when other data are lacking.

Table 1 provides descriptive characteristics of the sample by study site, ranked according to the prevalence of obesity. The Human Development Index (HDI) of the study sites ranged from 0.509 in Kenya to 0.929 in Australia. The average age of the sample was 10.4 years, and the prevalence of obesity ranged from 5.4% in Finland to 23.7% in China. Level of parental education also varied among the study sites; with the proportion of the sample with parents having at least a bachelor's degree ranging from 12.9% in South Africa to 73.4% in India.

All ISCOLE data were collected under a standardized research protocol using the same instrumentation at all study sites. Data included objectively measured indicators of adiposity and obesity (body mass index (BMI), waist circumference, body fat), lifestyle behaviors related to obesity (diet, physical activity, sleep, etc.), demographics and family health history, the home and neighborhood environment, and the school environment. All information was entered remotely (anthropometry, questionnaires, etc.) or uploaded (accelerometry) on a secure web-based data entry platform. ISCOLE employed a rigorous quality assurance and quality control program. This program included comprehensive in-person training and certification of all investigators and staff, random remote source data verification, in-person site monitoring visits, and data cleaning and final source data verification [7].

Table 1. Descriptive characteristics of the study sample from the International Study of Childhood Obesity, Lifestyle and the Environment (ISCOLE).

Study Site	HDI *	Boys (*n*)	Girls (*n*)	Age (year) **	NW (%)	OV (%)	OB (%)	Parent Education (%)		
								1	2	3
China (Tianjin)	**0.687**	**293**	**259**	**9.9 (0.4)**	**58.9**	**17.4**	23.7	33.0	44.4	22.6
Brazil (Sao Paulo)	0.718	287	297	10.5 (0.5)	56.3	22.8	20.9	24.3	52.8	22.9
United States (Baton Rouge)	0.910	281	370	10.0 (0.6)	58.8	22.4	18.7	8.9	44.6	46.6
Portugal (Porto)	0.809	358	419	10.4 (0.3)	52.8	29.7	17.5	46.7	32.8	20.5
Canada (Ottawa)	0.908	239	328	10.5 (0.4)	69.3	18.9	11.8	2.0	27.7	70.4
South Africa (Cape Town)	0.619	223	327	10.3 (0.7)	73.6	15.6	10.7	48.0	39.0	12.9
Australia (Adelaide)	0.929	243	285	10.7 (0.4)	62.1	27.5	10.4	11.4	47.7	40.9
India (Bangalore)	0.547	292	328	10.4 (0.5)	66.3	23.4	10.3	4.8	21.7	73.4
United Kingdom (Bath)	0.863	237	288	10.9 (0.5)	69.7	20.6	9.7	3.0	51.6	45.4
Kenya (Nairobi)	0.509	262	301	10.2 (0.7)	78.9	14.6	6.6	13.9	45.7	40.4
Colombia (Bogota)	0.710	454	465	10.5 (0.6)	77.2	17.1	5.8	31.8	50.7	17.5
Finland (Helsinki)	0.882	253	283	10.5 (0.4)	76.3	18.3	5.4	2.8	55.1	42.1

* Human Development Index [10]; ** Mean (SD); NW: normal weight; OV: overweight; OB: obese. Parent education levels are 1 <high school and some high school, 2 completed high school and some post-secondary (e.g., vocational diploma or certificate); 3 bachelor degree and post-graduate.

3. Advances in Scientific Methodology Related to the Assessment of Physical Activity, Sleep, Dietary Behavior, and the Neighborhood, Home and School Environments

Mounting a multi-national study of the scale of ISCOLE required the development of novel methods and the adaptation of existing tools that could be applied in sites that ranged considerably in level of human development. This section summarizes some of the methodological advances that were developed during the planning and implementation of ISCOLE. As described above, we have made all of our protocols and algorithms publicly available, and we have summarized our contributions to the use of accelerometry in large studies in detail elsewhere [11,12].

3.1. Physical Activity

A major strength of ISCOLE was the objective assessment of physical activity and sedentary behavior using a waist-mounted accelerometer protocol that was deployed in all study sites [7,11]. Awake-time wear protocols typically require the participants to remove their accelerometer before going to bed and then to reapply it in the morning upon waking. Concerns about wear time compliance have led some investigators to adopt a wrist-mounted rather than a waist-mounted protocol [13]. For example, the U.S. National Health and Nutrition Examination Survey (NHANES) switched from a waist-mounted to a wrist-mounted protocol between the 2005–2006 and 2011–2012 cycles of the survey [13]. In ISCOLE, we chose to attempt to improve wear time compliance by using a waist-mounted 24-h protocol rather than moving to a wrist-mounted protocol [7,14].

The 24-h protocol employed in ISCOLE resulted in impressive increases in wear time in comparison to previous studies. The average wear time in ISCOLE was 22.8 h per day [8]. Given that NHANES used a wake-only protocol, no direct comparisons can be made for total wear time. However, we conducted a study comparing the US ISCOLE site with the 2003–2006 NHANES (that used the waist mounted protocol), and the awake wear time in ISCOLE was 14.7 h per day compared to 13.7 h per day in NHANES, which represents a one hour per day improvement when using the 24-h protocol [14].

Using a 7-day protocol allowed us to estimate the reliability of accelerometer-determined physical activity and sedentary behavior [15]. The estimated minimum number of days needed to achieve a reliability of $G \geq 0.8$ ranged from 5 to 9 for boys and 3 to 11 for girls for light physical activity; 5 to 9 and 3 to 10 for moderate-to-vigorous intensity physical activity; 5 to 10 and 4 to 10 for total activity counts; and 7 to 11 and 6 to 11 for sedentary time, respectively [15]. The results demonstrate that, in most cases, close to seven days of monitored time is required to achieve adequate reliability; and future studies should take this into account when designing their protocols.

3.2. Sleep

The availability of seven days of 24-h accelerometry data in ISCOLE provided an opportunity to develop algorithms to objectively identify the sleep period [16,17]. Over several months, we developed a fully automated algorithm for identifying the nocturnal total sleep episode time in two stages. The first step was to develop and validate an initial algorithm against expert visual inspection of the data [16]. The initial algorithm combined aspects of the Sadeh algorithm [18] for sleep–wake scoring, made use of the inclinometer function in the accelerometer, and built upon the framework of the publicly available non-wear algorithm developed by the National Cancer Institute [19]. The initial algorithm identified sleep onset (i.e., 'bedtime') and sleep offset (i.e., 'waking') times. The second step was to refine the algorithm by adding the ability to identify disrupted nocturnal sleep episodes (and exclude episodes of nighttime non-wear/wakefulness) and avoid misclassification of daytime non-wear or sedentary behavior as sleep [17]. Compared with sleep logs, we achieved acceptable levels of accuracy (<10% mean absolute percent difference) [17]. The Pennington Biomedical Research Center (PBRC) hosts public web-based access to both the original [20] and refined [21] algorithms. As a companion to the sleep algorithms, we have published a full catalog of nocturnal sleep-related variables in ISCOLE [22].

3.3. Dietary Behavior

The primary dietary information used in ISCOLE was collected using a Food Frequency Questionnaire (FFQ) adapted from the Health Behavior in School-aged Children Survey [23]. The ISCOLE FFQ asks about the consumption of 23 food items, and was adapted for use in each of the 12 study sites [7]. We conducted a reliability and validity study in three culturally different study sites (Finland, US, and Colombia) [24]. Reliability correlation coefficients from two surveys completed ~5 weeks apart ranged from 0.37 to 0.78 and gross misclassification for all food groups was <5%. Validity correlation coefficients were below 0.5 for 22/23 food groups and gross misclassification was <5% for 22/23 food groups. Over- or underestimation did not appear for 19/23 food groups [24].

To identify dietary patterns, principal components analyses (PCA) were carried out using weekly portions as input variables [25]. Both site-specific and pooled data showed that dietary behaviors in ISCOLE to be well defined by two component solutions. We labelled the first component as the "unhealthy diet pattern", which included sugar-sweetened sodas, fast foods, ice cream, fried food, French fries, potato chips, and cakes. The second component we characterized as the "healthy diet pattern", which included dark-green vegetables, orange vegetables, fish, cheese, whole grains and fruits. Figure 1 presents the loadings for the two principal components.

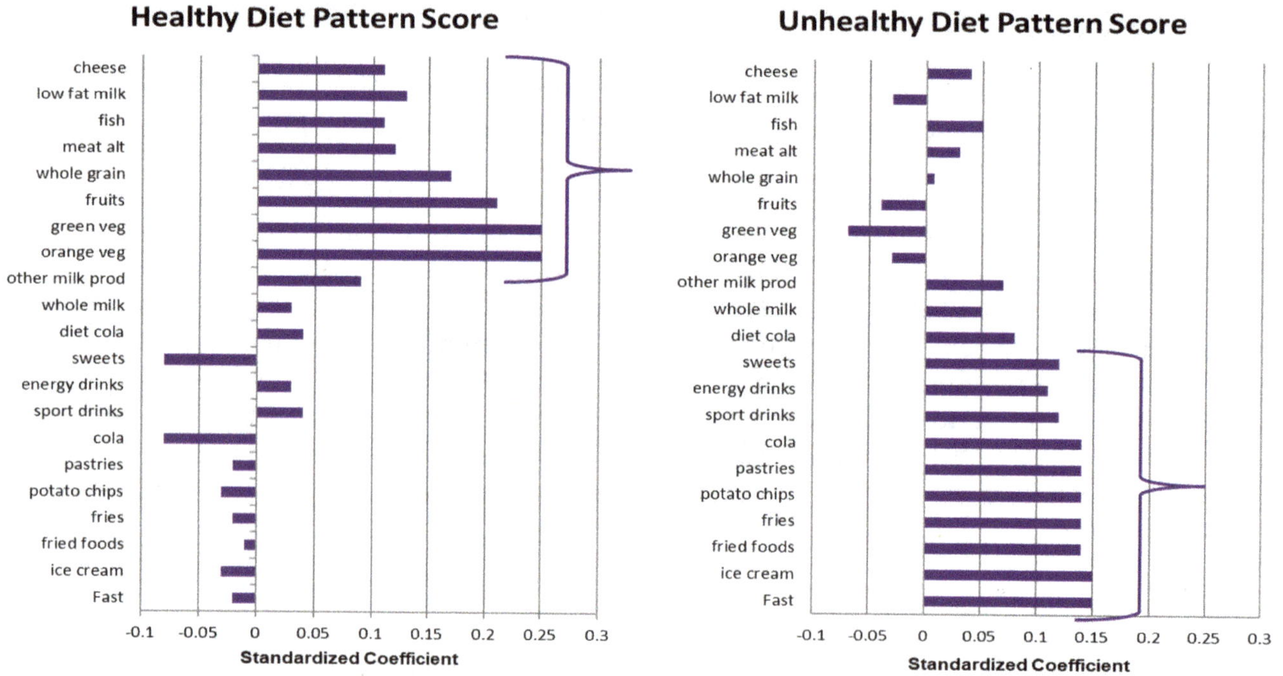

Figure 1. Principal component loadings for the healthy and unhealthy diet pattern scores in the International Study of Childhood Obesity, Lifestyle and the Environment (ISCOLE) (all sites combined), from Mikkila et al. [25].

3.4. Neighborhood, Home and School Environments

Information on several aspects of the neighborhood, home and school environments were collected in ISCOLE using a variety of approaches. A neighborhood and home environment questionnaire, which was based on the Neighborhood Impact on Kids (NIK) survey [26], was completed by parents/guardians. The school environment was assessed using two approaches. First, a school administrator questionnaire, which covered school facilities, healthy eating and physical activity policies, extracurricular activities, frequency of physical education and breaks (recess), and availability of healthy and unhealthy food, was completed by a school official [7]. Second, a school audit of the physical environment was performed at each participating school by one of the study staff. Each site completed a reliability audit (simultaneous audits by two independent, certified data collectors) for a minimum of two schools or at least 5% of their school sample [27]. For the assessed environmental features, inter-rater reliability (kappa) ranged from 0.37 to 0.96; 18 items (42%) were assessed with almost perfect reliability (K = 0.80–0.96), and a further 24 items (56%) were assessed with substantial reliability (K = 0.61–0.79) [27]. These results suggest that the ISCOLE school audit can be used to conduct reliable objective audits of the school environment across diverse, international school settings. However, the administration of the school audit tool can be challenging in some contexts, such as in countries where snow may cover or change aspects of the school environment. Furthermore, research is required to validate these tools under different environmental conditions.

4. Epidemiological Transitions in Obesity and Related Behaviors

The theory of epidemiologic transition characterizes long-term changes in patterns of morbidity and mortality away from causes related to undernutrition and infectious diseases towards chronic 'man-made' diseases as countries become more developed [28]. Related to the concept of epidemiological transition, theories about parallel nutritional and physical activity transitions have been described [29,30]. The nutrition transition is characterized by a shift away from traditional diets that were based on staple grains, local legumes, and fruits and vegetables, towards a diet comprised of more animal-based food products and processed food high in saturated fats and sugar [29]. The physical activity transition is characterized by long-term shifts in physical activity patterns away from necessity (acquiring food, water and shelter, escaping predation, procreation or transport in settings with low motor vehicle availability) towards a largely inactive lifestyle in high-income countries where physical activity has been successfully engineered out of our everyday lives. In high-income countries, humans no longer need to be physically active out of necessity but instead act out of choice to be physically active because of enjoyment, maintenance of body weight, employment, and the prevention of chronic diseases [30]. Whereas in lower-middle income countries where car availability remains relatively low in comparison to high income countries, physical activity could be more reflective of purposeful transport rather than leisure pursuits. These parallel transitions in nutrition and physical activity may contribute to the increased chronic disease burden associated with the epidemiological transition, such as higher rates of obesity, type 2 diabetes, cardiovascular disease, and many cancers.

A review of studies from Western developed countries published between 1990 and 2005 concluded that there was a significant inverse association between socio-economic status and obesity and that positive associations had all but disappeared [31]. However, little is known about how indicators of childhood obesity vary across levels of socio-economic status among countries at different levels of the human development index (HDI). ISCOLE was uniquely positioned to answer this question. Our results demonstrated that BMI and percent body fat were positively associated with family income in countries with low HDI, negatively associated in countries at high HDI, with no association in countries with an HDI in the midrange [32]. Similar patterns were observed for the association between HDI and the prevalence of obesity (Figure 2), reflecting variability in the stages of nutrition and physical activity transitions among countries.

In addition to obesity, we tested for socio-economic gradients in physical activity, dietary patterns and sleep duration in ISCOLE [33–35]. In girls, time spent in moderate-to-vigorous physical activity was negatively associated with family income at the 10th and 50th percentiles HDI (all $p < 0.012$); and positively related with family income at the 90th percentile ($p = 0.044$) [35]. In boys, time spent in moderate-to-vigorous physical activity was also negatively associated with family income at the 10th and 50th percentiles of HDI (both $p < 0.001$) [35]. These results are consistent with the existence of a physical activity transition. A parallel analysis of dietary patterns demonstrated that lower family income was associated with a higher "unhealthy" dietary pattern score and a lower "healthy" dietary pattern score in many countries; however, the pattern was not reflective of a nutrition transition in dietary patterns in these counties [34]. Finally, we also explored the association between sleep duration and family income [33]. No significant associations were observed in any site, and the summary odds ratio was also not significant (OR = 0.94; 95% Confidence Interval (CI) = 0.60 – 1.47) [33].

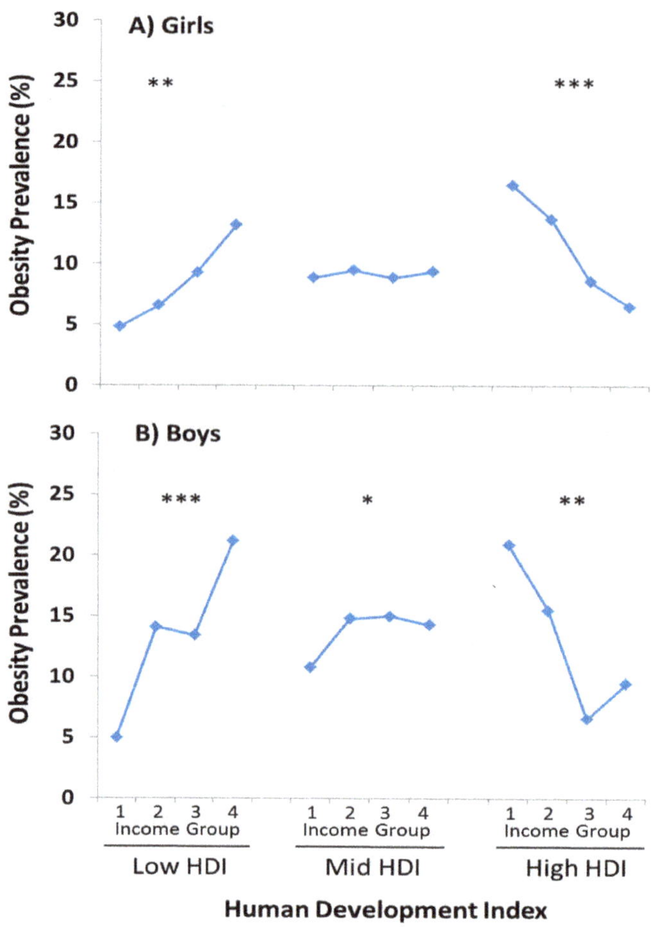

Figure 2. Income gradients in obesity prevalence across levels of HDI in (**A**) girls and (**B**) boys from ISCOLE. Low, middle and high human development index (HDI) correspond to the 10th, 50th and 90th percentiles of the ISCOLE sample (HDI = 0.52, 0.72 and 0.91, respectively). Tests for linear trend are indicated: * $p < 0.05$; ** $p < 0.001$; *** $p < 0.0001$. Figure is adapted from Broyles et al. [32].

In summary, in ISCOLE, we found evidence of epidemiological transitions in obesity and physical activity, but not for dietary patterns and sleep duration. Furthermore, research is required to better characterize country-level changes in these behaviors using temporal surveillance data in countries undergoing rapid economic and social development.

5. Correlates of Obesity and Lifestyle Behaviors at Multiple Levels

5.1. The Socio-Ecological Model

The socio-ecological model is a variant of the root Ecological Systems Theory firstly developed by Bronfenbrenner [36]. Socio-ecological models have been proposed as frameworks to think about the influences of factors at several levels (individual, social, physical and policy environments) on obesity, physical activity and dietary intake [37–39]. ISCOLE was designed to help answer some questions about the contributions of factors at multiple levels of the socio-ecological model to childhood obesity and related behaviors. Our study was a nested design, with individuals (Level 1) nested within schools (Level 2), which were in turn nested within study sites (Level 3). This design necessitated the use of multi-level mixed models for data analysis. This approach also allowed us to partition the percentage of the variance in several variables that is explained by factors at all three levels. The multilevel model is highly elegant in its statistical formulation [40], as well as its versatility [41] which made it a valid model to use with the hierarchical system of information gathered from different levels as in ISCOLE—individuals nested within schools which are nested within research sites. Furthermore, within-level as well as cross-level interactions were considered as per the ISCOLE framework, and these were modeled and statistically tested to verify their substantive tenability.

We undertook an analysis that estimated the proportion of the variance in several key variables at the study site, school and individual levels [42]. The proportion of the variance in BMI and waist circumference explained at the individual level is greater than 90%; the proportion of the variance explained in dietary patterns, sleep, physical activity and sedentary time at the individual level ranges between 66% and 88%, while the proportion of the variance in in-school physical activity and in-school sedentary behavior explained at the site and school levels is between 46% and 75%, with less of a contribution from individual-level factors [42]. These results suggest that interventions that target policy and environmental changes for increasing school-based physical activity and reducing in-school sedentary behavior may enhance obesity intervention efforts.

5.2. Obesity

Several analyses have been undertaken to identify the correlates of obesity in ISCOLE. Our first investigation involved determining the associations between several lifestyle traits (healthy diet patterns, unhealthy diet patterns, moderate-to-vigorous physical activity, TV viewing time, and sleep duration) and the presence of obesity [8]. The odds ratios for obesity (per standard deviation of the predictor variable) were 0.51 (95% CI: 0.45–0.57) for moderate-to-vigorous physical activity, 0.79 (95% CI: 0.72–0.86) for sleep duration, and 1.11 (95% CI: 1.04–1.19) for TV viewing time, while the diet pattern scores were not related to obesity [8]. The results were consistent in boys and girls. These findings led to an in-depth examination of the associations among obesity and accelerometer-derived measures of physical activity and sedentary behavior [43]. In the overall sample, the odds ratios for obesity (per standard deviation of each predictor variable) were significant for sedentary time (1.19; 1.08–1.30), moderate-to-vigorous physical activity (0.49; 95% CI, 0.44–0.55), and vigorous physical activity (0.41; 0.37–0.46). Furthermore, the associations of moderate-to-vigorous physical activity and vigorous physical activity with obesity were significant in all 12 sites, whereas the association between sedentary time and obesity was significant in five of the 12 sites [43].

Active school transport is one potential opportunity for children to accumulate physical activity during the day. Thus, we examined the association between active school transport and indicators of adiposity in ISCOLE [44]. After adjusting for several covariates, children who reported active school transport were less likely to be obese (odds ratio = 0.72, 95% CI: 0.60–0.87) and had a lower BMI z-score, percent body fat and waist circumference (all $p < 0.05$) compared with those who reported motorized travel [44]. Furthermore, the associations between active school transport and obesity did not differ by country or by sex.

Although we found that dietary patterns were not related to obesity in ISCOLE [8], we further explored the association between specific dietary behaviors and obesity. For example, frequent breakfast consumption was associated with lower BMI z-scores compared with occasional ($p < 0.0001$) and rare ($p < 0.0001$) consumption, as well as lower percentage body fat compared with occasional ($p < 0.0001$) and rare ($p < 0.0001$) consumption [45]. These associations differed significantly across study sites, and further research is required to understand these differences. We also explored the association between soft drink consumption and obesity [46]. There was a significant linear trend for increasing BMI z-scores across increasing consumption of regular soft drinks in boys ($p = 0.049$), but not in girls. On the other hand, there was no significant linear trend across categories of diet soft drink consumption in boys, but there was a graded, positive association in girls for BMI z-score ($p = 0.0002$) [46].

Evidence from high-income countries has identified associations between gestational diabetes and birth weight with subsequent childhood obesity. We explored these associations in the multi-national sample from ISCOLE. Compared to children with mothers who did not experience gestational diabetes, children with mothers who experienced gestational diabetes had an odds ratio of 1.53 (95% CI: 1.03–2.27) for obesity, 1.73 (95% CI: 1.14–2.62) for central obesity, and 1.42 (95% CI: 0.90–2.26) for high percentage body fat [47]. Furthermore, the odds ratios for obesity were 1.45 (95% CI: 1.10–1.92) for those with birthweight of 3500–3999 g and 2.08 (95% CI: 1.47–2.93) for those with birthweight ≥4000 g, compared with those with birthweight of 2500–2999 g [48]. The positive association between birth weight and obesity was linear in girls, whereas it was U-shaped in boys. We further explored the association between birthweight and obesity by examining interactions with physical activity and sedentary behavior. Interestingly, the positive association between birthweight and obesity was significant among children with either low moderate-to-vigorous physical activity or high sedentary time, but not among children with either high moderate-to-vigorous physical activity or low sedentary time [49].

Building upon the evidence supporting the inter-generational transmission of obesity, we found that parental overweight was associated with childhood overweight in the overall ISCOLE sample [50]. Furthermore, parental education was differentially associated with childhood overweight across the ISCOLE study sites, and more research is required to understand the context-specific associations between parental education and childhood overweight and obesity.

5.3. *Physical Activity and Sedentary Behavior*

Current public health recommendations call for children and youth to accumulate at least 60 min of moderate-to-vigorous physical activity every day [51]. In ISCOLE, 4.8% of children achieved ≥60 min of moderate-to-vigorous physical activity for all seven days of the week, while 25.5% attained the recommendation ≥5 days [52]. Furthermore, a total of 18.8% of the sample did not accumulate ≥60 min of moderate-to-vigorous on any of the monitored days [52]. There was variability in compliance to the guidelines across sites: the mean number of days of compliance ranged from 1.8 days per week in the United States to 3.5 days per week in Colombia [52]. Given the availability of 24-h, time-stamped accelerometry data and detailed information about the start and stop times for each student's school in ISCOLE, we were able to differentiate between before-school, during-school and after-school physical activity and sedentary behavior.

Physical education classes are an important opportunity for physical activity in children and youth. In ISCOLE, approximately 25% of participants reported attending physical education classes on three or more days per week [53]. After adjusting for several covariates, children who took physical education classes were more likely to have higher levels of physical activity and shorter time in spent in sedentary behavior both in and out of school during the school week [53].

We also found that children who used active school transportation had significantly higher weekday moderate-to-vigorous physical activity and significantly lower light physical activity before school compared with children who used motorized transport to school [54]. On average, children who used active transportation accumulated 6.0 (95% CI: 4.7–7.3) min more moderate-to-vigorous physical activity per day than children who used motorized transportation. There was wide variability in the prevalence of active school transportation across study sites, which varied from 5.2% in India to 79.4% in Finland [55]. We found wide variability in the correlates that were associated with active school transport across study sites. Longer trip duration (≥16 min vs. ≤15 min) was associated with lower odds of active school transportation in eight sites; whereas individual and neighborhood factors were associated with active school transportation in three sites or less [55].

In ISCOLE, we also investigated home and neighborhood correlates of physical activity. Across sites, children with at least one piece of electronic media in their bedroom had lower levels of moderate-to-vigorous physical activity than those who did not ($p < 0.001$) [56]. More frequent physical activity in the home and yard, ownership of more frequently used play equipment, and higher social support for physical activity were also associated with higher moderate-to-vigorous physical activity ($p < 0.0001$). However, association between play equipment ownership and moderate-to-vigorous physical activity varied across study sites ($p_{\text{interaction}} < 0.01$), suggesting that cultural differences should be studied further when developing interventions or making recommendations [56].

Aspects of the neighborhood social environment (collective efficacy and perceived crime) were also studied in ISCOLE as potential correlates of moderate-to-vigorous physical activity [57]. Collective efficacy was inversely associated with moderate-to-vigorous physical activity among children in low/lower-middle-income countries (β = −1.96; 95% CI: −3.72, −0.19) while it was positively associated with moderate-to-vigorous physical activity among children in high-income countries (β = 1.86; 95% CI: 0.76, 2.96) [57]. Perceived crime was significantly associated with lower moderate-to-vigorous physical activity (β = −2.12; 95% CI: −3.18, −1.06) among children in high-income countries but was not significantly associated with moderate-to-vigorous physical activity among children from low/lower-middle-income countries or upper-middle-income countries [57]. These results demonstrate heterogeneity in associations between aspects of the neighborhood environment and physical activity that need to be taken into account when developing strategies that target these correlates in different settings.

In addition to physical activity, we also investigated associations of 21 potential correlates with accelerometer-determined sedentary time and self-reported TV viewing time [58]. Boys reported greater TV viewing time than girls, while in 9 of 12 sites, girls engaged in more objectively-measured sedentary time than boys. Common correlates of sedentary time and TV viewing time included excess weight status, not meeting physical activity recommendations, and having a TV in the bedroom [58].

The associations between sleep and movement behaviors are currently of great interest [59]. In ISCOLE, sleep duration was negatively associated with moderate-to-vigorous physical activity and sedentary time, while sleep efficiency was negatively related to moderate-to-vigorous physical activity and positively associated with sedentary time [60]. The availability of time-stamped accelerometry data allowed us to examine temporal associations between sleep, physical activity and sedentary time [61]. Results showed that the relationships between sleep and physical activity and sedentary time are bi-directional. For example, for each one standard deviation (SD) unit increase in sleep duration, sedentary behavior was 0.04 SD units lower the following day, while light physical activity and moderate-to-vigorous physical activity were 0.04 and 0.02 SD units higher, respectively. Sleep duration was 0.02 SD units lower and 0.04 SD units higher for each one SD unit increase in sedentary time and moderate-to-vigorous physical activity, respectively [61]. While these results highlight the interactions between sleep and movement behaviors, the small effect sizes suggest that the clinical implications may be modest.

5.4. *Dietary Patterns*

As previously described, "healthy" and "unhealthy" dietary pattern scores were derived from FFQ data in ISCOLE [25]. Figure 3 presents the mean dietary scores across study sites. The results demonstrate variability in dietary pattern scores across countries, with the highest healthy dietary pattern score found in Canada, while the lowest is found in Colombia. Finland had the lowest unhealthy dietary pattern score while South Africa had the highest.

We explored the potential home and school environments as correlates of dietary patterns [62]. Here, we found that more meals eaten outside home and school were associated with higher unhealthy diet pattern scores. Furthermore, low availability of empty-calorie foods at home was found to be more important than high availability of wholesome foods at keeping unhealthy diet pattern scores low. The availability of wholesome foods at home was positively associated with the healthy diet pattern scores, while food availability at school was not associated with the dietary patterns [62]. In the ISCOLE sample, the home food environment was more significant than the school food environment in predicting the child's dietary patterns.

Given the availability of objective measures of sleep in ISCOLE, coupled with the FFQ data, we were able to study the association between sleep and dietary variables [60,63]. Both sleep duration and sleep efficiency were negatively associated with the unhealthy diet pattern score [60]. Interestingly, shorter sleep duration was associated with higher intake of regular soft drinks, while earlier bedtimes were associated with lower intake of regular soft drinks and higher intake of energy drinks and sports drinks [63]. More research is required to better understand the underlying mechanisms that might link beverage consumption to sleep patterns.

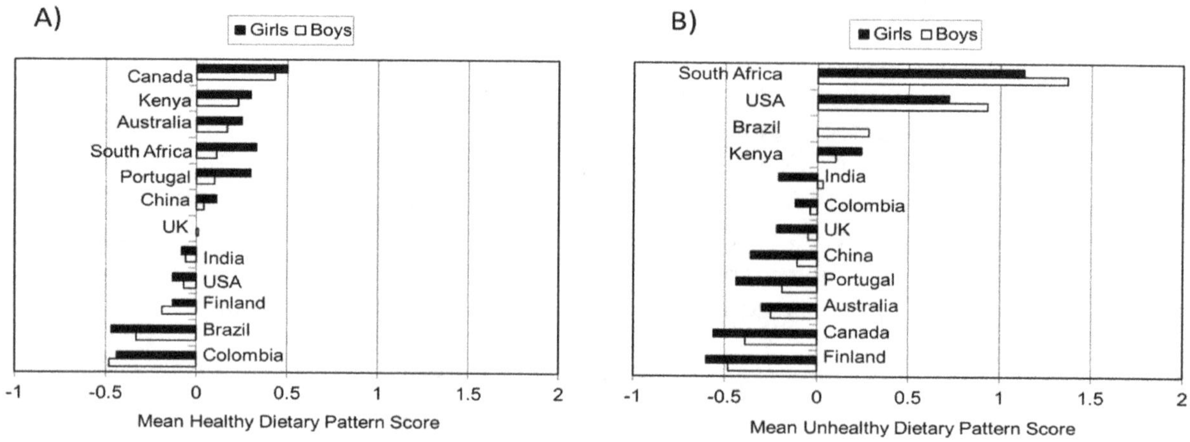

Figure 3. Mean dietary pattern scores across ISCOLE study sites. (**A**) presents the mean scores for the "healthy dietary pattern" and (**B**) presents the mean scores for the "unhealthy dietary pattern". Data were obtained from Mikkila et al. [25].

5.5. Higher-Order Correlates

Given that ISCOLE data were collected across multiple seasons in several geographical regions of the world, we were able to explore associations with other potential "higher-order" correlates of obesity and lifestyle behaviors. For example, we explored the association between moon phase, sleep and physical activity using data from 33,710 24-h accelerometer recordings of sleep and activity [64]. While differences in moderate-to-vigorous physical activity, light physical activity, and sedentary time between moon phases were negligible and non-significant (<2 min/day), sleep duration was significantly shorter (~5 min/night) during the full moon phase compared to the new moon phase [64]. Despite the statistical significance of the association between moon phase and sleep duration, the magnitude of the difference is unlikely to be clinically important.

The associations of weather with physical activity and sedentary time were explored using data from the Australian and Canadian ISCOLE sites [65]. Daily maximal temperature was significantly associated with physical activity and sedentary time in both Australia and Canada, and daily rainfall was negatively associated with physical activity in Australia and positively associated with sedentary time in Canada [65]. The results from both countries indicated that the best levels of physical activity and sedentary time occurred in a range between 20° and 25° Celsius. These results highlight the importance of taking weather into account in the development of intervention and surveillance strategies related to physical activity and sedentary behavior.

The associations of outdoor time with BMI, physical activity, sedentary time and dietary patterns were also explored in ISCOLE [66,67]. Time spent outside and dietary patterns were assessed by questionnaire, while time spent in physical activity and sedentary behavior were determined by accelerometry [7]. Time spent outside was not associated with BMI z-scores; however, each additional hour per day spent outdoors was associated with higher moderate-to-vigorous and light physical activity, and lower sedentary time [67]. Effect sizes were generally weaker in lower-middle-income countries. However, the evaluation of the Ciclovia in Colombia to promote physical activity outside on the streets was associated with higher moderate-to-vigorous and light physical activity, and lower sedentary time on Sundays [68]. Furthermore, time spent outdoors was positively associated with higher healthy dietary pattern scores, but there was no association with the unhealthy dietary pattern scores [66]. Similar patterns were observed in boys and girls, and across study sites. Research using longitudinal study designs is required to elucidate the mechanisms behind these observed associations.

6. The 24-h Movement Behavior Cycle in Relation to Integrated Guidelines and Novel Analytical Techniques

The focus of physical activity guidelines in public health has typically been on the promotion of moderate-to-vigorous physical activity. However, there has been increasing interest in understanding the health impacts associated with multiple movement behaviors (i.e., sedentary behavior, light activity, moderate-to-vigorous activity, and sleep) [59]. Canada has recently released *24-h Movement Guidelines for Children and Youth,* which attempts to integrate these movement behaviors [69]. For example, the guidelines recommend that 10 year-old children should accumulate at least 60 min of moderate-to-vigorous physical activity per day, sleep between 9 and 11 h per night, engage in no more than two hours of recreational screen time per day, spend several hours per day in light physical activity, while minimizing the time they spend sitting [69].

Figure 4 presents estimates of the mean proportions (%) of the day spent in sleep, sedentary behavior, and total physical activity (light, moderate and vigorous) in children across the 12 ISCOLE sites [70]. The mean proportions of the day spent in the different behaviors is remarkably similar across countries given the expanded axes of the ternary plot, as one would predict from the proportion of the variance in these variables that is explained at the site level [42]. The mean time spent in the movement behaviors ranges from 508 min in Portugal to 579 in the United Kingdom for sleep, from 486 min in Australia to 573 min in China for sedentary time, and from 336 min in China to 406 min in Kenya for total physical activity [70]. In addition to these three variables that constitute a 24-h day, mean levels of moderate-to-vigorous physical activity ranges from 43 min in China to 69 min in Finland [70].

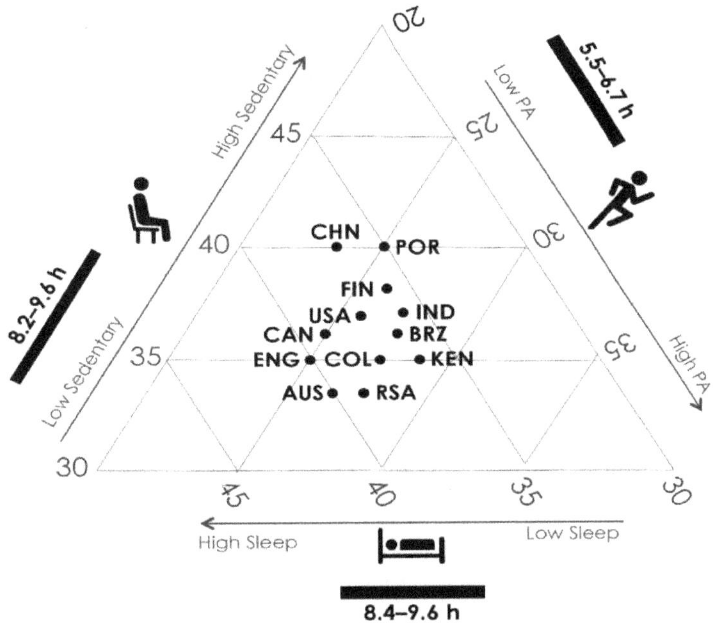

Figure 4. Ternary plot of the average proportions of the 24-h day spent in sleep (bottom axis), sedentary behaviour (left axis) and total physical activity (right axis) in the 12 ISCOLE countries. The black bars represent the range of time (h/day) spent in the various movement behaviours. For sedentary behavior, follow the direct horizontal line to the left axis; for physical activity, follow the lines sloping upwards from left to right to the right axis; for sleep, follow the lines sloping downwards from left to right to the bottom axis. Chinese (CHN) children, for example, spend on average 37% of the day sleeping, 40% of the day sedentary and 23% in physical activity. Compositional means are from Dumuid et al. [70]. AUS = Australia; BRZ = Brazil; CAN = Canada; CHN = China; COL = Colombia; ENG = England; FIN = Finland; IND = India; KEN = Kenya; POR = Portugal; RSA = Republic of South Africa; USA = United States.

Associations between meeting combinations of the 24-h guidelines and obesity [71], health-related quality of life [72], and dietary patterns [73] have been explored in ISCOLE. Overall, the proportion of the sample meeting the overall recommendations (all three behaviors: moderate-to-vigorous physical activity, recreational screen time, and sleep duration) was 7%; individually, 44% of the sample met the physical activity recommendation, 39% met the screen time recommendation, and 42% met the sleep duration recommendation [71]. Meeting all three of the recommendations was associated with much lower odds of obesity (odds ratio = 0.28; 95% CI: 0.18–0.45) [71], higher health-related quality of life scores (51.2 vs. 50.0; $p < 0.05$) [72], higher healthy dietary pattern scores (0.18 vs. −0.01; $p < 0.001$), and lower unhealthy dietary pattern scores (−0.31 vs. −0.02; $p < 0.001$) [73].

A day is constrained by the 24-h period, which presents some challenges for the analysis of multiple movement behaviors together in relation to other health parameters such as obesity [74,75]. Traditional analyses that use Euclidian operations such as linear regression fail to account for the Aitchison geometry of the constrained space [75], and therefore compositional analysis approaches have been proposed as an alternative [76]. Noting the lack of suitable analytical techniques available to handle the analysis of 24-h movements behaviors, Dumuid et al. [77] developed a novel method for predicting change in a continuous outcome based on relative changes within a composition, and for calculating associated confidence intervals to allow for statistical inference. Using data from ISCOLE, we demonstrated the application of compositional multiple linear regression to estimate adiposity from children's 24-h movement behaviors [77]. Furthermore, ISCOLE presented a unique opportunity to compare the results of traditional vs. compositional isotemporal substitution analyses in the associations between 24-h movement behaviors and obesity. The results of this investigation demonstrated that both compositional and traditional models estimated an unfavorable association with percentage body fat when time was reallocated from moderate-to-vigorous physical activity to any other behavior (sleep, sedentary behavior, light physical activity). However, unlike traditional models, compositional models found the differences in adiposity were (A) not necessarily symmetrical when an activity was being displaced, or displacing another movement behavior; (B) not linearly related to the durations of time reallocated; and (C) varied depending on the starting composition [75].

In an attempt to better understand the associations between lifestyle variables and obesity, Dumuid et al. [78] undertook a compositional cluster analysis in which the input variables including sedentary time, light, moderate and vigorous physical activity, sleep duration, TV viewing time, and healthy and unhealthy diet pattern scores were subjected to cluster analysis. Four clusters emerged and were labelled as: (A) Junk Food Screenies; (B) Actives; (C) Sitters; and (D) All-Rounders. Measures of adiposity varied across the clusters, and were highest in the Sitters and lowest in the Actives [78].

In addition to obesity, we have applied compositional data analysis to study the association between 24-h movement behaviors and health-related quality of life [70]. Relative to the other movement behaviors, the association was strongest with moderate-to-vigorous physical activity. Furthermore, this association was moderated by country-level HDI; the association between the moderate-to-vigorous physical activity and health-related quality of life was stronger among countries with a high HDI compared to countries with a lower HDI [70].

7. Other Novel Contributions of ISCOLE

In addition to the work described above, ISCOLE has made several other significant contributions to the literature.

7.1. Body Composition

The majority of the research conducted to date on associations between anthropometry and body fat in children has been in high-income countries, and there is a lack of data on associations in children from low- and middle-income countries. We explored the association between BMI and body fat (from bioelectric impedance) in ISCOLE [79]. Correlations between BMI and total body fat (kg) were >0.90 in all study sites, while correlations between BMI and percentage body fat (%) ranged from 0.76 to 0.96.

Boys from India had higher percentage body fat than boys from several other countries at all levels of BMI, whereas Kenyan girls had lower levels of percentage body fat than girls from several other countries at all levels of BMI. Boys and girls from Colombia had higher values of percentage body fat at low levels of BMI, while Colombian boys at moderate and high levels of BMI also had higher values of percentage body fat than boys in other countries [79].

Given the difficulty in measuring height and weight in some field situations, we explored the utility of using mid-upper-arm circumference as an index of adiposity in ISCOLE [80]. Correlations between mid-upper-arm circumference and percentage body fat were 0.86 in girls ($p < 0.001$) and 0.88 in boys ($p < 0.001$) [80]. Furthermore, results from receiver operating characteristic (ROC) curves demonstrated areas under the curve (AUCs) for the prediction of obesity ≥0.97 in both boys and girls, suggesting that mid-upper-arm circumference may be a good screening tool for obesity and excess adiposity in resource-limited settings.

7.2. Identification of Physical Activity Thresholds

We used ROC analyses to estimate the optimal thresholds of moderate-to-vigorous physical activity that were related to the identification of obesity in ISCOLE [43]. The results indicated that the optimal thresholds were 55 (95% CI: 50–64) minutes per day in the total sample, 65 (95% CI: 55–75) minutes per day in boys, and 49 (95% CI: 43–62) minutes per day in girls [43]. These thresholds are comparable to the global physical activity recommendation, which call for children to accumulate at least 60 min per day of moderate-to-vigorous physical activity [51].

Given the recent interest in the health effects associated with sedentary behavior, and the possible interaction between sedentary behavior and physical activity on health outcomes [81], we attempted to identify the optimal thresholds of moderate-to-vigorous physical activity at different levels of sedentary behavior [82]. The results showed that the optimal thresholds of moderate-to-vigorous physical activity to predict obesity ranged from 37.9 to 75.9 min per day in boys and from 32.5 to 62.7 min per day in girls across levels of sedentary behavior [82]. The incorporation of sedentary behavior did not alter or improve the prediction of obesity in this sample, suggesting that the current physical activity guidelines may apply broadly to all children, regardless of their level of sedentary behavior.

7.3. Inequality in Lifestyle and Obesity

Most studies examining associations between obesity and movement behaviors such as physical activity, sedentary behavior, and sleep duration have focused on average values, despite important within and between country variability in these behaviors. Using data from the accelerometers in smartphones in a sample of adults distributed across 111 countries, Althoff et al. [83] found that country-level inequality in physical activity (quantified using the Gini coefficient applied to the accelerometer steps/day data) was a better correlate of obesity prevalence than average physical activity volume (mean steps/day). We explored this issue in ISCOLE, and expanded the focus to include sedentary behavior and sleep as potential correlates of obesity [84].

Our results showed that average moderate-to-vigorous physical activity (hours/day) was a better correlate of obesity than moderate-to-vigorous physical activity inequality ($r = -0.77$ vs. $r = 0.00$, $p = 0.03$) [84] (see Figure 5). Along the same lines, average sedentary time (hours/day) was also a better correlate of obesity than sedentary time inequality ($r = 0.52$ vs. $r = 0.32$, $p = 0.05$). The differences in associations for mean vs. inequality measures for screen time and sleep period time were not statistically significant [84]. Although there is promise in further exploring associations between inequality in lifestyle behaviors and health outcomes, our results suggest that mean estimates of behavior are still important correlates of obesity in children.

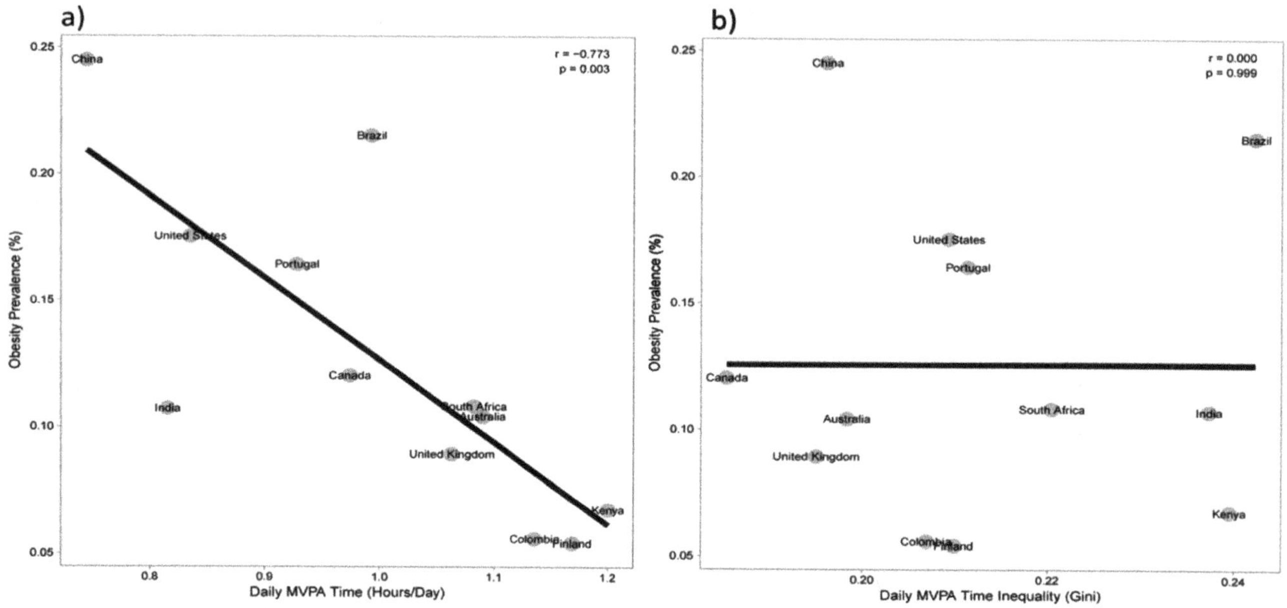

Figure 5. Association between moderate-to-vigorous physical activity (MVPA) and obesity. (**a**) shows the correlation between average MVPA and obesity, while (**b**) shows the correlation between MVPA inequality (Gini coefficient) and obesity. Boys and girls are combined for analysis. Correlation coefficients were compared using a Steiger's Z-test ($p = 0.029$), adapted from Chaput et al. [84].

8. Summary of Research Contributions

As described above, ISCOLE has made many significant research contributions related to understanding global patterns of obesity across countries at different levels of human development and identifying correlates of obesity, physical activity, sedentary behavior, and dietary intake. Furthermore, ISCOLE generated several important methodological advances to the field over the course of the study. Table 2 provides a summary of the major research contributions made by ISCOLE related to the global childhood obesity epidemic. The results from ISCOLE can help inform the development of interventions targeting promising correlates of obesity in different settings. Some findings were robust across all study sites; while other findings were limited to either higher or lower income countries. A careful examination of the patterns of results across countries will be required to deploy the most effective intervention in a given setting.

Table 2. Major research contributions of the International Study of Childhood Obesity, Lifestyle and the Environment (ISCOLE) to understanding the global obesity epidemic.

Research Area	Major Contribution
Global Patterns of Obesity and Related Behaviors	• There is evidence for global epidemiological transitions in obesity and physical activity across countries at different levels of human development; however, there is less evidence for epidemiological transitions in dietary behaviors and sleep duration • Inequality in lifestyle behaviors is not a better correlate of obesity than mean levels of lifestyle behaviors in countries at different levels of human development
Correlates of Obesity	• The proportion of the variance in BMI and waist circumference explained at the individual level is greater than 90%, with the remainder being explained at the school and site levels • Moderate-to-vigorous physical activity is a robust correlate of obesity across all study sites; active school transportation was also related to a lower odds of obesity • Sedentary behavior and TV viewing are both related to a higher odds of obesity • General dietary patterns (healthy/unhealthy) are not related to obesity; however, regular breakfast consumption was related to a lower odds of obesity; regular soft drink consumption was related to a higher odds of obesity in boys and diet soft drink consumption was related to a higher odds of obesity in girls • Parental overweight, gestational diabetes and high birth weight are related to a higher odds of obesity; high moderate-to-vigorous activity and low sedentary time seem to negate the effects of birthweight on childhood obesity • Meeting all three 24-h movement guidelines (moderate-to-vigorous physical activity, TV viewing, sleep) was associated with much lower odds of obesity
Correlates of Physical Activity & Sedentary Behavior	• Participation in physical education classes is associated with higher levels of moderate-to-vigorous physical activity and less sedentary behavior • Active transportation to school is associated with higher weekday moderate-to-vigorous physical activity and lower light physical activity before school • There is wide variability in the correlates of active school transport across study sites. Longer trip duration was associated with lower odds of active school transportation in eight sites; whereas individual and neighborhood factors were associated with active school transportation in three sites or less • Children with at least one piece of electronic media in their bedroom had lower levels of moderate-to-vigorous physical activity • More frequent physical activity in the home and yard, ownership of more frequently used play equipment, and higher social support for physical activity were associated with higher moderate-to-vigorous physical activity; the association between play equipment ownership and moderate-to-vigorous physical activity varied across sites • Collective efficacy was inversely associated with moderate-to-vigorous physical activity among children in low/lower-middle-income countries, while it was positively associated with moderate-to-vigorous physical activity among children in high-income countries. • Perceived crime was significantly associated with lower moderate-to-vigorous physical activity in high-income countries but not in low/lower-middle-income countries or upper-middle-income countries • Common correlates of sedentary time and TV viewing time were excess weight status, not meeting physical activity recommendations, and having a TV in the bedroom • Greater time spent outdoors was associated with higher moderate-to-vigorous and light physical activity, and lower sedentary time
Correlates of Dietary Intake	• More meals eaten outside home and school was associated with higher unhealthy diet pattern scores • Low availability of empty-calorie foods at home was more important than high availability of wholesome foods for a lower unhealthy diet pattern • Availability of wholesome foods at home was positively associated with a healthy diet pattern; food availability at school was not associated with the dietary patterns • Sleep duration and sleep efficiency were negatively associated with an unhealthy diet • Shorter sleep duration was associated with higher intake of regular soft drinks, while earlier bedtimes were associated with lower intake of regular soft drinks and higher intake of energy drinks and sports drinks • Meeting all three 24-h movement guidelines (moderate-to-vigorous physical activity, TV viewing, sleep) was associated with higher healthy dietary pattern scores and lower unhealthy dietary pattern scores
Methodological Advances	• Creation and validation of an automated algorithm to determine sleep parameters from 24-h waist-worn accelerometry • Development and application of a novel compositional data analysis approach to be used with 24-h movement behavior data • Adaptation and reliability assessment of a school environmental audit tool • Adaptation and validation of a food frequency questionnaire for use in different cultural settings

9. A Platform for International Training, Data Entry, and Data Quality for Multi-Country Research Studies

In addition to its scientific contributions, ISCOLE provided a platform for research capacity development around the world. The study was governed by a standardized protocol implemented using strict quality control procedures, including in-person and online study personnel training, site visits, and remote source data verification. All investigators shared responsibility for quality control. A major component of study management was a shared website, which allowed access to all study documents, training materials, remote data entry, accelerometer data uploads, and real-time data validation. This system, based on a common data model, facilitated timely communication and data transfers between the sites and coordinating center. The enrollment target for ISCOLE was 6000 children; however, the final sample size was 7372. We believe the successful recruitment and high data quality are the result of well trained and prepared research staff and co-ownership and investigator investment in the study. Over 240 people have worked on ISCOLE, including senior and junior faculty, post-doctoral fellows, students, and research staff. To date, 25 students (12 doctoral, 10 masters and 3 undergraduate) from 10 countries have used ISCOLE as the foundation for their thesis. ISCOLE has had a tremendous impact on developing research capacity in countries spanning a wide range of HDI.

10. Strengths and Limitations

There are several strengths and limitations associated with the design and implementation of ISCOLE. Marked strengths of the study include the implementation of a standardized research protocol using the same instruments (adapted to the local context as required) and equipment at all study sites, and the inclusion of research sites and investigators from countries that varied widely in human development [7]. Furthermore, the deployment of a web-based data collection and staff training infrastructure that allowed for real-time data entry and verification increased the assurance of quality data. The publication of the study questionnaires, protocols and data algorithms in peer-reviewed journals, which allows for transparency and reproducibility of the results, is another strength of the study. Such resources are also immensely beneficial to other researchers interested in similar or related research. The timely and thorough publication and presentation of ISCOLE findings helped maximize the dissemination and impact of the research, including, but not limited to the notable scientific and methodological advances discussed in this paper. ISCOLE also contributed markedly to capacity building via the personal skill development of research trainees.

There are several limitations of ISCOLE that warrant discussion. First, the fundamental design of ISCOLE is a cross-sectional study, which limits inferences about cause-and-effect relationships. Second, the ISCOLE study sites represent urban and semi-urban populations, and the samples do not include children from rural areas. The decision to exclude rural samples was based on logistical limitations related to data collection; further research is required to better understand urban-rural differences in the correlates of obesity and related behaviors in multi-national studies. This is of particular importance in low- and middle-income countries where the majority of people live in rural environments. We deployed a rigorous research protocol; however, the assessment of dietary intake in free-living children remains a challenge. We used a validated and widely used FFQ to assess dietary intake patterns; however, the FFQ was short and we were unable to precisely quantify dietary intake (kcals, macronutrients, etc.). Furthermore, research is required to develop better methods of dietary assessment in children.

11. A Transparent Model for Public-Private Research Partnerships

ISCOLE was funded by the Coca-Cola Company through a research contract with PBRC. PBRC, in turn, executed sub-contracts with each of the study site institutions. With the exception of requiring that the study be global in nature, the funder had no role in the design and conduct of the study;

collection, management, analysis and interpretation of the data, preparation of manuscripts, and the decision whether to publish the results or not. The overall study design, protocol, and all study procedures were developed solely by the principal investigators, co-investigators and research staff. During the period of the research contract (2011–2014), the research team provided regular updates to the funder about the study progress on a quarterly basis. These reports focused on the achievement of operational milestones such as completion of protocols, staff training, field site implementation, achieving recruitment targets, remote site monitoring, and progress on data management.

Given the increased scrutiny associated with industry-sponsored research, we took several precautions to ensure the integrity of the study methods and results. First, we established an External Advisory Board that was charged with assessing the overall progress, rigor and objectivity of ISCOLE, as well as providing an unbiased assessment of the science and the role of the sponsor. Second, we published the design and methods of ISCOLE in an open-access journal, and included the questionnaires and survey instruments in an online appendix [7]. Third, we have made our accelerometer manual of procedures and algorithms freely available online so that they can be tested, replicated and utilized by other scientists [14,16,17]. Fourth, wherever possible, we have published the results from ISCOLE in open-access, peer-reviewed journals so that they can be freely available to a wide audience. Furthermore, all scientific presentations and publications have clearly acknowledged the funding source and the role of the funder. To date, we have published more than 100 scientific papers that have all undergone peer-review and have been found worthy to make significant contributions to the extant literature. Moreover, the large number of students and young researchers who were engaged in ISCOLE highlights the research capacity building that occurred across low-, middle- and high-income countries. Finally, we have declared our data available upon reasonable request for researchers who wish to replicate or challenge our research findings.

Despite our concerted efforts to ensure transparency and rigor in the design and conduct of ISCOLE, we experienced skepticism about the role of the sponsor. We have received several Freedom of Information requests for access to emails from the study investigators and the sponsor. To date, we have provided emails to several media organizations and the US Right to Know organization. This correspondence was the subject of a manuscript that attempted to understand the relationship between "an industry sponsor and public health academics" [85]. The primary conclusion of the study in the first line of the conclusions section is that "Overall, apart from influencing the total number of study sites, we found no evidence of Coca-Cola exerting 'hard power' over the Pennington PIs, where the funder directly changes core methodological principles or points in the research" [85]. The authors tried to make the case that the funder was involved in the study design since they negotiated the number of study sites with the principal investigators as we developed the budget. However, we maintain that the overall study design was not impacted by the number of study sites, i.e., whether the study included 12, 13 or 14 countries; rather, this was purely a budgetary issue, where the budget largely drove the number of study sites that could be recruited [86]. The selection of study sites was at the discretion of the principal investigators. While the funder made suggestions about potential sites to include in order to ensure global representation, the final slate of study sites was selected solely by the principal investigators, and did not include specific sites recommended by the funder.

In summary, the ISCOLE investigators acted in good faith while developing and executing the ISCOLE protocol. Despite a high level of scrutiny (and review of thousands of our emails) from the media and other organizations, we have conducted ISCOLE with transparency and integrity and we are immensely proud of it. We hope that such scrutiny of our work will not dissuade other researchers from developing appropriately managed and transparent public-private partnerships to tackle important public health issues. We feel that ISCOLE represents a successful and transparent model for future public-private partnerships with academics.

12. Conclusions

ISCOLE was a collaboration of scientists, students and staff from 12 countries ranging widely in levels of human and economic development. Using a model of shared ownership, ISCOLE surpassed all recruitment and quality control goals. To date, more than 100 peer-reviewed papers have been published from ISCOLE. In addition to being an engine of research capacity development, ISCOLE has made many significant contributions to our understanding of the global childhood obesity epidemic in a short period of time. The findings of ISCOLE could, in turn, inform global efforts, such as the World Health Organization Global Action Plan on Physical Activity 2018–2030 [87], and the achievement of the United Nation's Sustainable Development Goals [88]. Furthermore, the results from ISCOLE can inform the development of culturally tailored interventions that can be deployed and tested across a range of settings, and we encourage future collaborations that will build upon ISCOLE to improve the health of children across the world.

Author Contributions: P.T.K. wrote the initial draft of the manuscript. All authors edited the manuscript, provided critical input, and approved the manuscript for publication.

Acknowledgments: We wish to thank the ISCOLE External Advisory Board and the ISCOLE participants and their families who made this study possible. The ISCOLE Research Group includes: Coordinating Center, Pennington Biomedical Research Center: Peter T. Katzmarzyk, PhD (Co-PI), Timothy S. Church, MD, PhD (Co-PI), Denise G. Lambert, RN (Project Manager), Tiago Barreira, PhD, Stephanie Broyles, PhD, Ben Butitta, BS, Catherine Champagne, PhD, RD, Shannon Cocreham, MBA, Kara Dentro, MPH, Katy Drazba, MPH, Deirdre Harrington, PhD, William Johnson, PhD, Dione Milauskas, BS, Emily Mire, MS, Allison Tohme, MPH, Ruben Rodarte MS, MBA; Data Management Center, Wake Forest University: Bobby Amoroso, BS, John Luopa, BS, Rebecca Neiberg, MS, Scott Rushing, BS; Australia, University of South Australia: Timothy Olds, PhD (Site Co-PI), Carol Maher, PhD (Site Co-PI), Lucy Lewis, PhD, Katia Ferrar, B Physio (Hon), Effie Georgiadis, BPsych, Rebecca Stanley, BAppSc (OT) Hon; Brazil, Centro de Estudos do Laboratório de Aptidão Física de São Caetano do Sul (CELAFISCS): Victor Keihan Rodrigues Matsudo, MD, PhD (Site PI), Sandra Matsudo, MD, PhD, Timoteo Araujo, MSc, Luis Carlos de Oliveira, MSc, Leandro Rezende, BSc, Luis Fabiano, BSc, Diogo Bezerra, BSc, Gerson Ferrari, MSc; Canada, Children's Hospital of Eastern Ontario Research Institute: Mark S. Tremblay, PhD (Site Co-PI), Jean-Philippe Chaput, PhD (Site Co-PI), Priscilla Bélanger, BSc, Mike Borghese, MSc, Charles Boyer, MA, Allana LeBlanc, MSc, Claire Francis, B.Sc.,Geneviève Leduc, PhD; China, Tianjin Women's and Children's Health Center: Pei Zhao, MD (Site Co-PI), Gang Hu, MD, PhD (Site Co-PI), Chengming Diao, MD, Wei Li, MD, Weiqin Li, MSc, Enqing Liu, MD, Gongshu Liu, MD, Hongyan Liu, MSc, Jian Ma, MD, Yijuan Qiao, MSc, Huiguang Tian, PhD, Yue Wang, MD, Tao Zhang, MSc, Fuxia Zhang, MD; Colombia, Universidad de los Andes: Olga Sarmiento, MD, PhD (Site PI), Julio Acosta, Yalta Alvira, BS, Maria Paula Diaz, Rocio Gamez, BS, Maria Paula Garcia, Luis Guillermo Gómez, Lisseth Gonzalez, Silvia Gonzalez, RD, Carlos Grijalba, MD, Leidys Gutierrez, David Leal, Nicolas Lemus, Etelvina Mahecha, BS, Maria Paula Mahecha, Rosalba Mahecha, BS, Andrea Ramirez, MD, Paola Rios, MD, Andres Suarez, Camilo Triana; Finland, University of Helsinki: Mikael Fogelholm, ScD (Site-PI), Elli Hovi, BS, Jemina Kivelä, Sari Räsänen, BS, Sanna Roito, BS, Taru Saloheimo, MS, Leena Valta; India, St. Johns Research Institute: Anura Kurpad, MD, PhD (Site Co-PI), Rebecca Kuriyan, PhD (Site Co-PI), Deepa P. Lokesh, BSc, Michelle Stephanie D'Almeida, BSc, Annie Mattilda R, MSc, Lygia Correa, BSc, Vijay D, BSc; Kenya, Kenyatta University: Vincent Onywera, PhD (Site Co-PI), Mark S. Tremblay, PhD (Site Co-PI), Lucy-Joy Wachira, PhD, Stella Muthuri, PhD; Portugal, University of Porto: Jose Maia, PhD (Site PI), Alessandra da Silva Borges, BA, Sofia Oliveira Sá Cachada, Msc, Raquel Nichele de Chaves, MSc, Thayse Natacha Queiroz Ferreira Gomes, MSc, Sara Isabel Sampaio Pereira, BA, Daniel Monteiro de Vilhena e Santos, PhD, Fernanda Karina dos Santos, MSc, Pedro Gil Rodrigues da Silva, BA, Michele Caroline de Souza, MSc; South Africa, University of Cape Town: Vicki Lambert, PhD (Site PI), Matthew April, BSc (Hons), Monika Uys, BSc (Hons), Nirmala Naidoo, MSc, Nandi Synyanya, Madelaine Carstens, BSc(Hons); United Kingdom, University of Bath: Martyn Standage, PhD (Site PI), Sean Cumming, PhD, Clemens Drenowatz, PhD, Lydia Emm, MSc, Fiona Gillison, PhD, Julia Zakrzewski, PhD; United States, Pennington Biomedical Research Center: Catrine Tudor-Locke, PhD (Site-PI), Ashley Braud, Sheletta Donatto, MS, LDN, RD, Corbin Lemon, BS, Ana Jackson, BA, Ashunti Pearson, MS, Gina Pennington, BS, LDN, RD, Daniel Ragus, BS, Ryan Roubion, John Schuna, Jr., PhD; Derek Wiltz. The ISCOLE External Advisory Board includes Alan Batterham, PhD, Teesside University, Jacqueline Kerr, PhD, University of California, San Diego; Michael Pratt, MD, Centers for Disease Control and Prevention, Angelo Pietrobelli, MD, Verona University Medical School.

References

1. NCD Risk Factor Collaboration (NCD-RisC). Worldwide trends in body-mass index, underweight, overweight, and obesity from 1975 to 2016: A pooled analysis of 2416 population-based measurement studies in 128.9 million children, adolescents, and adults. *Lancet* **2017**, *390*, 2627–2642. [CrossRef]
2. Riddoch, C.; Edwards, D.; Page, A.S.; Froberg, K.; Anderssen, S.A.; Wedderkopp, N.; Brage, S.; Cooper, A.R.; Sardinha, L.B.; Harro, M.; et al. The European youth heart study—Cardiovascular disease risk factors in children: Rationale, aims, study design, and validation of methods. *J. Phys. Act. Health* **2005**, *2*, 115–129. [CrossRef]
3. Moreno, L.A.; De Henauw, S.; Gonzalez-Gross, M.; Kersting, M.; Molnar, D.; Gottrand, F.; Barrios, L.; Sjostrom, M.; Manios, Y.; Gilbert, C.C.; et al. Design and implementation of the healthy lifestyle in Europe by nutrition in adolescence cross-sectional study. *Int. J. Obes.* **2008**, *32* (Suppl. 5), S4–S11. [CrossRef]
4. Ahrens, W.; Bammann, K.; Siani, A.; Buchecker, K.; De Henauw, S.; Iacoviello, L.; Hebestreit, A.; Krogh, V.; Lissner, L.; Marild, S.; et al. The IDEFICS cohort: Design, characteristics and participation in the baseline survey. *Int. J. Obes.* **2011**, *35* (Suppl. 1), S3–S15. [CrossRef] [PubMed]
5. Van Stralen, M.M.; te Velde, S.J.; Singh, A.S.; De Bourdeaudhuij, I.; Martens, M.K.; van der Sluis, M.; Manios, Y.; Grammatikaki, E.; Chinapaw, M.J.; Maes, L.; et al. EuropeaN energy balance research to prevent excessive weight gain among youth (ENERGY) project: Design and methodology of the energy cross-sectional survey. *BMC Public Health* **2011**, *11*, 65. [CrossRef]
6. Janssen, I.; Katzmarzyk, P.T.; Boyce, W.F.; Vereeken, C.; Mulvihill, C.; Roberts, C.; Currie, C.; Pickett, W. Comparison of overweight and obesity prevalence in school-aged youth from 34 countries and their relationships with physical activity and dietary patterns. *Obes. Rev.* **2005**, *6*, 123–132. [CrossRef]
7. Katzmarzyk, P.T.; Barreira, T.V.; Broyles, S.T.; Champagne, C.M.; Chaput, J.P.; Fogelholm, M.; Hu, G.; Johnson, W.D.; Kuriyan, R.; Kurpad, A.; et al. The International study of childhood obesity, Lifestyle and the environment (ISCOLE): Design and methods. *BMC Public Health* **2013**, *13*, 900. [CrossRef]
8. Katzmarzyk, P.T.; Barreira, T.V.; Broyles, S.T.; Champagne, C.M.; Chaput, J.P.; Fogelholm, M.; Hu, G.; Johnson, W.D.; Kuriyan, R.; Kurpad, A.; et al. Relationship between lifestyle behaviors and obesity in children ages 9–11: Results from a 12-country study. *Obesity* **2015**, *23*, 1696–1702. [CrossRef]
9. LeBlanc, A.G.; Katzmarzyk, P.T.; Barreira, T.V.; Broyles, S.T.; Chaput, J.P.; Church, T.S.; Fogelholm, M.; Harrington, D.M.; Hu, G.; Kuriyan, R.; et al. Are participant characteristics from ISCOLE study sites comparable to the rest of their country? *Int. J. Obes. Suppl.* **2015**, *5*, S9–S16. [CrossRef]
10. United Nations Development Programme. *Sustainability and Equity: A Better Future for All*; Human Development Report 2011; Palgrave Macmillan: New York, NY, USA, 2011.
11. Tudor-Locke, C.; Barreira, T.V.; Schuna, J.M.; Katzmarzyk, P.T. Unique contributions of ISCOLE to the advancement of accelerometry in large studies. *Int. J. Obes. Suppl.* **2015**, *5*, S53–S58. [CrossRef]
12. Tudor-Locke, C.; Mire, E.F.; Dentro, K.N.; Barreira, T.V.; Schuna, J.M., Jr.; Zhao, P.; Tremblay, M.S.; Standage, M.; Sarmiento, O.L.; Onywera, V.; et al. A model for presenting accelerometer paradata in large studies: ISCOLE. *Int. J. Behav. Nutr. Phys. Act.* **2015**, *12*, 52. [CrossRef]
13. Troiano, R.P.; McClain, J.J.; Brychta, R.J.; Chen, K.Y. Evolution of accelerometer methods for physical activity research. *Br. J. Sports Med.* **2014**, *48*, 1019–1023. [CrossRef]
14. Tudor-Locke, C.; Barreira, T.V.; Schuna, J.M., Jr.; Mire, E.F.; Chaput, J.P.; Fogelholm, M.; Hu, G.; Kuriyan, R.; Kurpad, A.; Lambert, E.V.; et al. Improving wear time compliance with a 24 h waist-worn accelerometer protocol in the international study of childhood obesity, lifestyle and the environment (ISCOLE). *Int. J. Behav. Nutr. Phys. Act.* **2015**, *12*, 172. [CrossRef]
15. Barreira, T.V.; Schuna, J.M.; Tudor-Locke, C.; Chaput, J.-P.; Church, T.S.; Fogelholm, M.; Hu, G.; Kuriyan, R.; Kurpad, A.; Lambert, E.V.; et al. Reliability of accelerometer-determined physical activity and sedentary behavior in school-aged children: A 12 country study. *Int. J. Obes. Suppl.* **2015**, *5*, S29–S35. [CrossRef]
16. Tudor-Locke, C.; Barreira, T.V.; Schuna, J.M., Jr.; Mire, E.F.; Katzmarzyk, P.T. Fully automated waist-worn accelerometer algorithm for detecting children's sleep-period time separate from 24 h physical activity or sedentary behaviors. *Appl. Physiol. Nutr. Metab.* **2014**, *39*, 53–57. [CrossRef]
17. Barreira, T.V.; Schuna, J.M., Jr.; Mire, E.F.; Katzmarzyk, P.T.; Chaput, J.P.; Leduc, G.; Tudor-Locke, C. Identifying children's nocturnal sleep using 24 h waist accelerometry. *Med. Sci. Sports Exerc.* **2015**, *47*, 937–943. [CrossRef]

18. Sadeh, A.; Sharkey, K.M.; Carskadon, M.A. Activity-based sleep-wake identification: An empical test of methodological issues. *Sleep* **1994**, *17*, 201–207. [CrossRef]
19. SAS Programs for Analyzing NHANES 2003-2004 Accelerometer Data. Available online: http://riskfactor.cancer.gov/tools/nhanes_pam/ (accessed on 15 April 2019).
20. Fully Automated Waist-worn Accelerometer Algorithm for Children's Sleep Period Time Separate From 24-h Physical Activity or Sedentary Behaviors. Available online: www.pbrc.edu/SleepPeriodTimeMacro (accessed on 15 April 2019).
21. Identifying Children's Nocturnal Sleep Using 24-h Waist Accelerometry. Available online: http://www.pbrc.edu/pdf/PBRCSleepEpisodeTimeMacroCode.pdf (accessed on 15 April 2019).
22. Tudor-Locke, C.; Mire, E.F.; Barreira, T.V.; Schuna, J.M.; Chaput, J.P.; Fogelholm, M.; Hu, G.; Kurpad, A.; Kuriyan, R.; Lambert, E.V.; et al. Nocturnal sleep-related variables from 24 h free-living waist-worn accelerometry: International Study of Childhood Obesity, Lifestyle and the Environment. *Int. J. Obes. Suppl.* **2015**, *5*, S47–S52. [CrossRef]
23. Currie, C.; Zanotti, C.; Morgan, A.; Currie, D.; de Looze, M.; Roberts, C.; Samdal, O.; Smith, O.R.F.; Barnekow, V. *Social Determinants of Health and Well-Being among Young People*; Health Behaviour in School-Aged Children (HBSC) Study: International Report from the 2009/2010 Survey; Health Policy for Children and Adolescents WHO Regional Office for Europe: Copenhagen, Denmark, 2012.
24. Saloheimo, T.; Gonzalez, S.A.; Erkkola, M.; Milauskas, D.M.; Meisel, J.D.; Champagne, C.M.; Tudor-Locke, C.; Sarmiento, O.; Katzmarzyk, P.T.; Fogelholm, M. The reliability and validity of a short food frequency questionnaire among 9–11 year olds: A multinational study on three middle-income and high-income countries. *Int. J. Obes. Suppl.* **2015**, *5*, S22–S28. [CrossRef]
25. Mikkila, V.; Vepsalainen, H.; Saloheimo, T.; Gonzalez, S.A.; Meisel, J.D.; Hu, G.; Champagne, C.M.; Chaput, J.P.; Church, T.S.; Katzmarzyk, P.T.; et al. An international comparison of dietary patterns in 9–11 year old children. *Int. J. Obes. Suppl.* **2015**, *5*, S17–S21. [CrossRef]
26. Saelens, B.E.; Sallis, J.F.; Frank, L.D.; Couch, S.C.; Zhou, C.; Colburn, T.; Cain, K.L.; Chapman, J.; Glanz, K. Obesogenic neighborhood environments, child and parent obesity: The neighborhood impact on kids study. *Am. J. Prev. Med.* **2012**, *42*, e57–e64. [CrossRef] [PubMed]
27. Broyles, S.T.; Drazba, K.T.; Church, T.S.; Chaput, J.P.; Fogelholm, M.; Hu, G.; Kuriyan, R.; Kurpad, A.; Lambert, E.V.; Maher, C.; et al. Development and reliability of an audit tool to assess the school physical activity environment across 12 countries. *Int. J. Obes. Suppl.* **2015**, *5*, S36–S42. [CrossRef] [PubMed]
28. Omran, A.R. The epidemiologic transition. A theory of the epidemiology of population change. *Milbank Mem. Fund Q.* **1971**, *49*, 509–538. [CrossRef] [PubMed]
29. Popkin, B.M. Nutritional patterns and transitions. *Pop. Dev. Rev.* **1993**, *19*, 138–157. [CrossRef]
30. Katzmarzyk, P.T.; Mason, C. The physical activity transition. *J. Phys. Act. Health* **2009**, *6*, 269–280. [CrossRef] [PubMed]
31. Shrewsbury, V.; Wardle, J. Socioeconomic status and adiposity in childhood: A systematic review of cross-sectional studies 1990–2005. *Obesity* **2008**, *16*, 275–284. [CrossRef]
32. Broyles, S.T.; Denstel, K.D.; Church, T.S.; Chaput, J.-P.; Fogelholm, M.; Hu, G.; Kuriyan, R.; Kurpad, A.; Lambert, E.V.; Maher, C.; et al. The epidemiological transition and the global childhood obesity epidemic. *Int. J. Obes. Suppl.* **2015**, *5*, S3–S8. [CrossRef]
33. Manyanga, T.; Barnes, J.D.; Tremblay, M.S.; Katzmarzyk, P.T.; Broyles, S.T.; Barreira, T.V.; Fogelholm, M.; Hu, G.; Maher, C.; Maia, J.; et al. No evidence for an epidemiological transition in sleep patterns among children: A 12-country study. *Sleep Health* **2018**, *4*, 87–95. [CrossRef]
34. Manyanga, T.; Tremblay, M.S.; Chaput, J.P.; Katzmarzyk, P.T.; Fogelholm, M.; Hu, G.; Kuriyan, R.; Kurpad, A.; Lambert, E.V.; Maher, C.; et al. Socioeconomic status and dietary patterns in children from around the world: Different associations by levels of country human development? *BMC Public Health* **2017**, *17*, 457. [CrossRef]
35. Barreira, T.V.; Broyles, S.T.; Tudor-Locke, C.; Chaput, J.-P.; Fogelholm, M.; Hu, G.; Kuriyan, R.; Kurpad, A.; Lambert, E.V.; Maher, C.; et al. Epidemiological transition in physical activity and sedentary time in children. *J. Phys. Act. Health* **2019**, in press.
36. Bronfenbrenner, U. *The Ecology of Human Development*; Harvard University Press: Cambridge, MA, USA, 1979.
37. Sallis, J.F.; Cervero, R.B.; Ascher, W.; Henderson, K.A.; Kraft, M.K.; Kerr, J. An ecological approach to creating active living communities. *Annu. Rev. Public Health* **2006**, *27*, 297–322. [CrossRef] [PubMed]

38. Story, M.; Kaphingst, K.M.; Robinson-O'Brien, R.; Glanz, K. Creating healthy food and eating environments: Policy and environmental approaches. *Annu. Rev. Public Health* **2008**, *29*, 253–272. [CrossRef]
39. Davison, K.K.; Birch, L.L. Childhood overweight: A contextual model and recommendations for future research. *Obes. Rev.* **2001**, *2*, 159–171. [CrossRef]
40. Goldstein, H. *Multilevel Statistical Models*, 3rd ed.; Oxford University Press: New York, NY, USA, 2003.
41. Corgeau, D. *Methodology and Epistemology of Multilevel Analysis: Approaches from Different Social Sciences*; Kluwer Academic Publishers: Dordrecht, The Netherlands, 2003.
42. Katzmarzyk, P.T.; Broyles, S.T.; Chaput, J.P.; Fogelholm, M.; Hu, G.; Lambert, E.V.; Maher, C.; Maia, J.; Olds, T.; Onywera, V.; et al. Sources of variability in childhood obesity indicators and related behaviors. *Int. J. Obes.* **2018**, *42*, 108–110. [CrossRef]
43. Katzmarzyk, P.T.; Barreira, T.V.; Broyles, S.T.; Champagne, C.M.; Chaput, J.-P.; Fogelholm, M.; Hu, G.; Johnson, W.D.; Kuriyan, R.; Kurpad, A.; et al. Physical activity, sedentary time and obesity in an international sample of children. *Med. Sci. Sports Exerc.* **2015**, *47*, 2062–2069. [CrossRef]
44. Sarmiento, O.L.; Lemoine, P.; Gonzalez, S.A.; Broyles, S.T.; Denstel, K.D.; Larouche, R.; Onywera, V.; Barreira, T.V.; Chaput, J.-P.; Fogelholm, M.; et al. Relationships between active school transport and adiposity indicators in school age children from low-, middle-and high-income countries. *Int. J. Obes. Suppl.* **2015**, *5*, S107–S114. [CrossRef]
45. Zakrzewski, J.K.; Gillison, F.B.; Cumming, S.; Church, T.S.; Katzmarzyk, P.T.; Broyles, S.T.; Champagne, C.M.; Chaput, J.P.; Denstel, K.D.; Fogelholm, M.; et al. Associations between breakfast frequency and adiposity indicators in children from 12 countries. *Int. J. Obes. Suppl.* **2015**, *5*, S80–S88. [CrossRef] [PubMed]
46. Katzmarzyk, P.T.; Broyles, S.T.; Champagne, C.M.; Chaput, J.P.; Fogelholm, M.; Hu, G.; Kuriyan, R.; Kurpad, A.; Lambert, E.V.; Maia, J.; et al. Relationship between soft drink consumption and obesity in 9–11 year old children in a multi-national study. *Nutrients* **2016**, *8*, 770. [CrossRef] [PubMed]
47. Zhao, P.; Liu, E.; Qiao, Y.; Katzmarzyk, P.T.; Chaput, J.P.; Fogelholm, M.; Johnson, W.D.; Kuriyan, R.; Kurpad, A.; Lambert, E.V.; et al. Maternal gestational diabetes and childhood obesity at age 9–11: Results of a multinational study. *Diabetologia* **2016**, *59*, 2339–2348. [CrossRef] [PubMed]
48. Qiao, Y.; Ma, J.; Wang, Y.; Li, W.; Katzmarzyk, P.T.; Chaput, J.P.; Fogelholm, M.; Johnson, W.D.; Kuriyan, R.; Kurpad, A.; et al. Birth weight and childhood obesity: A 12-country study. *Int. J. Obes. Suppl.* **2015**, *5*, S74–S79. [CrossRef]
49. Qiao, Y.; Zhang, T.; Liu, H.; Katzmarzyk, P.T.; Chaput, J.P.; Fogelholm, M.; Johnson, W.D.; Kuriyan, R.; Kurpad, A.; Lambert, E.V.; et al. Joint association of birth weight and physical activity/sedentary behavior with obesity in children ages 9–11 years from 12 countries. *Obesity* **2017**, *25*, 1091–1097. [CrossRef] [PubMed]
50. Muthuri, S.K.; Onywera, V.O.; Tremblay, M.S.; Broyles, S.T.; Chaput, J.P.; Fogelholm, M.; Hu, G.; Kuriyan, R.; Kurpad, A.; Lambert, E.V.; et al. Relationships between parental education and overweight with childhood overweight and physical activity in 9–11 year old children: Results from a 12-country study. *PLoS ONE* **2016**, *11*, e0147746. [CrossRef]
51. World Health Organization. *Global Recommendations on Physical Activity for Health*; World Health Organization: Geneva, Switzerland, 2010.
52. Gomes, T.N.; Katzmarzyk, P.T.; Hedeker, D.; Fogelholm, M.; Standage, M.; Onywera, V.; Lambert, E.V.; Tremblay, M.S.; Chaput, J.P.; Tudor-Locke, C.; et al. Correlates of compliance with recommended levels of physical activity in children. *Sci. Rep.* **2017**, *7*, 16507. [CrossRef]
53. Silva, D.A.S.; Chaput, J.P.; Katzmarzyk, P.T.; Fogelholm, M.; Hu, G.; Maher, C.; Olds, T.; Onywera, V.; Sarmiento, O.L.; Standage, M.; et al. Physical education classes, physical activity, and sedentary behavior in children. *Med. Sci. Sports Exerc.* **2018**, *50*, 995–1004. [CrossRef]
54. Denstel, K.D.; Broyles, S.T.; Larouche, R.; Sarmiento, O.L.; Barreira, T.V.; Chaput, J.-P.; Church, T.S.; Fogelholm, M.; Hu, G.; Kuriyan, R.; et al. Active school transport and weekday physical activity in 9–11 year old children from 12 countries. *Int. J. Obes. Suppl.* **2015**, *5*, S100–S106. [CrossRef] [PubMed]
55. Larouche, R.; Sarmiento, O.L.; Broyles, S.T.; Denstel, K.D.; Church, T.S.; Barreira, T.V.; Chaput, J.P.; Fogelholm, M.; Hu, G.; Kuriyan, R.; et al. Are the correlates of active school transport context-specific? *Int. J. Obes. Suppl.* **2015**, *5*, S89–S99. [CrossRef]
56. Harrington, D.M.; Gillison, F.; Broyles, S.T.; Chaput, J.P.; Fogelholm, M.; Hu, G.; Kuriyan, R.; Kurpad, A.; LeBlanc, A.G.; Maher, C.; et al. Household-level correlates of children's physical activity levels in and across 12 countries. *Obesity* **2016**, *24*, 2150–2157. [CrossRef]

57. Sullivan, S.M.; Broyles, S.T.; Barreira, T.V.; Chaput, J.P.; Fogelholm, M.; Hu, G.; Kuriyan, R.; Kurpad, A.; Lambert, E.V.; Maher, C.; et al. Associations of neighborhood social environment attributes and physical activity among 9-11 year old children from 12 countries. *Health Place* **2017**, *46*, 183–191. [CrossRef]
58. LeBlanc, A.G.; Katzmarzyk, P.T.; Barreira, T.V.; Broyles, S.T.; Chaput, J.P.; Church, T.S.; Fogelholm, M.; Harrington, D.M.; Hu, G.; Kuriyan, R.; et al. Correlates of total sedentary time and screen time in 9-11 year-old children around the world: The international study of childhood obesity, lifestyle and the environment. *PLoS ONE* **2015**, *10*, e0129622. [CrossRef]
59. Chaput, J.P.; Carson, V.; Gray, C.E.; Tremblay, M.S. Importance of all movement behaviors in a 24 hour period for overall health. *Int. J. Environ. Res. Public Health* **2014**, *11*, 12575–12581. [CrossRef]
60. Chaput, J.P.; Katzmarzyk, P.T.; LeBlanc, A.G.; Tremblay, M.S.; Barreira, T.V.; Broyles, S.T.; Fogelholm, M.; Hu, G.; Kuriyan, R.; Kurpad, A.; et al. Associations between sleep patterns and lifestyle behaviors in children: An international comparison. *Int. J. Obes. Suppl.* **2015**, *5*, S59–S65. [CrossRef]
61. Lin, Y.; Tremblay, M.S.; Katzmarzyk, P.T.; Fogelholm, M.; Hu, G.; Lambert, E.V.; Maher, C.; Maia, J.; Olds, T.; Sarmiento, O.L.; et al. Temporal and bi-directional associations between sleep duration and physical activity/sedentary time in children: An international comparison. *Prev. Med.* **2018**, *111*, 436–441. [CrossRef]
62. Vepsalainen, H.; Mikkila, V.; Erkkola, M.; Broyles, S.T.; Chaput, J.P.; Hu, G.; Kuriyan, R.; Kurpad, A.; Lambert, E.V.; Maher, C.; et al. Association between home and school food environments and dietary patterns among 9–11-year-old children in 12 countries. *Int. J. Obes. Suppl.* **2015**, *5*, S66–S73. [CrossRef]
63. Chaput, J.P.; Tremblay, M.S.; Katzmarzyk, P.T.; Fogelholm, M.; Hu, G.; Maher, C.; Maia, J.; Olds, T.; Onywera, V.; Sarmiento, O.L.; et al. Sleep patterns and sugar-sweetened beverage consumption among children from around the world. *Public Health Nutr.* **2018**, *21*, 2385–2393. [CrossRef]
64. Chaput, J.P.; Weippert, M.; LeBlanc, A.G.; Hjorth, M.F.; Michaelsen, K.F.; Katzmarzyk, P.T.; Tremblay, M.S.; Barreira, T.V.; Broyles, S.T.; Fogelholm, M.; et al. Are children like werewolves? Full moon and its association with sleep and activity behaviors in an international sample of children. *Front. Pediatr.* **2016**, *4*, 24. [CrossRef] [PubMed]
65. Lewis, L.K.; Maher, C.; Belanger, K.; Tremblay, M.; Chaput, J.P.; Olds, T. At the mercy of the gods: Associations between weather, physical activity, and sedentary time in children. *Pediatr. Exerc. Sci.* **2016**, *28*, 152–163. [CrossRef]
66. Chaput, J.P.; Tremblay, M.S.; Katzmarzyk, P.T.; Fogelholm, M.; Mikkila, V.; Hu, G.; Lambert, E.V.; Maher, C.; Maia, J.; Olds, T.; et al. Outdoor time and dietary patterns in children around the world. *J. Public Health (Oxf)* **2018**, *40*, e493–e501. [CrossRef]
67. Larouche, R.; Mire, E.F.; Belanger, K.; Barreira, T.V.; Chaput, J.P.; Fogelholm, M.; Hu, G.; Lambert, E.V.; Maher, C.; Maia, J.; et al. Relationships between outdoor time, physical activity, sedentary time, and body mass index in children: A 12-country study. *Pediatr. Exerc. Sci.* **2018**, *31*, 118–129. [CrossRef]
68. Triana Reyes, C.A.; Bravo-Balado, A.; Gonzalez, S.A.; Bolivar, M.A.; Lemoine, P.; Meisel, J.D.; Grijalba, C. Active streets for children: The case of the ciclovia of Bogota. *PLoS ONE* **2019**, in press.
69. Tremblay, M.S.; Carson, V.; Chaput, J.P.; Connor Gorber, S.; Dinh, T.; Duggan, M.; Faulkner, G.; Gray, C.E.; Gruber, R.; Janson, K.; et al. Canadian 24 h movement Guidelines for children and youth: An integration of physical activity, sedentary behaviour, and sleep. *Appl. Physiol. Nutr. Metab.* **2016**, *41*, S311–S327. [CrossRef] [PubMed]
70. Dumuid, D.; Maher, C.; Lewis, L.K.; Stanford, T.E.; Martin Fernandez, J.A.; Ratcliffe, J.; Katzmarzyk, P.T.; Barreira, T.V.; Chaput, J.P.; Fogelholm, M.; et al. Human development index, children's health-related quality of life and movement behaviors: A compositional data analysis. *Qual. Life Res.* **2018**, *27*, 1473–1482. [CrossRef] [PubMed]
71. Roman-Vinas, B.; Chaput, J.P.; Katzmarzyk, P.T.; Fogelholm, M.; Lambert, E.V.; Maher, C.; Maia, J.; Olds, T.; Onywera, V.; Sarmiento, O.L.; et al. Proportion of children meeting recommendations for 24 h movement guidelines and associations with adiposity in a 12-country study. *Int. J. Behav. Nutr. Phys. Act.* **2016**, *13*, 123. [CrossRef] [PubMed]
72. Sampasa-Kanyinga, H.; Standage, M.; Tremblay, M.S.; Katzmarzyk, P.T.; Hu, G.; Kuriyan, R.; Maher, C.; Maia, J.; Olds, T.; Sarmiento, O.L.; et al. Associations between meeting combinations of 24 h movement guidelines and health-related quality of life in children from 12-countries. *Public Health* **2017**, *153*, 16–24. [CrossRef] [PubMed]

73. Thivel, D.; Tremblay, M.S.; Katzmarzyk, P.T.; Fogelholm, M.; Hu, G.; Maher, C.; Maia, J.; Olds, T.; Sarmiento, O.L.; Standage, M.; et al. Associations between meeting combinations of 24-hour movement recommendations and dietary patterns of children: A 12-country study. *Prev. Med.* **2018**, *118*, 159–165. [CrossRef] [PubMed]
74. Chastin, S.F.; Palarea-Albaladejo, J.; Dontje, M.L.; Skelton, D.A. Combined effects of time spent in physical activity, sedentary behaviors and sleep on obesity and cardio-metabolic health markers: A novel compositional data analysis approach. *PLoS ONE* **2015**, *10*, e0139984. [CrossRef] [PubMed]
75. Dumuid, D.; Stanford, T.E.; Pedisic, Z.; Maher, C.; Lewis, L.K.; Martin-Fernandez, J.A.; Katzmarzyk, P.T.; Chaput, J.P.; Fogelholm, M.; Standage, M.; et al. Adiposity and the isotemporal substitution of physical activity, sedentary time and sleep among school-aged children: A compositional data analysis approach. *BMC Public Health* **2018**, *18*, 311. [CrossRef] [PubMed]
76. Pedisic, Z. Measurement issues and poor adjustments for physical activity and sleep undermine sedentary behaviour research—The focus should shift to the balance between sleep, sedentary behaviour, standing and activity. *Kinesiology* **2014**, *46*, 135–146.
77. Dumuid, D.; Stanford, T.E.; Martin-Fernandez, J.A.; Pedisic, Z.; Maher, C.A.; Lewis, L.K.; Hron, K.; Katzmarzyk, P.T.; Chaput, J.P.; Fogelholm, M.; et al. Compositional data analysis for physical activity, sedentary time and sleep research. *Stat. Methods Med. Res.* **2017**, *27*. [CrossRef] [PubMed]
78. Dumuid, D.; Olds, T.; Lewis, L.K.; Martin-Fernandez, J.A.; Barreira, T.; Broyles, S.; Chaput, J.P.; Fogelholm, M.; Hu, G.; Kuriyan, R.; et al. The adiposity of children is associated with their lifestyle behaviours: A cluster analysis of school-aged children from 12 nations. *Pediat.r Obes.* **2018**, *13*, 111–119. [CrossRef]
79. Katzmarzyk, P.T.; Barreira, T.V.; Broyles, S.T.; Chaput, J.P.; Fogelholm, M.; Hu, G.; Kuriyan, R.; Kurpad, A.; Lambert, E.V.; Maher, C.; et al. Association between body mass index and body fat in 9–11-year-old children from countries spanning a range of human development. *Int. J. Obes. Suppl.* **2015**, *5*, S43–S46. [CrossRef] [PubMed]
80. Chaput, J.-P.; Katzmarzyk, P.T.; Barnes, J.D.; Fogelholm, M.; Hu, G.; Kuriyan, R.; Kurpad, A.; Lambert, E.V.; Maher, C.; Maia, J.; et al. Mid-upper arm circumference as a screening tool for identifying children with obesity: A 12-country study. *Pediatric. Obes.* **2017**, *12*, 439–445. [CrossRef]
81. Ekelund, U.; Steene-Johannessen, J.; Brown, W.J.; Fagerland, M.W.; Owen, N.; Powell, K.E.; Bauman, A.; Lee, I.M. Does physical activity attenuate, or even eliminate, the detrimental association of sitting time with mortality? A harmonised meta-analysis of data from more than 1 million men and women. *Lancet* **2016**, *388*, 1302–1310. [CrossRef]
82. Chaput, J.-P.; Barnes, J.D.; Tremblay, M.S.; Fogelholm, M.; Hu, G.; Lambert, E.V.; Maher, C.; Maia, J.; Olds, T.; Onywera, V.; et al. Thresholds of physical activity associated with obesity by level of sedentary behaviour in children. *Pediatr. Obes.* **2018**, *13*, 450–457. [CrossRef]
83. Althoff, T.; Sosic, R.; Hicks, J.L.; King, A.C.; Delp, S.L.; Leskovec, J. Large-scale physical activity data reveal worldwide activity inequality. *Nature* **2017**, *547*, 336–339. [CrossRef]
84. Chaput, J.P.; Barnes, J.D.; Tremblay, M.S.; Fogelholm, M.; Hu, G.; Lambert, E.V.; Maher, C.; Maia, J.; Olds, T.; Onywera, V.; et al. Inequality in physical activity, sedentary behaviour, sleep duration and risk of obesity in children: A 12-country study. *Obes. Sci. Pract.* **2018**, *4*, 229–237. [CrossRef] [PubMed]
85. Stuckler, D.; Ruskin, G.; McKee, M. Complexity and conflicts of interest statements: A case-study of emails exchanged between Coca-Cola and the principal investigators of the International Study of Childhood Obesity, Lifestyle and the Environment (ISCOLE). *J. Public Health Pol.* **2018**, *39*, 49–56. [CrossRef] [PubMed]
86. Katzmarzyk, P.T.; Church, T.S. Letter to the editors. *J. Public Health Pol.* **2018**, *39*, 254–257. [CrossRef] [PubMed]
87. World Health Organization. *Global Action Plan on Physical Activity 2018–2030: More Active People for a Healthier World*; World Health Organization: Geneva, Switzerland, 2018.
88. United Nations. *Transforming Our World: The 2030 Agenda for Sustainable Development*; United Nations: New York, NY, USA, 2015.

11

Intake Levels of Fish in the UK Paediatric Population

Sibylle Kranz [1,*,†], Nicholas R. V. Jones [2] and Pablo Monsivais [2,‡]

1 Centre for Exercise, Nutrition and Health Sciences, University of Bristol, Bristol BS8 1TH, UK
2 UKCRC Centre for Diet and Activity Research (CEDAR), Cambridge CB2 0QQ, UK; nrvj2@cantab.net (N.R.V.J.); pm491@medschl.cam.ac.uk (P.M.)
* Correspondence: Sibylle.kranz@virginia.edu
† Current address: Department of Kinesiology, University of Virginia, Charlottesville 22904, USA.
‡ Current address: Department of Nutrition and Exercise Physiology, Washington State University, Spokane, WA 99210, USA.

Abstract: The United Kingdom (UK) is an island and its culture, including diet, is heavily influenced by the maritime resources. Dietary guidance in the UK recommends intake of fish, which provides important nutrients, such as long-chain omega-3 polyunsaturated fatty acids (*n*-3 PUFA). This study was designed to describe the fish intake habits of UK children using a nationally representative sample. Dietary and socio-demographic data of children 2–18 (N = 2096) in the National Diet and Nutrition Survey Rolling Program (NDNS) Years 1–4 (2008–2012) were extracted. Average nutrient and food intakes were estimated. Logistic regression models were used to predict the meeting of fish intake recommendations, controlling for age, sex, income, total energy intake, and survey year. All analyses were conducted using survey routines and dietary survey weights. In this nationally representative study, 4.7% of children met the fish and 4.5% the oily fish intake recommendations; only 1.3% of the population met both recommendations. Fish intake levels did not significantly change with children's increasing age. Higher vegetable but lower meat consumption predicted meeting the fish intake recommendations, indicating that children eating fish have better diet quality than non-consumers. Further research is needed to explore how intake behaviours can be changed to improve children's diet quality.

Keywords: fish intake; diet quality; nutrition monitoring; NDNS-RP; child nutrition

---

1. Introduction

Fish contains very specific nutrients, including eicosapentanoic acid (EPA) and docosahexaenoic acid (DHA), which are considered critical, as these long-chain n(omega)-3 polyunsaturated fatty acids (PUFA) have important roles in health [1], such as heart health [2], brain [3], and eye development [4–6]. Since EPA and DHA are not easily synthesized in the human body and the conversion rate from medium-chain *n*-3 fatty acids, such as alpha linoleic acid (ALA), is only approximately 1% [7], dietary intake of fish is considered part of a healthy diet [8–10].

Public health guidance recommends the consumption of fish, especially oily fish (i.e., salmon, herring, anchovy, smelt, and mackerel). The *Dietary Guidelines for Americans* [11] and United Kingdom (UK) Scientific Advisory Committee on Nutrition (SACN) [12] both suggest the consumption of two servings of fish (140 g each) per week, one serving of which should be from oily fish. This is equivalent to a calculated daily average minimum of 40 g of fish, of which 20 g should be from oily fish. Meeting these intake recommendations would contribute approximately 450 mg of EPA/DHA, which is considered as the adequate intake level by the two agencies. The Joint Food and Agriculture Organization (FAO) and World Health Organization (WHO) Expert Consultation on Fats and Fatty Acids in Human Nutrition provide a similar recommendation, namely 300 mg/day EPA and DHA, of which at least 200 mg/day should be DHA [13].

Studies of children's diets in Germany indicated that children consuming even small amounts of fish had significantly improved long-chain n-3 PUFA consumption levels compared to non-consumers [14]. A study of national fish consumption trends in American children reported overall low intake of fish; moreover, only one of the three most frequently consumed fish species was an oily variety [15]. Likewise, another analysis of the diets of one through five year old American children found very low intake of fish and long-chain n-3 PUFA [16].

The countries of the UK (England, Wales, Scotland, and Northern Ireland) are geographically maritime—islands surrounded by waters that are traditionally harvested for fish and seafood. Although slightly varied between these four countries, the historic diet culture in the UK includes many fish- and seafood-based dishes, such as baked or pickled fish, seafood salads or pies, and smoked/dried fish. The most recognized dishes internationally include "fish and chips" (battered and deep fried cod, haddock or plaice served with large-cut potato fries), "kippers" (salted and smoked herring), or smoked mackerel. These dishes are found on the menu of most eateries in the UK. They are offered as low-cost street-food but also in higher-end restaurants as "traditional fare".

The national dietary intake guidance for the UK is issued by the Food Standards Agency in form of the "The Eatwell Plate" and reflects the SACN recommendations for fish and oily fish [17]. Survey data shows that fish intake is recognized as a healthy choice by young people, although opinions somewhat vary [18]. Despite the relatively high availability of fish and seafood and consistent public health guidance to consume more fish, just like American children, UK children may not meet the intake recommendation.

The primary goal of this study was to use nationally representative data to examine the fish and seafood consumption of children in the UK, and to compare reported consumption levels with the intake recommendations for total fish and oily fish. A secondary goal was to examine the association of fish intake to other indicators of diet quality, in this case vegetable and meat intake.

2. Materials and Methods

2.1. Population Sample

Data from 2–18 year-old children (N = 2096) of the survey years 1–4 of the National Diet and Nutrition Survey rolling programme (NDNS-RP, 2008–2012) were included in this study. Children's age was used to stratify the population in three distinct age groups: 2–5 year olds, 6–11 year olds, and 12–18 year olds. All analyses were conducted for the total sample, as well as separately for those who reported consuming any fish. NDNS is publicly available and de-identified data, thus this study does not fall under the scope of research in human subjects.

Dietary, demographic, and socioeconomic data were obtained from the dataset. Demographic and socio-economic data (sex, race/ethnicity, and income) were used to describe the sample. Income was not available for 21 (1%) children in the sample, leaving N = 2075 children for whom the household income was categorized and equalised using a method previously used [16]. Income was coded as missing when household income was not provided.

2.2. Nutritional Variables

To estimate dietary intake, four consecutive 24-h estimated diet diaries (records) were collected from participants. Participants kept dietary intake records for four consecutive days. Dietary intake data collection was conducted year-round. No information as to the season of the data collected here is available. Weekend days were over-sampled in year one of the survey and under-sampled in the remaining years of the dataset used here, thus providing a fair estimate of usual daily intake of the participants. Each participant aged 12 and older was instructed on how to complete his or her own diary using household measures (i.e., measuring cups and spoons) and information from product packages to estimate the amounts of food and drink consumed. Children 16 and older were asked to estimate the portions of food and drink consumed by referring to a photo booklet of commonly-consumed items. For children younger than 12, parents or care-givers were asked to complete the diary, with information from the child. By the second or third diary day, survey staff met with the participant to review the diary days completed so far and provide feedback for improving the quality of diet data collection for the remaining diary days. Daily average food group and nutrient consumptions are reported in the dataset. Completed diaries were coded and entered by trained survey staff. Data were entered into the MRC-Human Nutrition Research dietary assessment system DINO (Diet IN Nutrients Out), an analysis system written in Microsoft Access. Nutrient intake assessed by DINO is based on a food composition database derived from UK food tables and supplemented with additional information from the food industry. Details of the use of DINO to estimate nutrient intakes in NDNS has been reported [19].

For the purpose of this study, total energy (kilocalories per day (kcal)), food group (in percent of total energy consumed for protein, fat, carbohydrates, and total sugars) and individual food items (in grams per 1000 kcal consumed or fruits and vegetables, total meat, red meat, white meat, eggs, nuts and seeds, total fish, white fish, oily fish, canned tuna, and shellfish) were calculated. This approach allows for comparison across age groups, which consume different levels of total energy and therefore increasing amounts of each food group with increasing age. Based on the reported diet, children were classified as "fish consumers" if they consumed any amount of fish or seafood (NDNS Variable 33 "White fish coated or fried", Variable 34 "Other white fish, shellfish and fish dishes", and Variable 35 "Oily fish") or as non-consumers otherwise. All data were reported for all children and disaggregated by age group for the total sample and the fish consumers and non-consumers separately. In the NDNS dataset, the n-3 PUFA are estimated as one variable, thus, no differentiation between the intake of long-chain n-3 PUFA, such as EPA and DHA, and short- or medium-chain PUFA can be made.

2.3. Statistical Analysis

All analyses were conducted using survey routines and the dietary survey weights to maintain the nationally representative character of the data. Analyses were conducted in STATA Version 13 (STATA Corporation, College Station, TX, USA). Mean consumption of food groups and nutrients was calculated for the total population and for each age group separately and reported as mean $\pm$ standard error. Intakes of macronutrients were expressed as percent energy and food groups were expressed on a gram (g) per-1000 kcal basis in order to facilitate comparisons across age groups. Since fish and seafood consumption was highly skewed, so median and interquartile range were estimated to describe the consumption in the population. Non-parametric test for trend across ordered groups was used to determine if consumption increased or decreased with increasing age across three age groups (2–5, 6–11, 12–18 years old). Significant differences in mean consumption between the group of children who consume fish and non-consumers was determined using the *lincom* command, the survey routine equivalent to the Student's T-test to compare means. Logistic regression modelling was employed to determine the contributors to children's odds of (a) meeting the dietary intake recommendation for total fish (40 g/day); (b) for oily fish (20 g/day); and (c) for any consumption of fish. All models controlled for age, sex, household income, total energy intake, and NDNS survey year. Statistical significance was assumed using a 95% level of significance.

3. Results

Based on the nature of this study, the demographic profile of the population included in the sample is representative of all children in the UK (data not shown). More than half of the population (55%, N = 1142) consumed any fish/seafood during the four days of dietary intake measurement (Table 1). Of those, 4.7% met the total fish intake recommendation, 4.5% the oily fish intake recommendation, and only 1.3% (N = 28 children) of 2–18 year olds met both (the total fish and the oily fish intake recommendations).

Table 1. Proportion of children meeting the recommended fish and seafood intake of the "Eatwell Plate" UK national intake recommendations in the National Diet and Nutrition Survey 2008–2012 in the total sample (N = 2075).

Characteristic	Total Sample (N = 2096)	2–5 Year Olds (N = 634)	6–11 Year Olds (N = 664)	12–18 Year Olds (N = 798)
Fish consumers [1]	54.9	62.9	58.3	45.5
Meet fish recommendation (≥40 g of fish/day)	4.2	2.5	4.6	5.3
Meet oily fish recommendation (≥20 g of fish/day)	4.0	2.4	4.8	4.7
Meet fish and oily fish recommendations	1.3	0.6	1.4	1.0

[1] Includes NDNS food groups "White fish coated or fried", "Other white fish, shellfish and fish dishes", and "Oily fish".

Fish and seafood intake was highly skewed, hence, both mean and standard error (SE) as well as median and interquartile range (IQR), the 25th and 75th percentile of intake, were calculated. Total fish and seafood consumption was low (mean ± SE = 10.41 ± 0.42; median and IQR: 3.78 g/day and 0; 16.5 g/day); oily fish consumption was even lower (mean ± SE = 1.78 ± 0.17; median and IQR: 0 g/day and 0; 0 g/day); the 90th percentile of oily fish intake was only 2.55 g/day.

Analysis of the average dietary intake of foods and food groups in the total sample and the subsamples of fish consumers, and those children meeting the intake recommendations, showed that children who consumed fish had better diet quality (Table 2). Those children consumed more vegetables and less meat. Most nutrient and food group intake vary with age in the total population, in that total energy, meat density (red and white meat density) and shellfish increased while percent of energy from added sugar, fruit and vegetable density, total- and white fish density decreased. Comparison of intake between fish consumers and non-consumers showed that children who consume fish have higher fruit and vegetable density in their diet and lower meat density.

Logistic regression models showed that neither household income nor ethnic group was associated with total fish or oily fish intake (data not shown) and subsequent modelling including age, sex, equalised household income, total energy consumed and NDNS survey year as covariates (Table 3).

Consuming any fish was strongly and positively associated with being in the medium or highest tertile of vegetable intake and negatively associated with eating the medium or highest tertile of meat (OR = 1.55, 95% CI 1.19–2.12; OR = 1.88, 95% CI 1.39–2.58; OR = 0.72, 95% CI 0.55–0.98; OR = 0.47' 95% CI 0.34–0.66, respectively). Consuming the recommended amount of two servings of fish was significantly and positively predicted by consuming the highest tertile of vegetables (OR = 2.51, 95% CI 1.30–4.84) and significantly but negatively associated with consuming the highest tertile of meat (OR = 0.32, 95% CI 0.16–0.64). The odds of meeting the intake recommendation for oily fish was increased with eating the highest tertile of vegetables (OR = 3.49, 95% CI 1.21–9.96) and the medium or highest tertile of meat consumption (OR = 2.84, 95% CI 1.20-6.75 and OR = 2.65, 95% CI 1.90–7.84, respectively).

Table 2. Estimated intakes of select food groups and foods † by children in the National Diet and Nutrition Survey 2008–2012 in the total sample and by age group (N = 2096).

	All Children	2–5 Year Olds	6–11 Year Olds	12–18 Year Olds	Test for Trend ‡ *p*-Value
Total sample (N = 2096)					
Total energy (kcal/day)	1554 ± 14	1205 ± 17	1608 ± 18	1801 ± 24	<0.001 ***
Protein (% energy/day)	14.8 ± 0.8	15.1 ± 0.1	14.4 ± 0.1	14.8 ± 0.1	0.172
Fat (% energy/day)	33.7 ± 0.1	33.8 ± 0.3	33.4 ± 0.2	33.8 ± 0.2	0.783
Carbohydrates (% energy/day)	51.2 ± 0.2	51.2 ± 0.3	52.2 ± 0.2	50.5 ± 0.3	0.011 *
Energy-adjusted intakes of food groups (g/1000 kcal consumed)					
Fruits and vegetables	126.3 ± 2.4	158.9 ± 5.1	129.4 ± 3.7	96.8 ± 2.7	<0.001 ***
Total meat	47.2 ± 0.8	37.7 ± 4.1	46.4 ± 1.1	44.8 ± 1.4	<0.001 ***
Red meat	30.6 ± 0.7	25.7 ± 1.2	30.6 ± 1.1	34.8 ± 1.2	<0.001 ***
White meat	16.6 ± 0.5	12.1 ± 0.7	15.8 ± 0.7	21.0 ± 0.8	<0.001 ***
Eggs	6.9 ± 0.4	6.8 ± 0.6	6.1 ± 0.6	7.6 ± 0.7	0.345
Nuts and seeds	0.6 ± 0.1	0.7 ± 0.6	0.6 ± 0.1	0.6 ± 0.1	0.263
Total fish	7.1 ± 0.3	7.9 ± 0.5	7.2 ± 0.5	6.2 ± 0.4	<0.001 ***
White fish	4.0 ± 0.2	4.9 ± 0.4	4.2 ± 0.4	2.3 ± 0.2	<0.001 ***
Oily fish	1.2 ± 0.1	1.1 ± 0.2	1.3 ± 0.2	1.1 ± 0.2	0.164
Canned tuna	1.6 ± 0.1	1.6 ± 0.3	1.1 ± 0.1	1.9 ± 0.3	0.152
Shellfish	0.6 ± 0.1	0.2 ± 0.1	0.6 ± 0.1	0.8 ± 0.2	<0.001 ***
Consumers of fish/seafood (N = 1142)					
Total energy (kcal/day)	1522 ± 18 ⊥	1211 ± 18	1621 ± 26	1776 ± 34	<0.001 ***
Protein (% energy/day)	15.1 ± 0.1 ⊥	15.3 ± 0.2 ⊥	14.7 ± 0.2 ⊥	15.2 ± 0.2 ⊥	0.812
Fat (% energy/day)	33.8 ± 0.2	33.7 ± 0.4	33.6 ± 0.3	34.2 ± 0.3	0.875
Carbohydrates (% energy/day)	50.9 ± 0.2 ⊥	51.0 ± 0.4	51.8 ± 0.3 ⊥	50.0 ± 0.4	0.055

Table 2. *Cont.*

	All Children	2–5 Year Olds	6–11 Year Olds	12–18 Year Olds	Test for Trend ‡ p-Value
Energy-adjusted intakes of food groups (g/1000 kcal consumed)					
Fruits and vegetables	135.3 ± 3.2 ⊥	162.9 ± 0.006.2	138.3 ± 4.1 ⊥	100.4 ± 3.7	<0.001 ***
Total meat	43.4 ± 1.1 ⊥	35.3 ± 1.8 ⊥	43.7 ± 1.5 ⊥	52.3 ± 2.0 ⊥	<0.001 ***
Red meat	27.6 ± 0.7 ⊥	23.6 ± 1.4 ⊥	28.4 ± 1.3 ⊥	31.2 ± 1.6 ⊥	<0.001 ***
White meat	15.8 ± 0.6	11.7 ± 1.0	15.3 ± 0.8	21.1 ± 1.3	<0.001 ***
Eggs	6.6 ± 0.5	7.0 ± 0.8	6.1 ± 0.9	6.9 ± 0.8	0.247
Nuts and seeds	0.7 ± 0.1 ⊥	0.7 ± 0.2	0.7 ± 0.2 ⊥	0.6 ± 0.2	0.153
Total fish	12.9 ± 0.4	12.6 ± 0.8	12.5 ± 0.6	13.7 ± 0.7	0.064
White fish	4.0 ± 0.2	7.8 ± 0.6	7.2 ± 0.5	5.0 ± 0.5	<0.001 ***
Oily fish	1.2 ± 0.1	1.8 ± 0.3	2.3 ± 0.3	2.5 ± 0.4	0.406
Canned tuna	1.6 ± 0.1	2.6 ± 0.5	1.9 ± 0.2	4.4 ± 0.5	<0.001 ***
Shellfish	0.6 ± 0.1	0.3 ± 0.1	1.1 ± 0.2	1.9 ± 0.4	<0.001 ***
Non-consumers of fish/seafood (N = 954)					
Total energy (kcal/day)	1594 ± 22 ⊥	1196 ± 30	1590 ± 25	1821 ± 34	<0.001 ***
Protein (% energy/day)	14.4 ± 0.12 ⊥	14.7 ± 0.2 ⊥	14.1 ± 0.2 ⊥	14.5 ± 0.2	0.314
Fat (% energy/day)	33.6 ± 0.2	34.0 ± 0.5	33.2 ± 0.4	33.6 ± 0.4	0.565
Carbohydrates (% energy/day)	51.5 ± 0.2 ⊥	51.4 ± 0.5	52.8 ± 0.4	50.9 ± 0.4	0.062
Energy-adjusted intakes of food groups (g/1000 kcal consumed)					
Fruits and vegetables	115.5 ± 3.7 ⊥	152.2 ± 8.7	116.9 ± 6.8 ⊥	93.8 ± 3.9	<0.001 ***
Total meat	51.9 ± 1.2 ⊥	41.8 ± 2.2 ⊥	50.1 ± 1.9 ⊥	58.8 ± 1.8 ⊥	<0.001 ***
Red meat	34.4 ± 1.1 ⊥	29.2 ± 1.9 ⊥	33.6 ± 1.8 ⊥	37.8 ± 1.7 ⊥	0.002 **
White meat	17.6 ± 0.7	12.6 ± 1.1	16.5 ± 1.1	21.0 ± 1.1	<0.001 ***
Eggs	7.1 ± 0.6	6.6 ± 1.0	6.0 ± 0.8	8.1 ± 1.0	0.945
Nuts and seeds	0.5 ± 0.1 ⊥	0.6 ± 0.2	0.3 ± 0.1 ⊥	0.6 ± 0.1	0.878

† Includes NDNS food groups "White fish coated or fried", "Other white fish, shellfish and fish dishes", and "Oily fish"; ‡ across ordered groups by age group; Asterisks indicate significant trend with increasing age * $p < 0.05$; ** $p < 0.01$; *** $p < 0.0001$; ⊥ significantly different between fish consumers and non-consumers.

Table 3. Association (odds ratios and 95% confidence intervals) of children's dietary characteristics for children, who (a) are fish consumers and (b) meet the fish intake recommendation of 280 g/week (or 40 g/day), and (c) meet the oily fish intake recommendation of 140 g/week (or 20 g/day) (N = 2096).

		Odds Ratio	95% Confidence Interval
(a) Consume any fish/seafood			
Tertile of vegetable	Lowest	1.00	
	Medium	1.55 **	1.19, 2.12
	Highest	1.88 ***	1.39, 2.58
Tertile of meat	Lowest	1.00	
	Medium	0.72 *	0.55, 0.98
	Highest	0.47 ***	0.34, 0.66
(b) Meet fish intake recommendation			
Tertile of vegetable	Lowest	1.00	
	Medium	0.99	0.45, 2.16
	Highest	2.51 **	1.30, 4.84
Tertile of meat	Lowest	1.00	
	Medium	0.55	0.27, 1.09
	Highest	0.32 **	0.16, 0.64
(c) Meet oily fish intake recommendation			
Total fish intake (g/day)		1.07 ***	1.05, 1.09
Tertile of vegetable	Lowest	1.00	
	Medium	1.89	0.67, 5.97
	Highest	3.47 **	1.21, 9.96
Tertile of meat	Lowest	1.00	
	Medium	2.84 **	1.20, 6.75
	Highest	2.65 *	1.90, 7.84

Values were significantly different at: * $p < 0.05$; ** $p < 0.01$; *** $p < 0.0001$, all models controlling for age, sex, total energy intake, equalized household income, and NDNS survey year.

4. Discussion

Recommendations for fish intake, especially those focussing on oily fish, are in part designed to promote adequate intakes of EPA and DHA in children and adults. Low intake of EPA/DHA is commonly observed in the Western diet [17] and might negatively affect children's brain development and function [18,19]. Data from observational studies indicated that low levels of EPA/DHA may be associated with rising prevalence of childhood developmental disorders, such as attention-deficit hyperactivity disorder and dyslexia [20]. Overall, EPA and DHA have a recognized role in health and disease prevention [1–6]. As our results show, the proportion of children in the UK meeting the intake recommendations for total fish and oily fish intake is extremely small. This is reason for concern.

Although small amounts of EPA and DHA can be found in foods other than fish, those foods (predominantly eggs and dark poultry meats) are also very high in saturated fatty acids [21]. Although we showed that a very large proportion of 2–18 year-old children in the UK fail to meet the intake recommendation for total fish and/or oily fish, we are not able to directly assess if children meet the targeted daily minimum consumption amounts for EPA and DHA because EPA and DHA are not reported separately from medium- and short-chain fatty acids in the NDNS data set. This particular problem with the UK national dietary data survey system has been noted previously [22]. It would be very beneficial for policy purposes if future releases of the NDNS nutrient data wold be modified to allow a direct measurement of the individual dietary fatty acids. However, it is noteworthy to point out that the measurement of EPA and DHA in free-living individuals is a challenge, due to tissue storage, conversion rate, and saturable plasma levels [20]. In the future, other approaches might be possible to better estimate fish intake, such as a metabolomic study of biomarkers of meat and fish intake [21].

Despite the lack of direct measurement of EPA and DHA intake levels in this sample, our analysis showed that the vast majority of 2–18 year old children in the UK fail to meet the intake recommendations for fish. Interestingly, the density of fish in the diet increased with increasing age for most categories of fish, but consumption of white fish dropped and oily fish remained almost the same in 12–18 year olds while intake of canned tuna and shellfish experienced a marked increase compared to the two younger age groups. While the similar findings in the US paediatric population [22] may be explained by the relatively low availability of affordable fish, especially oily fish, the same phenomenon in the UK must have different reasons and begs to be explored further. In the US, especially young children from low-income households may have limited access to fish, due to their mothers dietary intake practices, which have been shown to be low in fish and other healthy items [23]. However, as the authors for that research report explain, there is severe lack of evidence on the possible venues to rectify the problem of low diet quality in low-income women. Some possible contributing factors may be the lack of access (i.e., family ability to obtain seafood from local vendors) and availability (i.e., the quantity and quality of food provided), the relatively higher cost of some oily fish compared to (for example) cheaper processed meats [23]. Also, parents' and carers' knowledge and ability to prepare fish, as well as their role-modelling of eating fish and seafood [24] may contribute. Other changes in local culture, such as the lack of family meals and a preference to consume foods from other cuisines are potential contributing to the low intake of fish in children. These phenomena may also be the underlying cause of reduction of fish intake in Mediterranean countries, which used to be traditionally high in fish intake [24,25]. A published research report for an intervention study to increase dietary EPA and DHA consumption of preschool-age children showed that the substitution of meats usually used for the lunch meal in child care settings can be replaced with oily fish [25]. Since oily fish, such as salmon, herring, and sardines, are so high in EPA and DHA that even a small increase in intake results in significantly improved intakes, adding fish to mixed dishes, such as pasta and sauce, may significantly improve children's EPA and DHA consumption.

One possible limitation of this study was the use of four estimated dietary records to estimate intake. Although this method has been accepted for large nutrition surveys, intake of rarely consumed foods, such as seafood, may be misrepresented using this somewhat short-term data collection method. On the other hand, the level of detail provided by multiple-day records is superior to diet information obtained from long-term food frequency questionnaires. Compared to the intake estimates used in US national surveys (using two 24-hour recalls), the use of four days of food records doubled the odds of capturing those rarely consumed foods. Ideally, future research on fish intake would include a biomarker of intake levels, such as trimethylamine-N-oxide [21].

One major strength of this study was the use of a nationally-representative data set, which allows generalizability of the results. Some might expect that younger children have different intake patterns than teenagers. However, the consumption levels of all fish and seafood types available in the dataset show that intake increases with age, with the exception of white fish.

A key finding was that only approximately 2% of the population met the recommendations for both total fish and oily fish intake. Interestingly, our data show that children who consumed any fish or seafood also had healthier eating patterns, characterized by higher vegetable intake but lower meat intake. This relationship between higher vegetable but lower meat intake showed a significant trend, in that the odds for meeting the fish intake recommendations were even better in the children consuming in the highest tertile of vegetable compared to the medium tertile. Likewise, the odds for meeting the intake recommendations were lower for the children consuming in the highest tertile for meat intake compared to the medium tertile of meat consumption. This finding suggests for the first time that in the UK paediatric population, fish intake may be a useful proxy for overall healthy eating patterns.

Results of this study indicate that programmes and policies to promote the consumption of fish in the UK are not heeded. Although some might recommend more frequent and larger amounts of fish intake in the paediatric population, even a small intake of predatory fish raises the concern for the possible nutrition-toxicity issues [26]. Supplying sufficient amounts of safe fish to meet EPA and DHA intake recommendations may also be at odds with the sustainability of marine ecosystems [27]. At the same time, exploring other dietary sources of EPA and DHA that are low-cost, widely available, and acceptable to children might be beneficial for all children, not only in the UK.

5. Conclusions

Our study indicates that children in the UK do not consume sufficient amounts of fish. However, due to the lack of data on the EPA and DHA consumption, it is not clear whether or not the low fish intake is associated with inadequate levels of these two important nutrients for brain development and functioning. Further research is needed to pursue this question and to identify the barriers to fish intake in a population of traditionally high fish- and seafood diets.

Acknowledgments: N.R.V.J. and P.M. were supported by the Centre for Diet and Activity Research (CEDAR), a UKCRC Public Health Research Centre of Excellence. Funding from the British Heart Foundation, Cancer Research UK, Economic and Social Research Council, Medical Research Council, the National Institute for Health Research, and the Wellcome Trust, under the auspices of the UK Clinical Research Collaboration, is gratefully acknowledged. The funders had no role in the design or conduct of the study or the writing of the manuscript. This research received no specific grant from any funding agency, commercial or not-for-profit sectors.

Author Contributions: S.K. is the primary author and led the analysis and writing. N.R.V.J. and P.M. contributed to analysis and writing. All authors have read and approved the final manuscript.

References

1. Yashodhara, B.M.; Umakanth, S.; Pappachan, J.M.; Bhat, S.K.; Kamath, R.; Choo, B.H. Omega-3 fatty acids: A comprehensive review of their role in health and disease. *Postgrad. Med. J.* **2009**, *85*, 84–90. [CrossRef] [PubMed]
2. Mozzaffarian, D.; Wu, J.H.Y. (*n*-3) fatty acids and cardiovascular health: Are effects of EPA and DHA shared or complementary? *J. Nutr.* **2012**, *142*, 614S–625S. [CrossRef] [PubMed]
3. Innis, S.M. Dietary omega 3 fatty acids and the developing brain. *Brain Res.* **2008**, *1237*, 35–43. [CrossRef] [PubMed]
4. Birch, E.E.; Garfield, S.; Castaneda, Y.; Hughbankswheaton, D.; Uauy, R.; Hoffman, D. Visual acuity and cognitive outcomes at 4 years of age in a double-blind, randomized trial of long-chain polyunsaturated fatty acid-supplemented infant formula. *Early Hum. Dev.* **2007**, *83*, 279–284. [CrossRef] [PubMed]
5. Jacques, C.; Levy, E.; Muckle, G.; Jacobson, S.W.; Bastien, C.; Dewailly, E.; Ayotte, P.; Jacobson, J.L.; Saint-Amour, D. Long-term effects of prenatal omega-3 fatty acid intake on visual function in school-age children. *J. Pediatr.* **2011**, *158*, 73. [CrossRef] [PubMed]
6. SanGiovanni, J.P.; Chew, E.Y. The role of omega-3 long-chain polyunsaturated fatty acids in health and disease of the retina. *Prog. Retin. Eye Res.* **2005**, *24*, 87–138. [CrossRef] [PubMed]
7. Gebauer, S.K.; Psota, T.L.; Harris, W.S.; Kris-Etherton, P.M. *N*-3 fatty acid dietary recommendations and food sources to achieve essentiality and cardiovascular benefits. *Am. J. Clin. Nutr.* **2006**, *83*, 1526S–1535S. [PubMed]
8. Institute of Medicine of the National Academy of Sciences. *Dietary Reference Intakes for Energy, Carbohydrate, Fiber, Fat, Fatty Acids, Cholesterol, Protein, and Amino Acids (Macronutrients)*; National Academy Press: Washington, DC, USA, 2002.
9. Flock, M.R.; Harris, W.S.; Kris-Etherton, P.M. Long-chain omega-3 fatty acids: Time to establish a dietary reference intake. *Nutr. Rev.* **2013**, *71*, 692–707. [CrossRef] [PubMed]
10. Scientific Advisory Committee for Nutrition (SCAN). *Advice on Fish Consumption: Benefits and Risks*; Food Standards Agency and the Department of Health: London, UK, 2004.
11. World Health Organization Study Group. Interim summary of conclusions and dietary recommendations on total fat and fatty acids. In Proceedings of the Joint FAO/WHO Expert Consultation on Fats and Fatty Acids in Human Nutrition, Geneva, Switzerland, 10–14 November 2008.

12. Kris-Etherton, P.M.; Taylor, D.S.; Yu-Poth, S.; Huth, P.; Moriarty, K.; Fishell, V.; Hargrove, R.L.; Zhao, G.; Etherton, T.D. Polyunsaturated fatty acids in the food chain in the United States. *Am. J. Clin. Nutr.* **2000**, *71*, 179S–188S. [PubMed]
13. Sichert-Hellert, W.; Wicher, M.; Kersting, M. Age and time trends in fish consumption pattern of children and adolescents, and consequences for the intake of long-chain *n*-3 polyunsaturated fatty acids. *Eur. J. Clin. Nutr.* **2009**, *63*, 1071–1075. [CrossRef] [PubMed]
14. Tran, N.L.; Barraj, L.M.; Bi, X.; Schuda, L.C.; Moya, J. Estimated long-term fish and shellfish intake—National health and nutrition examination survey. *J. Expo. Sci. Environ. Epidemiol.* **2013**, *23*, 128–136. [CrossRef] [PubMed]
15. Keim, S.A.; Branum, A.M. Dietary intake of polyunsaturated fatty acids and fish among US children 12–60 months of age. *Matern. Child. Nutr.* **2013**, *11*, 987–998. [CrossRef] [PubMed]
16. Maguire, E.R.; Monsivais, P. Socio-economic dietary inequalities in UK adults: An updated picture of key food groups and nutrients from national surveillance data. *Br. J. Nutr.* **2014**, *113*, 1–9. [CrossRef] [PubMed]
17. Van Elst, K.; Bruining, H.; Birtoli, B.; Terreaux, C.; Buitelaar, J.K. Food for thought: Dietary changes in essential fatty acid ratios and the increase in autism spectrum disorders. *Neurosci. Biobehav. Rev.* **2014**, *45C*, 369–378. [CrossRef] [PubMed]
18. Rosales, F.J.; Reznick, J.S.; Zeisel, S.H. Understanding the role of nutrition in the brain and behavioral development of toddlers and preschool children: Identifying and addressing methodological barriers. *Nutr. Neurosci.* **2009**, *12*, 190–202. [CrossRef] [PubMed]
19. Simopoulos, A.P. The importance of the ratio of omega-6/omega-3 essential fatty acids. *Biomed. Pharmacother.* **2002**, *56*, 365–379. [CrossRef]
20. Schuchardt, J.P.; Huss, M.; Stauss-Grabo, M.; Hahn, A. Significance of long-chain polyunsaturated fatty acids (PUFAs) for the development and behaviour of children. *Eur. J. Pediatr.* **2010**, *169*, 149–164. [CrossRef] [PubMed]
21. Butler, G. Manipulating dietary PUFA in animal feed: Implications for human health. *Proc. Nutr. Soc.* **2014**, *73*, 87–95. [CrossRef] [PubMed]
22. Pot, G.K.; Prynne, C.J.; Roberts, C.; Olson, A.; Nicholson, S.K.; Whitton, C.; Teucher, B.; Bates, B.; Henderson, H.; Pigott, S.; et al. National diet and nutrition survey: Fat and fatty acid intake from the first year of the rolling programme and comparison with previous surveys. *Br. J. Nutr.* **2012**, *107*, 405–415. [CrossRef] [PubMed]
23. Jones, N.R.; Conklin, A.I.; Suhrcke, M.; Monsivais, P. The growing price gap between more and less healthy foods: Analysis of a novel longitudinal UK dataset. *PLoS ONE* **2014**, *9*, e109343. [CrossRef] [PubMed]
24. Santiago-Torres, M.; Adams, A.K.; Carrel, A.L.; Larowe, T.L.; Schoeller, D.A. Home food availability, parental dietary intake, and familial eating habits influence the diet quality of urban Hispanic children. *Child. Obes.* **2014**, *10*, 408–415. [CrossRef] [PubMed]
25. Huss, L.R.; McCabe, S.D.; Dobbs-Oates, J.; Burgess, J.; Behnke, C.; Santerre, C.R.; Kranz, S. Development of child-friendly fish dishes to increase young children's acceptance and consumption of fish. *Food Nutr. Sci.* **2013**, *4*, 78–87. [CrossRef]
26. Mahaffey, K.R.; Clickner, R.P.; Jeffries, R.A. Methylmercury and omega-3 fatty acids: Co-occurrence of dietary sources with emphasis on fish and shellfish. *Environ. Res.* **2008**, *107*, 20–29. [CrossRef] [PubMed]
27. Brunner, E.J.; Jones, P.J.; Friel, S.; Bartley, M. Fish, human health and marine ecosystem health: Policies in collision. *Int. J. Epidemiol.* **2009**, *38*, 93–100. [CrossRef] [PubMed]

12

The Association between Parent Diet Quality and Child Dietary Patterns in Nine- to Eleven-Year-Old Children from Dunedin, New Zealand

Brittany Davison [1], Pouya Saeedi [1], Katherine Black [1], Harriet Harrex [1], Jillian Haszard [1], Kim Meredith-Jones [2], Robin Quigg [3], Sheila Skeaff [1], Lee Stoner [4], Jyh Eiin Wong [5] and Paula Skidmore [1,*]

1 Department of Human Nutrition, University of Otago, Dunedin 9054, New Zealand; brittany_davison@hotmail.com (B.D.); pouya.saeedi@otago.ac.nz (P.S.); katherine.black@otago.ac.nz (K.B.);harriet.harrex@otago.ac.nz (H.H.); jillian.haszard@otago.ac.nz (J.H.); sheila.skeaff@otago.ac.nz (S.S.)
2 Department of Medicine, University of Otago, Dunedin 9054, New Zealand; kim.meredith-jones@otago.ac.nz
3 Cancer Society Social and Behavioural Research Unit, Department of Preventive and Social Medicine, Dunedin School of Medicine, University of Otago, Dunedin 9054, New Zealand; robin.quigg@otago.ac.nz
4 Department of Exercise and Sports Science, University of North Carolina, Chapel Hill, NC 27519, USA; stonerl@email.unc.edu
5 School of Healthcare Sciences, Faculty of Health Sciences, Universiti Kebangsaan Malaysia, Kuala Lumpur 50300, Malaysia; wjeiin@ukm.edu.my
* Correspondence: paula.skidmore@otago.ac.nz

Abstract: Previous research investigating the relationship between parents' and children's diets has focused on single foods or nutrients, and not on global diet, which may be more important for good health. The aim of the study was to investigate the relationship between parental diet quality and child dietary patterns. A cross-sectional survey was conducted in 17 primary schools in Dunedin, New Zealand. Information on food consumption and related factors in children and their primary caregiver/parent were collected. Principal component analysis (PCA) was used to investigate dietary patterns in children and diet quality index (DQI) scores were calculated in parents. Relationships between parental DQI and child dietary patterns were examined in 401 child-parent pairs using mixed regression models. PCA generated two patterns; 'Fruit and Vegetables' and 'Snacks'. A one unit higher parental DQI score was associated with a 0.03SD (CI: 0.02, 0.04) lower child 'Snacks' score. There was no significant relationship between 'Fruit and Vegetables' score and parental diet quality. Higher parental diet quality was associated with a lower dietary pattern score in children that was characterised by a lower consumption frequency of confectionery, chocolate, cakes, biscuits and savoury snacks. These results highlight the importance of parental modelling, in terms of their dietary choices, on the diet of children.

Keywords: children; parents; diet quality; dietary patterns

---

1. Introduction

Good dietary habits need to be developed during childhood, not only to improve short-term health and but also to avoid carrying unhealthy habits into adulthood, which is also associated with negative health outcomes in long term, such as increased risk of cardiovascular disease [1,2]. One key area associated with children's dietary intake is the influence of parental diet [3–5]. Previous research in this area initially focused heavily on the relationships between parental and child consumption of fruit and vegetables [6]. More recent studies have looked at different food groups and/or nutrients, including a review that showed associations between child and parent intake of energy and total fat [7–9]. However, it is unrealistic to assume that foods are eaten in isolation. Instead, it is important to recognise that people consume meals and that there are synergistic relationships between food and nutrients [10]. To consider the diet as a whole, dietary patterns can be used. These take into account the combinations of foods consumed and have been increasingly used alongside individual dietary intake data. Dietary patterns can be derived theoretically or empirically [11].

Theoretical dietary patterns are used to determine how closely people adhere to a diet. For example, the Healthy Eating Index (HEI) is used to measure how well an individual's diet conforms to the US Healthy Food Pyramid [12]. Empirically derived dietary patterns use statistical techniques, such as principal component analysis (PCA), to derive data driven patterns specific to the population of interest [11]. There is little research investigating the relationship between parent and child dietary patterns, particularly with regards to empirically derived dietary patterns. Only three studies have investigated the association between parent and child diet quality, all of which used theoretical methods to determine dietary patterns [7,13,14]. All found positive relationships between parent and child diet quality.

The limited current literature provides an indication that dietary quality is associated between parents and children, although theoretically derived patterns based on the national nutrition guidelines differ between countries. Consequently, any significant relationships found using a particular country specific index may not be applicable to other populations. Secondly, there is a lack of research investigating the relationship between parent and child diets using empirically derived dietary patterns. The objective of the current study was to determine whether a higher parent DQI score based on the New Zealand Food and Nutrition Guidelines is associated with more healthful dietary patterns in New Zealand children aged 9–11.

2. Materials and Methods

2.1. Study Design and Participants

The present study analysed data collected as part of the Physical activity, Exercise, Diet And Lifestyle Study (PEDALS), which was a cross-sectional survey conducted in Dunedin, New Zealand between April and December 2015. Thirty out of 55 primary schools in the greater Dunedin area were invited to participate. The remaining schools were not invited as they had less than 15 Year 5 and 6 pupils on the school roll. In New Zealand, Year 5 and 6 students are typically between 9–11 years old. School principals were sent study invitation packs and if they agreed to participate, the research team visited the school to present at a Year 5 and 6 assembly. Eligible students were given packs to take home, containing letters of information and consent forms for themselves and their parents. Written parental consent and written child assent were both required in order for both the child and parent to participate. The study was conducted in accordance with the Declaration of Helsinki, and all procedures involving human subjects were approved by the University of Otago Human Ethics Committee

2.2. Data Collection

Participating children completed two questionnaires during class time, with assistance for reading questions given from the research team when necessary. The first questionnaire contained questions about the child (date of birth, age, sex, and year at school), their food and drink consumption, and known correlates of these. The second questionnaire focused on physical activity and its correlates. Trained research assistants also measured children's height, weight, waist circumference, handgrip strength, body composition, blood pressure and arterial stiffness. Cardiovascular fitness was assessed using the 20 metre shuttle run test. Child participants also received accelerometers to wear for seven days. The children were given two further questionnaires and an accelerometer to take home to their primary caregiver/parent/guardian. The parent questionnaire covered similar topics to the children's questionnaires. Questions on ethnicity, socio-economic status (SES), height, weight, education and health behaviours were also included. SES was assessed using the New Zealand Deprivation Index Score (NZDep13), which combines nine variables from the 2013 census, reflecting eight dimensions of deprivation, including owning a house and access to a car [15]. The deprivation index is an ordinal scale ranging from one (least deprived) to ten (most deprived). School decile is determined by the deprivation level, as measured by NZDep13, of students attending the school, with the lowest decile rating reflecting the 10% of schools nationwide with students mostly from high deprivation areas. School decile was divided into 'Low' (Deciles 1 to 4) 'Middle' (Deciles 5 to 8) and 'High' (Deciles 9 and 10).

The PEDALS Food Frequency Questionnaire (FFQ) was used to assess the children's usual dietary intake. This was a 28-item non-quantitative FFQ, which incorporates questions from the Health Behaviour in School-Age Children Questionnaire [16]. The PEDALS FFQ has been shown to have acceptable relative validity and reproducibility in this age group [16]. The food items included were fruits, vegetables, milk (standard (full fat), light/semi-skimmed (contains around 1.5 g fat per 100 mL) and trim/skimmed (contains around 0.1 g fat per 100 mL), cheese, yoghurt, ice cream, processed meats, other meats, fish, fruit juice, fizzy drinks (diet and standard), breakfast cereals, bread (white and brown/wholemeal), rice, pasta, potato, potato chips, hot chips, biscuits, bakery food, snack bars, lollies/sweets, chocolate, tomato sauce/ketchup and sandwich spreads. Participants reported their usual intake from seven categories ranging from 'Never' to 'Every day, more than once.'

Included in the second parent questionnaire was a dietary habits questionnaire (DHQ), which was used to assess parental dietary intake and eating habits, and was used in the 2008–2009 Adult Nutrition Survey in New Zealand [17]. This DHQ focused on food choices made over the previous four weeks. Nineteen questions were included, beginning with ten questions assessing intake of red and processed meat, chicken, fish and shellfish, hot chips, soft drinks and energy drinks, fruit juice and confectionery. Participants reported consumption from one of six categories: never; less than once a week; one to two times per week; three to four times a week; five to six times a week; seven or more times per week. There were five questions on dietary practices, such as removing fat from meat and chicken, adding salt to food, and choosing low fat and salt varieties over standard varieties. Lastly, there were four questions on type of milk, butter or margarine, bread and cooking fat used most often. Information was also collected on the highest level of education obtained by the parent participant and answers were collapsed into three groups—Secondary education until around minimum school leaving age (15 to 16 years) or equivalent, further secondary school completion (usually around 18 years), and post-secondary education.

Missing data were imputed for certain questions from the questionnaires. For responses to be imputed, at least 75% of each set of questions, where a question had at least four sub-questions, needed to have been completed and 'worst-case scenario' responses were entered. For these analyses, the only data that were imputed were for the FFQ and the DHQ. The FFQ was considered a question, and each item within it a sub-question. Thirty-five data points (0.25% of the total) were imputed for the entire FFQ dataset. The DHQ was also considered a question, and each item within it a sub-question. Seventy-two data points (0.85% of the total) were imputed for the entire DHQ dataset.

2.3. Statistical Analysis

Participants (child and parent pair) were excluded if they did not have complete information on all variables of interest for this analysis. For descriptive analyses, ethnicity was categorised into three groups, as in previous New Zealand surveys [17]: 'Māori'; 'Pacific People'; and 'New Zealand European and Other' (NZEO) were prioritised in that order. NZEO includes those who identify as New Zealand European, as well as other groups that were too small for individual analysis, such as Indian and Korean. Due to the small number of Māori and Pacific Island participants in the sample, ethnicity was further condensed to two groups: 'Māori and Pacific People' and 'NZEO' when included in multivariate analysis. Child body mass index (BMI) was calculated using measured height and weight, z-scores calculated using World Health Organisation (WHO) growth charts and categorised using the WHO categorization [18]. Self-reported height and weight were used to calculate parent BMI. A BMI < 25 was categorized as healthy, 25–29.9 was overweight, and $\geq$ 30 was obese. Twenty-eight food items from the PEDALS FFQ were aggregated into 21 groups based on similarity in nutritional profile. Children's dietary pattern scores were derived using PCA with varimax orthogonal rotation. Determining the number of components (patterns) was based on eigenvalues >1 and identification of the elbow in the scree plot [19]. Once the patterns had been identified, food groups within these patterns with factor loadings $\geq$0.2 were considered significant when naming the patterns. Skew was removed from the distribution of the scores and then scores were standardized. A dietary quality index (DQI) for parents was calculated from the DHQ data. This was slightly modified from that developed by Wong et al. for New Zealand adolescents aged 16–18 years [20]. The only modifications made to the adult index, compared to the published adolescent index, were the exclusion of the items assessing frequency of consumption of confectionery, fruit juice, processed meat, and type of cooking fat (which loaded very lowly on the index), and the inclusion of two items assessing frequency of adding salt and consumption of reduced-salt foods. This adult DQI showed good validity in the 3993 adult participants from the 2008–2009 New Zealand Adult Nutrition Survey (unpublished data). A 5-point scoring system was used, with scores ranging from 0 to 4. A response that matched a more positive dietary habit was assigned a higher score. The total diet quality score was a summation of scores from 15 items and ranged from 0 to 60.

Mixed regression models were used to investigate associations, with school as a random effect. These were used to determine the difference between boys' and girls' dietary pattern scores and male and female parent DQI scores. Both unadjusted and adjusted models were run for the association between parent DQI score and child dietary patterns. Adjustment was made for parent age, sex and BMI; child age, sex, ethnicity and BMI z-score; and level of deprivation (NZDep13). We also ran an additional model that included parental education, but as the addition of this variable made no difference to any results this is not shown.

Interaction terms between the DQI score and (a) who completed the DQI (mother or father) and (b) sex of the child were included to determine whether associations between dietary patterns and DQI were moderated by the sex of the parent or the child. If an interaction term was significant, then stratified results were also determined. If not significant, then the interaction term was removed from the model. Regression coefficients (95% CI) and P values are presented. Two-sided p values of < 0.05 were considered statistically significant. All statistical analysis used Stata 14.1 (StataCorp, College Station, TX, USA).

3. Results

Overall, complete demographic, questionnaire and anthropometric data was obtained from 401 child–parent pairs. Figure 1 provides an overview of school, student and parent recruitment. Seventeen of 30 invited schools took part, with 470 students available on data collection days. Of these, 468 students took part in PEDALS. The majority of students (57%) attended high decile schools (8–10) (Table 1). The mean age of the child participants was 10.2 years. The majority of child participants were of NZEO ethnicity, with 9% identifying as Māori and 3% as Pacific People. Based on the WHO BMI categories, 16% of child participants were overweight and 11% were obese. Parent participants were on average 41.6 years old and the majority of those completing the parental questionnaires were female (83.5%). Overall, 50% of parents were overweight or obese (70% of fathers and 46% of mothers). Forty-seven percent of fathers and 44% of mothers were in the lowest NZDep13 categories (1–3).

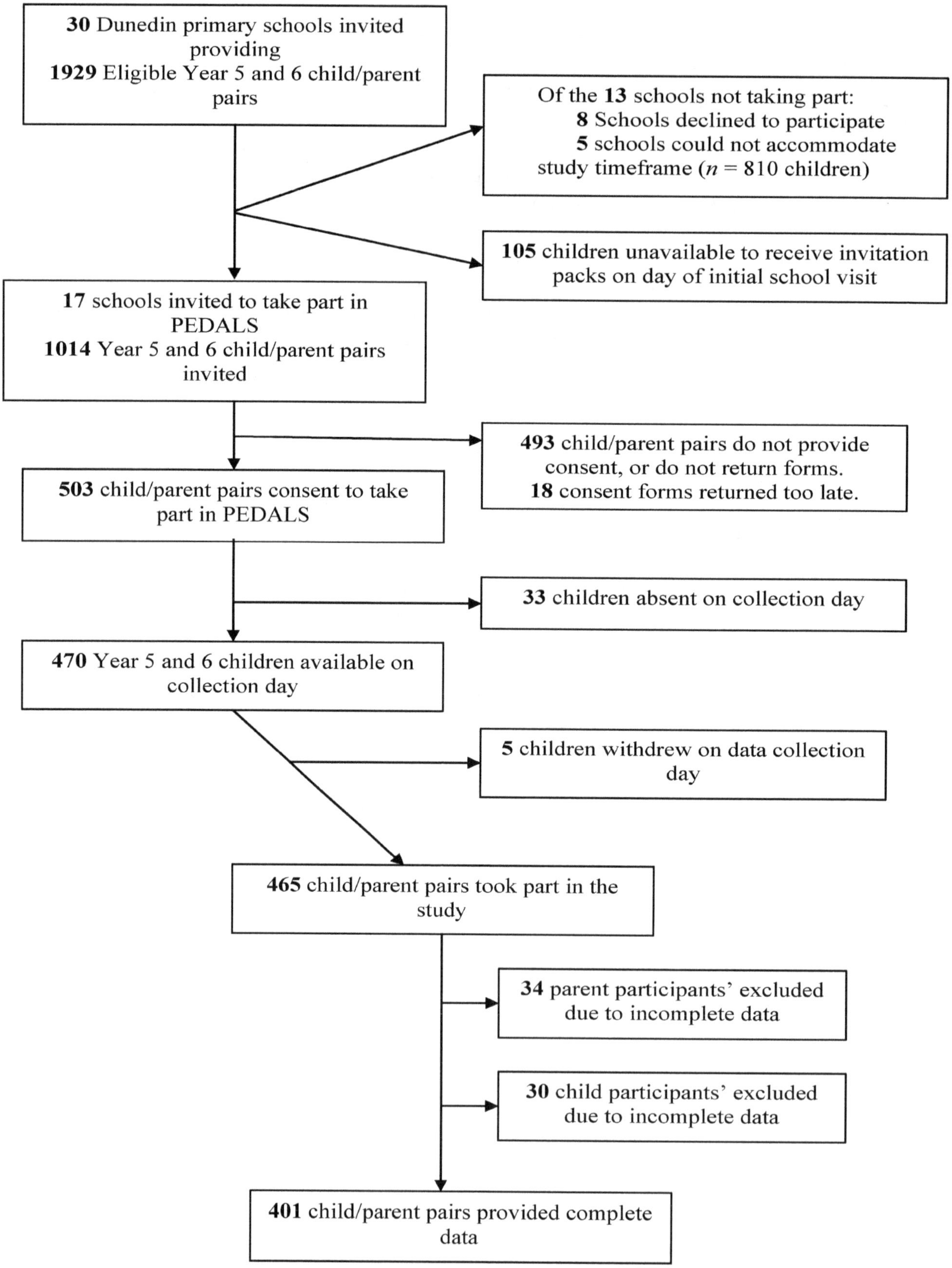

Figure 1. Recruitment flowchart for PEDALS.

Table 1. Characteristics of child and parent PEDALS participants.

Characteristic	Total Children (n = 401)		Boys (n = 198)		Girls (n = 203)		Total Parents (n = 401)		Fathers (n = 66)		Mothers (n = 335)	
	n	(%)	n	(%)	n	(%)	n	(%)	n	(%)	n	(%)
Age (years) *	10.2	0.6	10.3	0.6	10.2	0.6	41.6	5.5	43.5	6.3	41.3	5.3
Ethnicity												
Māori	36	9	23	12	13	6	21	5	2	3	19	6
Pacific	11	3	4	2	7	4	4	1	0	0	4	1
NZEO	354	88	171	86	183	90	376	94	64	97	312	93
BMI †												
Underweight/normal	292	73	144	73	148	73	201	50	20	30	181	54
Overweight	66	16	27	13	39	19	133	33	33	50	100	30
Obese	43	11	27	14	16	8	67	17	13	20	54	16
School Year												
Year 5	227	57	104	53	123	61			37	56	190	57
Year 6	174	43	94	47	80	39			29	44	145	43
School decile												
Low (1–3)	26	6	13	7	13	6			6	9	20	6
Medium (4–7)	147	37	67	34	80	39			28	42	119	36
High (8–10)	228	57	118	59	110	55			32	49	196	58
NZDep13 §												
Low (1–3)	180	45	99	50	81	40			31	47	149	44
Medium (4–6)	151	38	66	33	85	42			18	27	133	40
High (7–10)	70	17	33	17	37	18			17	26	53	16
DQI score ‖ (range from 0–60)							43	7	40	6	44	7

* Presented as mean and standard deviation; † World Health Organisation (WHO) criteria used to derive and allocate BMI categories; ‡ Ratings given to schools in New Zealand to determine government funding; deciles range from 1 (low) to 10 (high). The lower the decile, the more funding received; § The New Zealand Deprivation Index 2013; ‖ Diet Quality Index.

Fruits and vegetables were consumed at least once every day by 66% and 56% of children, respectively. Four percent of children consumed fizzy drinks, 4% consumed diet fizzy drinks, 5% consumed lollies/sweets and 5% consumed chocolate every day. Three percent of parents consumed fizzy drink and 5% consumed confectionery every day. Only 1% or less consumed red meat, hot chips or processed meat every day. Standard milk was the most commonly consumed milk by parents (42%) and light grain bread was the most commonly consumed bread (48%).

PCA produced two dietary patterns that explained 37% of the total variance. The patterns were a 'Snacks' pattern and a 'Fruit and Vegetables' pattern (Table 2). The 'Snacks' pattern loaded positively for ice cream, non-dairy drinks, white bread, pasta and noodles, salty snacks, sweet baked items, lollies/sweets, sweet snacks and sandwich spreads. The 'Fruit and Vegetables' pattern loaded positively for fruits, vegetables, trim milk, standard milk, cheese, yoghurt, processed meats, other meats, breakfast cereals and brown/wholemeal bread.

Boys had a significantly higher 'Snacks' pattern score compared to girls 0.13 (SD = 1.0) compared to −0.12 (SD = 1.0), $p = 0.005$. There was no significant difference between boys and girls for 'Fruit and Vegetables' pattern scores ($p = 0.384$). The mean parent DQI score was 43 (SD = 7), with a possible highest score of 60. The mean score for mothers was 44 (SD = 7), four points higher than the mean father score of 40 (SD = 6) ($p < 0.001$). After adjustment for confounders there was a significant inverse relationship between the 'Snacks' pattern score and parent DQI scores, with a one unit increase in parental diet quality score associated with a 0.03SD (CI: 0.02, 0.04) decrease in the child 'Snacks' pattern score (Table 3). There was no significant relationship between the 'Fruit and Vegetables' pattern and DQI score. None of the included interaction terms included in the models were significant (data not shown).

Table 2. Factor loadings (orthogonal varimix rotation) of food items/groups in two identified dietary patterns in 9–11 year-old children in PEDALS.

Food Items/Group	Snacks	Fruit and Vegetables
Fruits	−0.10	0.33
Vegetables (including potato) *	−0.01	0.36
Trim milk (green) [including on cereals, milo, hot chocolate]	−0.03	0.31
Milk (blue) [including on cereals, milo, hot chocolate]	0.02	0.29
Cheese	0.00	0.33
Yoghurt	0.01	0.33
Ice cream	0.28	0.02
Processed meat (such as meat pies, sausage, sausage roll, salami, luncheon, bacon, ham)	0.12	0.25
Other meats (such as mince, beef, chicken)	0.12	0.27
Fish (including canned tuna or salmon, fish cakes, fish fingers, fish pie, battered fish)	0.18	0.14
Non-dairy drinks †	0.31	0.02
Breakfast cereals	0.00	0.25
White bread	0.26	−0.05
Brown /Wholemeal bread	−0.12	0.32
Rice, rice based dishes	0.16	0.10
Pasta (such as spaghetti, macaroni), noodles	0.24	0.12
Salty snacks ‡	0.40	−0.05
Biscuits, cakes, muffins, doughnuts, fruit pies	0.35	−0.04
Lollies/sweets	0.33	−0.09
Sweet snacks §	0.33	0.02
Spreads ǀǀ	0.29	0.02
Eigen value	5.36	2.60
Variance explained	25.5%	12.4%

* Vegetables: "vegetables" + "Potato (such as mashed, boiled)"; † Non-dairy drinks: "Fruit juice (such as Orange juice, Apple juice, Raro, Refresh, Keri, Twist, Ribena"; + "Diet fizzy drinks (such as Diet Coke, Pepsi Max, Sprite Zero and any other "light" or "sugar free" varieties)" + "Fizzy drinks (such as Coke, Pepsi, Sprite, L&P, Fanta, Ginger Beer)"; ‡ Salty snacks: "Potato chips, potato snacks, corn chips" + "Hot chips, wedges, French fries"; § Sweet snacks: "Snack bars (such as muesli bar, fruit bar, rice bubble bar)" + "Chocolate, Chocolate bars"; ǀǀ Spreads: "Tomato sauce, Ketchup" + "Peanut butter, Nutella" + "Jam, honey".

Table 3. Associations between children dietary patterns and parent Diet Quality Index Scores.

	DQI Score					
		Unadjusted			Adjusted *	
	β	(95% CI)	*p*	β	(95% CI)	*p*
'Snacks'	−0.04	−0.05, −0.02	<0.001	−0.03	−0.04, −0.02	<0.001
'Fruit and Vegetables'	0.01	−0.002, 0.03	0.091	0.01	−0.001, 0.03	0.060

* Adjusted for parent age, sex and BMI, and child age, sex, ethnicity and BMI z-score, and level of deprivation (NZDep13).

4. Discussion

This is the first study globally to investigate the relationship between parental and child dietary patterns using theoretical and empirical methods of derivation, respectively. The results indicate that there is an inverse association between parent diet quality and the child 'Snacks' pattern.

In this study, 66% of children consumed fruit at least once daily, whereas only 4% had fizzy drinks every day, suggesting that this sample of children had relatively healthy diets. However, it cannot be concluded whether or not the children were reaching the recommended three servings of vegetables and two servings of fruit per day as this information cannot be derived from a non-quantitative FFQ. Data from a nationally representative New Zealand study conducted in 2008–2009 shows that only 30% of 5–9 years old and less than 38% of 10–14 years old were achieving both recommendations [21]. As the sample from the current study had relatively low levels of deprivation and the children were mainly from the NZEO group, it is possible that a higher proportion of children were having five servings of fruit and vegetables per day compared to the national average. However, this is purely speculation, given the nature of the FFQ used in this study.

Two dietary patterns were derived from the child FFQ data using PCA: 'Snacks' and 'Fruit and Vegetables'. Though empirically derived dietary patterns are specific to the population of interest, similarities across studies are commonly seen, allowing for comparisons between populations. The 'Snacks' pattern and 'Fruit and Vegetables' patterns derived in this study resemble patterns in other studies with similar aged children across the Western world [22–24]. Whilst the naming of the patterns varies, the foods contributing the most to these patterns are comparable. For example, Oellingrath et al. [23] derived a 'Varied Norwegian' pattern in 924 children aged 9–10 years, which is similar to the 'Fruit and Vegetables' pattern derived in this study. Food groups that loaded positively in both of these patterns included fruit, vegetables, potatoes, cheese, yoghurt and brown bread. The results from this study show that boys have a higher 'Snacks' score compared to the girls. This finding is also similar to the Oellingrath et al. study [23] who found that boys had a higher score for their 'Snacking' pattern. It is not surprising that in both studies, boys had a more frequent consumption of treat and junk type foods that taste good due to their high fat and/or sugar content, as previous research has suggested that taste is a major influence in boys' food preference and food choice [24]. Conversely, girls report to be more influenced by how healthy foods are than how they taste [25,26].

In the current study, parents' diet quality was negatively associated with the children's 'Snacks' pattern. This suggests that if parents have a poorer quality diet, their children's overall diet consists of a more frequent consumption of less healthful foods. Though there are no other studies investigating the relationship between theoretically and empirically derived dietary patterns in parents and children, there is other evidence to suggest that diet quality are closely positively related between parents and children [7,13]. We found that adjustment for parental education had no real effect on any analyses but this is likely to be due to that fact that 71% of participating parents had post-secondary school level education.

Using an a priori dietary score to measure dietary quality in children is controversial, as some investigators believe further validation and longitudinal research is needed before these can be used in epidemiological studies [27]. The rationale behind this is that it is unknown which study designs and settings are most appropriate when utilising a priori scores to determine paediatric disease risk [27]. The use of PCA, and derivation of multiple also allows for investigation of the relationship between parental diet quality and different aspects of the child diet.

It is likely that the overall diets of 9–12 year-old children are associated with their parent's diets due to the lack of autonomy children have at this age in regard to dietary choices. Children in this age range consume at least two-thirds of their meals at home and are provided with nearly all of their food by their parents [13]. The literature convincingly suggests that many individual foods consumed by children are influenced by their parent's intakes [6–9]. At this age, parents are considered to be one of the strongest influences on children's diets [28–30]. It is therefore interesting that in the current study only certain combinations of foods and drinks that loaded strongly in the patterns were significantly associated with parent diet quality ('Snacks' pattern), while others were not ('Fruit and Vegetables' pattern). It may be that associations are attenuated as some parental questionnaires were completed by the child's male caregiver. The non-quantitative nature of the child FFQ may also explain these results. However, it may also be because the snack type foods are the ones that children may have more autonomy over, rather than those provided in main meals.

It is important to remember that the cross-sectional nature of this study means that directions of relationships cannot be measured. However, if we could assume that the parental diet influences the diet of their child, then improving parent diet quality has the potential to positively change children's diets. Data from the 2014–2015 New Zealand Health Survey shows that approximately 64% of adults consume three or more servings of vegetables daily and 57% consume two or more servings of fruit daily [31]. If more New Zealand parents can reach these targets, then the likelihood of their children also doing this may be increased. However, given the fact that significant relationships were only seen for the "Snacks" pattern, a focus on reducing consumption of less healthy foods by parents may be a more effective strategy.

As children grow into adolescents, the association between parents' and children's diets may weaken due to increased autonomy and greater influences outside of the home, such as school, jobs and social activities [32]. Previous research showing that the odds ratio for healthy diet agreement between parents and children falling from 4.05 for 2–10 years old, to 1.55 for children and adolescents older than 10 years [9]. Such findings highlight how the influences of children's diets change during the transition from childhood to adolescence, making this a key time to optimise food intake. Previous research shows that while dietary habits track from childhood into adolescence and adulthood [1], healthy eating habits also decline, particularly during the transition from childhood to adolescence [33]. Therefore, by providing a family environment that optimizes the development of healthy eating before adolescence, the effects of a decline in healthy eating during adolescents may be less marked. More recent research [34] has also shown that parental influence is also associated with healthier diet behaviours in adolescence. However, it may well be that this is due to maintenance or adaptation of already learned behaviours, rather than learning new behaviours.

Some limitations of this study include the use of a FFQ to measure the children's dietary intake, which only measures frequency, not amounts. In addition to this, the FFQ was relatively short with only 28 items, meaning the entire diet may not have been extensively covered. Despite this, the FFQ was found to be a valid tool for ranking participants according to food group intake [15] and was an appropriate method for this study, where multiple questionnaires were being administered. The DHQ was previously validated in almost 4000 adults so was suitable to be used in this study (unpublished data). Furthermore, although the sample of participants in PEDALS is representative of the Dunedin population it is not nationally representative, as there is a lower proportion of Māori and Pacific people in Dunedin, compared to the whole of New Zealand [33]. This is also reflected in the high proportion of those from higher decile schools and areas of low neighbourhood deprivation and the lower levels of overweight and obesity compared to national level data [35]. However, the schools who were not chosen to take part, or who declined participation, were not markedly different in decile from those who participated and the majority of schools not participating were those of higher deciles. Also, the sample is representative of the population of the South Island of New Zealand [35] and as the majority of New Zealanders are of 'New Zealand European or Other' ethnicity, the results of the current study are likely to be applicable to the majority of New Zealand children.

This study has several strengths, in particular the use of dietary patterns, rather than selected food groups. This is advantageous as dietary patterns look at the diet as a whole. All PCA analyses require some potentially subjective decisions to be made, but this was minimised through the use of standardised methods to group foods and naming patterns in a similar way to previous studies. Sufficient children were recruited into the PEDALS Study to meet the requirements for PCA. At least ten participants per food group entered into PCA are required in order to obtain robust results [36] and the study sample more than met this. Lastly, all questionnaires used were previously tested and validated in similar populations to this sample.

5. Conclusions

The current study found an association between parental diet quality and selected children's dietary patterns. Parents with a poor diet quality were more likely to have children that had a frequent consumption of 'Snacks'. This highlights the need for further investigation into the relationship between parent and child dietary patterns, as poor childhood diet quality remains prevalent in large parts of the world.

Acknowledgments: The authors would like to thank all participating schools for providing appropriate space for us to carry out our data collection, access to the students during class time, and assisting with supervision of students during data collection. We also thank all students and parents who participated in the study and all those who were involved in data collection and processing. PEDALS was funded by the National Heart Foundation of New Zealand (Grant number 1618) and The University of Otago (Grant number ORG 0114-1015).

Author Contributions: B.D., P.S., S.S., K.B. and J.H. were responsible for the development of this particular study and performing data analyses. P.S. is the principal investigator for the overall PEDALS project and was responsible for conception and design of the project and oversaw questionnaire design, data collection and data processing. S.P., H.H., K.M.J., R.Q., L.S. and J.E.W. contributed to the design of the project, including questionnaire design, data collection and processing. B.D. wrote the first draft, under the supervision of PMLS. All authors provided critical review and revision of the manuscript and have read and approved the final version of the manuscript.

References

1. Craigie, A.M.; Lake, A.A.; Kelly, S.A.; Adamson, A.J.; Mathers, J.C. Tracking of obesity-relatedbehaviours from childhood to adulthood: A systematic review. *Maturitas* **2011**, *70*, 266–284. [CrossRef] [PubMed]
2. Kaikkonen, J.E.; Mikkilä, V.; Raitakari, O.T. Role of childhood food patterns on adult cardiovascular disease risk. *Curr. Atheroscler. Rep.* **2014**, *16*, 1–15. [CrossRef] [PubMed]
3. Patrick, H.; Nicklas, T.A. A review of family and social determinants of children's eating patterns and diet quality. *J. Am. Coll. Nutr.* **2005**, *24*, 83–92. [CrossRef] [PubMed]
4. Crockett, S.J.; Sims, L.S. Environmental influences on children's eating. *J. Nutr. Educ.* **1995**, *27*, 235–249. [CrossRef]
5. Wardle, J.; Cooke, L. Genetic and environmental determinants of children's food preferences. *Br. J. Nutr.* **2008**, *99*, S15–S21. [CrossRef] [PubMed]
6. Pearson, N.; Biddle, S.J.H.; Gorely, T. Family correlates of fruit and vegetable consumption in children and adolescents: A systematic review. *Public Health Nutr.* **2009**, *12*, 267–283. [CrossRef] [PubMed]
7. Robinson, L.N.; Rollo, M.E.; Watson, J.; Burrows, T.L.; Collins, C.E. Relationships between dietary intakes of children and their parents: A cross-sectional, secondary analysis of families participating in the Family Diet Quality Study. *J. Hum. Nutr. Diet.* **2015**, *28*, 443–451. [CrossRef] [PubMed]
8. Wolnicka, K.; Taraszewska, A.M.; Jaczewska-Schuetz, J.; Jarosx, M. Factors within the family environment such as parents' dietary habits and fruit and vegetable availability have the greatest influence on fruit and vegetable consumption by Polish children. *Public Health Nutr.* **2015**, *18*, 2705–2711. [CrossRef] [PubMed]
9. Wang, Y.; Beydoun, M.A.; Li, J.; Liu, Y.; Moreno, L.A. Do children and their parents eat a similar diet? Resemblance in child and parental dietary intake: Systematic review and meta-analysis. *J. Epidemiol. Community Health* **2011**, *65*, 177–189. [CrossRef] [PubMed]
10. Michels, K.B.; Schulze, M.B. Can dietary patterns help us detect diet–disease associations? *Nutr. Res. Rev.* **2005**, *18*, 241–248. [CrossRef] [PubMed]
11. Newby, P.K.; Tucker, K.L. Empirically derived eating patterns using factor or cluster analysis: A review. *Nutr. Rev.* **2004**, *62*, 177–203. [CrossRef] [PubMed]
12. Lazarou, C.; Newby, P.K. Use of dietary indexes among children in developed countries. *Adv. Nutr.* **2011**, *2*, 295–303. [CrossRef] [PubMed]
13. Beydoun, M.; Wang, Y. Parent-child dietary intake resemblance in the United States: Evidence from a large representative survey. *Soc. Sci. Med.* **2009**, *68*, 2137–2144. [CrossRef] [PubMed]
14. Robson, S.M.; Couch, S.C.; Peugh, J.L.; Glanz, K.; Zhou, C.; Sallis, J.F.; Saelens, B.F. Parent diet quality and energy intake are related to child diet quality and energy intake. *J. Acad. Nutr. Diet.* **2016**, *116*, 984–990. [CrossRef] [PubMed]
15. Atkinson, J.; Salmond, C.; Crampton, C. *NZDep2013 Index of Deprivation User's Manual*; University of Otago: Wellington, New Zealand, 2014.
16. Saeedi, P.; Skeaff, S.A.; Eiin Wong, J.; Skidmore, P.M.L. Reproducibility and relative validity of a short food frequency questionnaire in 9–10 year-old children. *Nutrients* **2016**, *8*, 1–13. [CrossRef] [PubMed]
17. A Focus on Nutrition: Key Findings of the 2008/09 New Zealand Adult Nutrition Survey. Available online: https://www.health.govt.nz/system/files/documents/publications/a-focus-on-nutrition-v2.pdf (accessed on 14 March 2017).
18. de Onis, M.; Onyango, A.W.; Borghi, E.; Siyam, A.; Nishida, C.; Siekmann, J. Development of a WHO growth reference for school-aged children and adolescents. *Bull. World Health Organ.* **2007**, *85*, 660–667. [CrossRef] [PubMed]

19. Osborne, J.; Costello, A. Best practices in exploratory factor analysis: Four recommendations for getting the most from your analysis. *Pan-Pacific Manag. Rev.* **2009**, *12*, 131–146.
20. Wong, J.E.; Skidmore, P.M.L.; Williams, S.M.; Parnell, W.R. Healthy dietary habits score as an indicator of diet quality in New Zealand Adolescents. *J. Nutr.* **2014**, *144*, 937–942. [CrossRef] [PubMed]
21. A National Survey of Children and Young People's Physical Activity and Dietary Behaviours in New Zealand: 2008/09. Available online: https://www.health.govt.nz/system/files/documents/publications/cyp-physical-activity-dietary-behaviours-08-09-keyfindgs.pdf (accessed on 14 March 2017).
22. Aranceta, J.; Perez Rodrigo, C.; Ribas, L.; Serra-Majem, L. Sociodemographic and lifestyle determinants of food patterns in Spanish children and adolescents: The enKid study. *Eur. J. Clin. Nutr.* **2003**, *57*, S40–S44. [CrossRef] [PubMed]
23. Oellingrath, I.M.; Svendsen, M.V.; Brantsæter, A.L. Eating patterns and overweight in 9- to 10-year-old children in Telemark County, Norway: A cross-sectional study. *Eur. J. Clin. Nutr.* **2010**, *64*, 1272–1279. [CrossRef] [PubMed]
24. Nu, C.T.; MacLeod, P.; Barthelemy, J. Effects of age and gender on adolescents' food habits and preferences. *Food Qual. Prefer.* **1996**, *7*, 251–262. [CrossRef]
25. Sweeting, H.N. Gendered dimensions of obesity in childhood and adolescence. *Nutr. J.* **2008**, *7*, 1–14. [CrossRef] [PubMed]
26. Weible, D. Gender-driven food choice: Explaining school milk consumption of boys and girls. *J. Consum. Policy* **2013**, *36*, 403–423. [CrossRef]
27. Marshall, S.; Burrows, T.; Collins, C.E. Systematic review of diet quality indices and their associations with health-related outcomes in children and adolescents. *J. Hum. Nutr. Diet.* **2014**, *27*, 577–598. [CrossRef] [PubMed]
28. Brug, J.; Tak, N.; te Velde, S.; Bere, E.; de Bourdeaudhuij, I. Taste preferences, liking and other factors related to fruit and vegetable intakes among schoolchildren: Results from observational studies. *Br. J. Nutr.* **2008**, *99*, S7–S14. [CrossRef] [PubMed]
29. Davison, K.K.; Birch, L.L. Childhood overweight: A contextual model and recommendations for future research. *Obes. Rev.* **2001**, *2*, 159–171. [CrossRef] [PubMed]
30. Koui, E.; Jago, R. Associations between self-reported fruit and vegetable consumption and home availability of fruit and vegetables among Greek primary-school children. *Public Health Nutr.* **2008**, *11*, 1142–1148. [CrossRef] [PubMed]
31. Ministry of Health. *Tier 1 Statistics 2014/15: New Zealand Health Survey*; Ministry of Health: Wellington, New Zealand, 2015.
32. Videon, T.M.; Manning, C.K. Influences on adolescent eating patterns: The importance of family meals. *J. Adolesc. Health* **2003**, *32*, 365–373. [CrossRef]
33. Birch, L.; Savage, J.S.; Ventura, A. Influences on the development of children's eating behaviours: From infancy to adolescence. *Can. J. Diet. Pract. Res* **2007**, *68*, S1–S56.
34. Draper, C.E.; Grobler, L.; Micklesfield, L.K.; Norris, S.A. Impact of social norms and social support on diet, physical activity and sedentary behaviour of adolescents: A scoping review. *Child Care Health Dev.* **2015**, *41*, 654–667. [CrossRef] [PubMed]
35. 2013 Census QuickStats about Culture and Identity. Available online: http://www.stats.govt.nz/Census/2013-census/profile-and-summary-reports/quickstats-culture-identity.aspx (accessed on 14 March 2017).
36. Floyd, F.; Wildaman, K. Factor analysis in the development and refinement of clinical assessment instruments. *Psychol. Assess.* **1995**, *7*, 286–299. [CrossRef]

13

The Family Mealtime Observation Study (FaMOS): Exploring the Role of Family Functioning in the Association between Mothers' and Fathers' Food Parenting Practices and Children's Nutrition Risk

Kathryn Walton [1,*], Emma Haycraft [2], Kira Jewell [3], Andrea Breen [3], Janis Randall Simpson [3] and Jess Haines [3]

1 Department of Translational Medicine, The Hospital for Sick Children, Toronto, ON M5G 0A4, Canada
2 School of Sport, Exercise and Health Sciences, Loughborough University, Loughborough, Leicestershire LE11 3TU, UK; e.haycraft@lboro.ac.uk
3 Department of Family Relations & Applied Nutrition, University of Guelph, Guelph, ON N1G 2W1, Canada; kjewell@uoguelph.ca (K.J.); abreen@uoguelph.ca (A.B.); rjanis@uoguelph.ca (J.R.S.); jhaines@uoguelph.ca (J.H.)
* Correspondence: kathryn.walton@sickkids.ca

Abstract: This cross-sectional study explores associations between mothers' and fathers' food parenting practices and children's nutrition risk, while examining whether family functioning modifies or confounds the association. Home observations assessed parents' food parenting practices during dinnertime ($n = 73$ families with preschoolers). Children's nutrition risk was calculated using NutriSTEP®. Linear regression models examined associations between food parenting practices and NutriSTEP® scores. An interaction term (family functioning × food parenting practice) explored effect modification; models were adjusted for family functioning to explore confounding. Among mothers, more frequent physical food restriction was associated with higher nutrition risk in their children ($\beta = 0.40$ NutriSTEP® points, 95% Confidence Interval (CI) = 2.30, 7.58) and among both mothers and fathers, positive comments about the target child's food were associated with lower nutrition risk (mothers: $\beta = -0.31$ NutriSTEP® points, 95% CI = −0.54, −0.08; fathers: $\beta = -0.27$ NutriSTEP® points, 95% CI = −0.75, −0.01) in models adjusted for parent education and child Body Mass Index (BMI) *z*-score. Family functioning did not modify these associations and they remained significant after adjustment for family functioning. Helping parents to use positive encouragement rather than restriction may help to reduce their children's nutrition risk.

Keywords: family meals; food parenting practices; preschoolers; nutrition risk; direct observation

---

1. Introduction

Nutrition plays a critical role in the growth, development, school readiness, subsequent academic achievement, and overall health status of young children [1]. Eating preferences and patterns are established early in life [2] and longitudinal research shows that food preferences and choices during the preschool years are strongly associated with dietary patterns and food choices later in life [3]. This stability of eating habits from early childhood to adulthood [4,5] suggests that young children's eating habits have important implications not only for children's current health, but also their risk of future chronic disease [6–8]. Despite the evidence that the preschool age is a key time for establishing healthy dietary patterns, few Canadian preschoolers are meeting dietary recommendations [9,10]. It is estimated that 11–30% have moderate risk for poor nutritional intake and 10–17% have high risk, as assessed by the Nutrition Screening Tool for Every Preschooler (NutriSTEP®), a validated measure used to assess eating habits and identify nutrition problems in preschool-aged children [11–13]. Nutrition risk can range from under- to overnutrition and, among preschoolers, is defined as the presence of characteristics that can lead to nutritional deficiencies including poor growth, under or over consumption of certain food groups, and difficulties chewing or swallowing [11].

Parents are the primary influence in young children's lives and there is evidence to suggest that parents' food parenting practices influence children's dietary intake [2,14–16] and their resulting risk of inadequate nutrition, i.e., their nutrition risk [13]. However, existing research exploring the influence of food parenting practices has produced equivocal results. For example, although early research demonstrated that restricting access to less healthful foods was associated with higher subsequent intakes of these foods [17], results from more recent studies suggest that parental restriction may be associated with healthier dietary intakes among young children [18].

Recent scientific reviews [19,20] have identified that these inconsistent findings may be due to the methodological limitations of existing research, including a reliance on parental report to assess food parenting. The validity of such reports is limited due to potential error through inaccurate recall or bias due to social desirability. Recent research has found inverse associations between parental report and observed feeding practices [21], as well as no associations at all [22–24]. Therefore, direct observation is needed to more accurately explore associations between food parenting practices and children's nutrition risk.

In addition to a reliance on parental-report measures, the current literature does not account for the feeding context, including the home environment, in which feeding interactions transpire and the presence of mothers and fathers during mealtimes. Family systems theory posits that individual or family behaviors must be understood within the global family context or system [25]. General family factors, such as family functioning, may moderate the associations of food parenting practices on children's nutrition risk because they influence how the feeding practices are experienced by the child [26]. Family functioning is defined by how family members manage daily routines, communicate and connect emotionally with one another [26]. There is some evidence that family functioning is associated with frequency of fast food consumption among adolescent females [27]; however, the mechanisms by which family functioning influences dietary intake remain largely unknown, especially among young children.

Although mothers have traditionally held the primary role in feeding children, fathers also play an important and increasingly more prominent role during feeding interactions [28]. Unfortunately, fathers have been underrepresented in existing feeding research [28,29]. Mothers and fathers have been found to differ in the food parenting practices they use [13,30], highlighting the need to explore the potentially differential relationship between their food parenting and their children's nutrition risk. Furthermore, the existing body of literature has been based on studies conducted outside of Canada where feeding and parenting norms may differ. To date, only two studies exploring food parenting practices among preschoolers have been conducted in Canada [13,31]; both used parental report of food parenting practices.

The overall aim of this study is to address the limitations of existing research through a cross-sectional study to examine the associations between mothers' and fathers' food parenting practices, assessed via direct observation in the home, and children's nutrition risk among a sample of Canadian families with preschool-aged children. We hypothesized that: (1) the children of parents who engage in controlling and pressuring food parenting would have higher NutriSTEP® nutrition risk scores and therefore poorer nutritional status than those whose parents do not use these food parenting practices; and (2) children whose parents use positive encouragement during meals would have lower NutriSTEP® nutrition risk scores than those whose parents do not use these food parenting practices. The second aim of this study was to examine whether family functioning modifies or confounds the association of food parenting practices and children's nutrition risk. We hypothesized that family functioning would moderate the association between controlling food parenting practices and children's nutrition risk. Compared to children from families with high family functioning, the positive associations between controlling food parenting practices and nutrition risk would be stronger among children from families with low family functioning.

2. Methods

2.1. Participants and Procedure

We recruited families to participate in the Family Mealtime Observation Study (FaMOS) through a variety of methods including Facebook, posters in daycare centers, visits to library story times and word of mouth. Families were eligible to participate if: (1) they had a child between the ages of 18 months and 5 years; (2) it was typical for the family to eat meals together; and (3) parent(s) were able to speak and respond to surveys in English. In families with more than one child within our target age range, the child with the closest birthday to the date of the first home visit was chosen to be the target child; in the case of twins, a coin was flipped to randomly choose the target child.

Once families were confirmed as eligible to participate, a research assistant (RA) visited each family in their home at a time that was convenient for the family. During this visit, parent(s) provided consent on behalf of themselves and their child(ren) to participate. All children in the family provided assent to be video-recorded and the target child provided additional assent to have their height and weight measured. Where possible, in two-parent homes, both parents were asked to be home during this initial visit. The parent(s) decided on which three mealtimes over the following days would be recorded. All observations collected were of the evening meal. The evening meal was chosen as it was identified by parents as the typical "family meal" and, in two-parent homes, the time when both parents usually ate with the target child. Families were reminded that we wanted to see "typical" family mealtime experiences and that there was no reason to do anything special on the nights they recorded their meal. In cases where English was the family's second language, families were reminded to speak English during the recorded mealtimes. Each family was provided with a video camera and tripod to record their meals and the RA assisted the parent(s) with the initial video camera set-up and placement to ensure that all family members were in-view of the recording and that their faces could be seen. The RA measured parents' and target children's heights using a calibrated stadiometer and weights using a calibrated electronic scale. Following the home visit, we emailed parents a link to a 15-min online questionnaire, which asked them to report on their food parenting practices and aspects of their home environment, and to complete a nutrition risk questionnaire for the target child. In two parent families, each parent was sent an individual link to the questionnaire to complete.

On the evenings that a family was scheduled to record, an RA called or texted the family 15 min prior to the scheduled start of their mealtime to remind them to turn on the camera. Families were asked to record their entire meal. Study staff was not present during mealtime recordings. One hour after the family meal, an RA called or texted the family to confirm that they were indeed able to record, and to note any atypical events that may have occurred during the meal (i.e., target child had an atypical temper tantrum during the meal, camera ran out of battery, etc.). If the family was unable to record, another date was chosen for recording.

Following the recording of the three meals, an RA visited the family home again to pick up the camera. During this second home visit, the RA confirmed that three observations were recorded on the camera and that the parent questionnaires had been completed. Families were provided a $50 grocery gift card for participating. This study was approved by the University of Guelph Research Ethics Board (REB#14OC033).

2.2. Measures

Observed food parenting practices: we used the Family Mealtime Coding System (FMCS) [23,32] to measure mothers' and fathers' feeding practices. The FMCS was created to reflect the Child Feeding Questionnaire [33] and seven of its subscales were used in the current study: pressure for target child to eat ("eat three more bites"), physical prompts for target child to eat (spoon feeding child or putting food on the utensil for child to pick up), verbal restriction of target child's food consumption ("you can't have any more"), physical restriction of target child's food consumption (moving a specific food away from child), food rewards to encourage target child to eat ("if you eat your peas, you can have ice cream"), non-food rewards to encourage target child to eat ("if you finish your meal, you can watch TV"), and positive comments about food (either comments about food in general, the parent's own food, or the target child's food, explored separately) [23]. All instances of each food parenting behavior were logged and frequencies of occurrence for each behavior were calculated for the mealtime observation. The FMCS has been found to be a reliable measure of food parenting practices among preschool aged children (inter-rater reliability >86.5%) [23,32].

Target Child's Nutrition Risk: we measured the target child's nutrition risk using the Nutrition Screening Tool for Every Preschooler (NutriSTEP®) [11]. NutriSTEP® was developed by registered dietitians and is a 17-item questionnaire used to assess eating habits and identify nutrition problems in preschool aged children (3–5 years) across five subscales: eating behaviours, dietary intake, parental concerns about food and activity, screen time duration, and the use of supplements [11]. The primary parent (parent who completed the questionnaire first) completed the NutriSTEP® questionnaire for the target child. NutriSTEP® has been validated against registered dietitians' assessment of children's nutritional status (based on medical and nutritional history, three-day food records and anthropometric measurements) among a large sample of ethnically and geographically diverse families in Canada [11]. Scores on NutriSTEP® and registered dietitians' ratings were correlated ($r = 0.48$, $p = 0.01$) and the questionnaire was found to be reliable when completed by parents on two separate occasions, 2–4 weeks apart (kappa >0.75) [11]. Individual questions are answered using a tailored Likert scale, which are then coded into a numerical score through the use of the designated NutriSTEP® coding system. These scores are then summed to generate a nutrition risk score for the target child (ranging from 0 to 68), with higher scores representing greater nutrition risk. For descriptive purposes, scores were tabulated to determine three levels of risk of poor nutrition based on the standardized NutriSTEP® cut-offs: low (scores ≤20), medium (scores 21–25), and high (scores >25) [11]. A medium score identifies a level of risk that can be managed by public health services and a high score indicates risk requiring further assessment by a registered dietitian. For regression analyses, NutriSTEP® scores were explored as a continuous variable.

2.3. Covariates and Moderating Variables

Parental Educational Attainment: as an indicator of socio-economic status, mothers and fathers reported their educational attainment individually on an eight-point Likert Scale ranging from eighth grade or less to Postgraduate Training or Degree. Responses were dichotomized to graduated college/university and less than a college/university education.

Child Body Mass Index (BMI): trained research assistants measured children's heights and weights during home visit 1, as described above. Based on the World Health Organization (WHO) growth charts, we calculated BMI z-scores using WHO Anthro Software (version 3.2.2, WHO, Geneva, Switzerland) to assess child weight adjusted for age and gender.

Family Functioning: we measured family functioning using the "general functioning" subscale of the McMaster Family Assessment Device (FAD) [34]. Because family functioning is a family-level variable, we used the primary parent's report of family functioning. The scale consists of statements about families to which participants indicated the degree to which they agreed on a four-point scale (strongly disagree to strongly agree) and includes items that measure the overall health/pathology of the family relating to six dimensions of family functioning: (a) problem solving; (b) communication; (c) roles; (d) affective responsiveness; (e) affective involvement; and (f) behavioral control. The FAD has been validated against experienced family therapists' clinical ratings and found to correspond with clinicians' ratings of healthy and unhealthy families; 'general functioning' subscale ($t(39) = 2.49$, $p < 0.05$) [35]. Test-retest reliability has also been reported for the 'general functioning' subscale when completed by participants one week later ($r = 0.71$) [35]. We averaged responses to each of the

12 items comprising the 'general functioning' subscale to create an overall score; higher scores indicate lower levels of family functioning [34]. In our sample, the Cronbach's alpha for this subscale was 0.86, indicating strong internal consistency. For descriptive purposes, a cut-off of 2.17 was used to distinguish high and low functioning families (<2.17 = high functioning, ≥ 2.17 = low functioning) [35]. For regression analyses, family functioning was explored as a continuous variable.

2.4. Data Analysis

Videos of the mealtime observations were coded using Noldus Observer XT 12.5 (Noldus Information Technology, Wageningen, The Netherlands). To reduce camera reactivity, only mealtimes two and three were coded; video one was used as a warm-up for families [23]. Videos were coded by two independent coders who received a standardized training (4 h in length) outlining use of the Observer XT software and the behaviors to code using the FMCS [23,32]. Prior to coding videos for the current study, coders were provided with five sample videos and were required to demonstrate reliability (kappa >0.8) in comparison to pre-determined codes. During analysis, coders met bi-weekly to discuss coding challenges and to code a video together to ensure adherence to the coding scheme. Detailed notes from these meetings were kept to document decisions. Both coders also conducted regular reviews of their own coding to ensure intra-rater reliability during the coding of the full sample. A random sample of 20% of the videos were coded by both coders to ensure reliability [36]. We calculated intra-rater and inter-rater reliability using Observer XT's reliability function. Our inter-rater reliability (kappa = 0.8) and intra-rater reliability (kappa = 0.82) were both excellent [37].

Analyses were run separately for mothers and fathers, as previous research has suggested differences in mothers' and fathers' food parenting practices [28]. For both the mothers and fathers, there were no statistically significant differences in food parenting practices used in videos 2 and 3; thus, scores for parenting practices were averaged across the two observations. We calculated descriptive and frequency statistics for each food parenting practice to understand the practices used during mealtimes, as well as Mann-Whitney U-tests of difference between mothers' and fathers' food parenting practices. We ran linear regression models to examine the association between food parenting practices and children's NutriSTEP® risk scores. To examine whether family functioning modifies the association between food parenting practices and NutriSTEP® risk scores, we ran linear regression models including an interaction term, created using centered variables (family functioning × food parenting practice). There was no evidence of modification by family functioning ($p > 0.05$ for the interaction terms; results not shown); thus, we then included family functioning in the model as a covariate to examine whether family functioning confounds the association between food parenting practices and NutriSTEP® risk scores. Based on previous research, all models were adjusted for parent educational attainment and child BMI *z*-score [38,39]. Additionally, we explored whether associations between food parenting practices and child nutrition risk score differed by child gender; results from stratified models showed no difference by child gender (results not shown). Statistical analyses were conducted using SPSS version 25 for Mac (PASW, IBM, New York, NY, USA).

3. Results

3.1. Participant and Family-Level Characteristics

Of the families who expressed interest in our study by completing our eligibility screener ($n = 112$), two were ineligible because they did not have a child within our target age range, three lived too far away for RAs to conduct home visits, one indicated that they did not speak English during mealtimes and 29 of the families did not follow-up to schedule a home visit. We scheduled and completed home visits with 77 families. We were unable to obtain video data from four families; one family found that the camera was too distracting for the target child, and three families spoke languages other than English during their meal recordings.

Thus, our final sample for analysis consisted of 73 families (137 parents; 74 mothers, 63 fathers). Most of the parents (n = 73) identified as the "primary parent" (by completing the questionnaire first) were mothers. The majority of parents in this study were married or living with a partner (94.5%; Table 1), 85.3% of parents reported having graduated from College or University or more (i.e., post-graduate degree), and 86.1% of families reported a total household income of ≥$50,000/year. Moreover, the majority of parents identified as "white" (84.6%). Most of the families in this study participated in family dinners seven days a week (83.6%) and 90.4% were considered to have high family functioning (scores <2.17).

Table 1. Parent and family-level characteristics of participants in the Family Mealtime Observation Study (FaMOS) (n = 73 Families; 137 Parents).

Parental Characteristics (n = 137)	
	***n* (%)**
Relation to Child	
Mother [i]	74 (54.0)
Father	63 (46.0)
Parental Age in years, mean (SD)	36.1 (9.5)
Parental Educational Attainment	
High School Education or Less	5 (3.7)
Some College or University	15 (11.0)
College Graduate	18 (13.2)
University Graduate	50 (36.8)
Post Graduate Training or Degree	48 (35.3)
Parent Race/Ethnicity	
White	115 (84.6)
Chinese	5 (3.7)
Latin American	6 (4.4)
Other (South Asian, Southeast Asian, West Indian, Black, Aboriginal/Indigenous)	10 (7.3)
Parent Birth Country	
Outside of Canada	18 (14.9)
Parental Weight Status (BMI, kg/m^2) [ii], mean (SD)	**26.9 (6.5)**
Underweight (BMI <18.5)	1 (0.7)
Normal Weight (BMI 18.5–24.9)	56 (43.8)
Overweight/Obese (BMI ≥25)	71 (55.5)
Family-Level Characteristics (n = 73)	
	***n* (%)**
Family Structure	
Married or living with a partner	69 (94.5)
Total Household Income	
<$49,999/year	10 (13.9)
$50,000–$99,999/year	25 (34.7)
≥$100,000/year	37 (51.4)
Family Functioning, mean SD	**1.62 (0.39)**
High (<2.17)	66 (90.4)
Low (≥2.17)	7 (9.6)
Family Dinners (days/week)	
Every day (7 days/week)	61 (83.6)
Most days (4–6 days/week)	9 (12.3)
Rarely (<3 days/week)	3 (4.1)

[i] One same-sex couple. [ii] Parent weight missing for pregnant mothers (n = 9). SD standard deviation; BMI: Body Mass Index.

The average age of the target child was 3.3 ± 1.1 years and 56.2% were female (Table 2). The majority of children (65.3%) were considered to have a healthy weight status and low nutrition risk (89.0%).

Table 2. Characteristics of children participating in the Family Mealtime Observation Study (FaMOS) (n = 73).

	n (%)
Child Age mean (SD) 3.3 years (1.1)	
Child Gender	
Female	41 (56.2)
Child Race/Ethnicity	
White	57 (78.1)
Other (including Latin American, Southeast Asian, Chinese, Black and West Indian)	16 (21.9)
Child Weight Status (BMI *z*-score) [i] mean (SD) 0.9 (1.9)	
Healthy Weight	47 (65.3)
At risk of Overweight	19 (26.4)
Overweight/Obese	6 (8.3)
NutriSTEP® Score mean (SD) 13.3 (5.2)	
Low risk (≤20)	65 (89.0)
Medium risk (21–25)	6 (8.2)
High risk (>25)	2 (2.7)

[i] Child weight missing for one child who declined measurement. SD: standard deviation; BMI: Body Mass Index.

3.2. *Exploration of Mealtime Videos and Food Parenting Practices*

The average meal length was 24.5 min. Our results suggest that, overall, mothers were more engaged in food parenting than fathers (Table 3). Mothers used significantly more controlling feeding practices (described as mean frequency of occurrence, times/meal); specifically, more verbal restriction (mothers: 1.31 times/meal ± 1.59; fathers: 0.63 times/meal ± 0.88; $p < 0.05$), food rewards (mothers: 0.75 times/meal ± 1.79; fathers: 0.49 ± 1.13, $p < 0.05$), and non-food rewards (mothers: 0.31 times/meal ± 0.57; fathers: 0.14 times/meal ± 0.36, $p < 0.05$) than fathers. Additionally, mothers used more positive encouragement, specifically towards the target child's food during meals, than fathers (mothers: 7.12 times/meal ± 5.31; fathers: 4.26 times/meal ± 3.45, $p < 0.05$).

Table 3. Descriptive and frequency statistics for mothers' and fathers' observed food parenting practices [a] with target child and Mann-Whitney *U*-tests of difference between mothers' and fathers' observed food parenting.

	Mothers (n = 74)			Fathers (n = 63)			Mann-Whitney *U*-Test *z*-Scores
	Mean (SD)	Minimum	Maximum	Mean (SD)	Minimum	Maximum	
Verbal Pressure to eat	4.37 (5.22)	0	37.5	3.03 (3.06)	0	11.5	−1.7
Physical Pressure to eat	2.31 (4.22)	0	21	1.63 (2.80)	0	13	−0.67
Verbal Restriction	**1.31 (1.59)**	**0**	**9.5**	**0.63 (0.88)**	**0**	**4**	**−3.13**
Physical Restriction	0.21 (0.43)	0	2	0.12 (0.35)	0	2	−1.29
Use of Food as Reward	**0.75 (1.79)**	**0**	**14.5**	**0.49 (1.13)**	**0**	**6.5**	**−2.00**
Use of Non-Food Rewards	**0.31 (0.57)**	**0**	**2.5**	**0.14 (0.36)**	**0**	**2**	**−2.02**
Positive comments about food in general	3.91 (3.29)	0	14	3.11 (2.96)	0	16	−1.42
Positive comments about own food	1.83 (1.47)	0	7.5	1.78 (1.54)	0	5.5	−0.42
Positive comments about target child's food	**7.12 (5.31)**	**0**	**25**	**4.26 (3.45)**	**0**	**14.5**	**−3.52**

[a] Measured by the Family Mealtime Coding System. Significant differences at $p < 0.05$ level are bolded. SD standard deviation.

3.3. *Exploration of Food Parenting Practices and Target Child's NutriSTEP® Risk Scores*

3.3.1. Mothers

Among mothers, more frequent physical restriction of food was associated with higher NutriSTEP® nutrition risk scores in their children (β = 0.40 NutriSTEP® points, 95% CI = 2.30, 7.58) and more frequent positive comments about the target children's food were associated with lower nutrition risk (β = −0.31 NutriSTEP® points, 95% CI = −0.54, −0.08) in models adjusted for parent educational attainment and child BMI *z*-score (Model 1; Table 4). These associations remained significant after adjustment for family functioning (Model 2; Table 4). No other significant associations between mothers' food parenting practices and the target child's nutrition risk scores were found.

Table 4. Linear Regression models examining associations of Observed Food Parenting Practices with NutriSTEP® Scores.

Observed Food Parenting Practice	Mothers (n = 74)		Fathers (n = 63)	
	Model 1	Model 2	Model 1	Model 2
	Effect Estimate (95% CI)		Effect Estimate (95% CI)	
Verbal Pressure to eat	−0.01 (−0.25, 0.22)	−0.01 (−0.24, 0.23)	0.03 (−0.37, 0.46)	0.04 (−0.36, 0.50)
Physical Pressure to eat	−0.05 (−0.36, 0.23)	−0.05 (−0.35, 0.24)	0.20 (−0.09, 0.80)	0.21 (−0.10, 0.80)
Verbal Restriction	0.28 (−0.68, 0.88)	0.30 (−0.68, 0.89)	0.13 (−0.73, 2.17)	0.15 (−0.67, 2.29)
Physical Restriction	**0.40 (2.30, 7.58)**	**0.41 (2.39, 7.72)**	0.03 (−3.00, 3.99)	0.06 (−2.88, 4.52)
Use of Food as Reward	−0.14 (−1.10, 0.26)	−0.14 (−1.10, 0.27)	−0.08 (−1.44, 0.79)	−0.08 (−1.45, 0.80)
Use of Non-Food Rewards	−0.16 (−3.59, 0.69)	−0.16 (−3.65, 0.67)	0.01 (−3.43, 3.64)	0.02 (−3.36, 3.79)
Positive comments about food in general	−0.16 (−0.63, 0.11)	−0.16 (−0.63, 0.11)	0.15 (−0.18, 0.67)	0.18 (−0.15, 0.73)
Positive comments about own food	−0.15 (−1.40, 0.29)	−0.15 (−1.40, 0.31)	−0.13 (−1.19, 0.42)	−0.14 (−1.24, 0.40)
Positive comments about target child's food	**−0.31 (−0.54, −0.08)**	**−0.31 (−0.54, −0.08)**	**−0.27 (−0.75, −0.01)**	−0.27 (−0.76, 0.00)

Dependent Variable: NutriSTEP® Risk Score, continuous Model 1. Adjusted for parent educational attainment, dichotomous and child BMI-z score, continuous Model 2. Adjusted for model 1 covariates and family functioning, continuous Estimates where the 95% Confidence Interval (CI) does not include 0.0 are bolded.

3.3.2. Fathers

Among fathers, more frequent positive comments about the target children's food were associated with lower nutrition risk (β = −0.27 NutriSTEP® points, 95% CI = −0.75, −0.01) in models adjusted for parent educational attainment and child BMI *z*-score (Mode 1; Table 4). The association remained similar, but not significant (CIs just overlapping 0) after adjustment for family functioning (Model 2; Table 4). Similar to our results with mothers, adjustment for family functioning did not otherwise change our results, and no other significant associations between fathers' food parenting practices and the target child's nutrition risk scores were found (Model 2; Table 4).

4. Discussion

In this sample of Canadian parents of preschool aged children, we observed that mothers' use of physical restriction was associated with higher nutrition risk for their child and both mothers' and fathers' use of positive comments towards the target child's food was associated with lower nutrition risk. Family functioning did not modify or confound these associations. To our knowledge, this is the first study to explore the associations of observed food parenting practices with preschool children's nutrition risk while considering the potential influence of family functioning on these associations.

Our finding that maternal use of physical restriction of food was associated with greater risk of nutritional inadequacy supports our hypothesis that controlling food parenting practices would be associated with increased nutrition risk. This finding is consistent with previous longitudinal research that suggests restriction undermines a child's ability to recognize their own hunger and satiety cues [40] and increases eating in the absence of hunger [14], thereby increasing the child's risk for overeating and potential for increased nutrition risk. Similar to previous observational studies, we observed fairly low levels of parental restriction [22,23,30,41,42]. It has been suggested that overt restriction (i.e., taking food away from a child or telling them to stop eating a certain food) may occur more often during less structured eating occasions such as snack time and that covert restriction may occur more during structured mealtimes (i.e., not bringing certain foods into the home or offering them at mealtimes) [43]. Future research should explore the association of restriction and children's dietary intake and eating behaviors throughout the day using a longitudinal study design to help tease out the directionality of the association. It is possible that the mothers in this sample were concerned about their child's nutritional intake and thus used more physical restriction during mealtimes.

Our finding that mothers' and fathers' positive comments about the target child's food were associated with lower nutrition risk among children also supports our initial hypotheses. Research by Holley and colleagues [44] found parental modeling and positive comments to be helpful in increasing children's consumption of disliked vegetables. Positive encouragement, without pressure, has also been related to lower reported levels of fussy eating and greater reports of food enjoyment in preschoolers [45]. Taken together, these results suggest that positive parental comments may be an effective method of both increasing intake of healthful foods and decreasing nutrition risk scores among preschool aged children. Future research should test the ability of interventions to teach parents to use positive encouragement rather than controlling feeding practices to improve dietary intake and reduce nutrition risk among preschoolers.

It has been argued that family dysfunction may diminish the impact of positive role modeling and intensify adverse impacts of controlling feeding practices during mealtimes [46]. However, our results suggest family functioning does not modify or confound the association between parents' food parenting practices and preschoolers' nutrition risk. Contrary to our hypotheses, the associations between controlling food parenting practices and greater nutrition risk were not stronger among children from families with low family functioning. Similarly, effect estimates did not change when family functioning was added to the analytic models. When it comes to reducing children's nutrition risk, our findings suggest that food parenting practices are an important avenue of intervention, regardless of level of family functioning. However, future research should seek to replicate our findings in populations with diverse levels of family functioning; it is possible that the limited variability of family functioning in our sample may have contributed to the null effects of family functioning on the associations explored.

Mothers', but not fathers', use of physical restriction was associated with children's nutrition risk. However, this finding is contrary to previous research using mother and father reports of food parenting. Among a sample of Canadian parents, Watterworth et al. [13] found that fathers, but not mothers, reported 'restriction for health' was associated with higher nutrition risk among children. Comparisons between the two studies are difficult due to Watterworth and colleagues' [13] use of parental report of food parenting practices, as previous research has found little association between observed and reported food parenting practices [21–24]. Mealtime observations only capture overt restriction and parents may use covert restriction, which would not be observed during mealtime videos, but can be captured in food parenting questionnaires. Future research should explore the use of mixed observational and parent-report methods in an attempt to more accurately capture both overt and covert restriction as well as the meaning behind the restriction (e.g., for health or weight control) [47].

We found that mothers used significantly more verbal restriction and food and non-food rewards than fathers during meals. Overall, we found that positive comments about the target child's food (e.g., "your broccoli looks delicious") was the most commonly used food parenting practice among both mothers and fathers, followed by verbal pressure to get the child to eat (e.g., "eat three more bites") for mothers and positive comments about food in general (e.g., "milk helps us grow strong bones and teeth") for fathers, which is similar to previous observational research [30]. Our findings suggest that mothers and fathers differ in the food parenting practices they use. While observational studies including fathers have been limited [28], the research exploring differences in mothers' and fathers' observed food parenting practices has produced conflicting results [23,30]. One U.K.- based study that used the FMCS [23] reported no significant differences in the frequency of mothers' and fathers' food parenting practices. However, similar to our findings, an American study by Orrell-Valente and colleagues [30] found that, overall, mothers used significantly more food parenting practices than fathers and they also tended to use praise more frequently. Interestingly, the study that showed no difference between mothers' and fathers food parenting [23] was conducted in the U.K., suggesting that food parenting practices could be regionally and culturally defined. These inconsistent results highlight the importance of exploring both mothers' and fathers' food parenting practices to further understand how parents may influence each other's food parenting practices and how this interaction between mothers and fathers may impact children's dietary intake. Harris et al., have pioneered work in this area and found that, compared to discordant mother-father pairs, Australian mother-father pairs who concordantly report low levels of pressure to eat had children with lower levels of pickiness [48]. Additional research is needed to understand the impact of concordance/discordance between mothers' and fathers' food parenting practices in Canada.

Our study had a number of key strengths. First, the inclusion of fathers in this study is fairly unique within studies exploring food parenting practices [13,28], or children's health in general [29]. This allowed for a more accurate analysis of the context in which preschoolers from primarily two-parent families are fed. Second, the use of direct observation allowed us to more accurately explore associations between food parenting practices and children's nutrition risk. Furthermore, these observations were conducted in the home, without the presence of an RA, to allow for typical mealtime interactions to occur. Many studies exploring food parenting practices have either been conducted in lab settings or in the home in the presence of an RA where interactions are more likely to be atypical. Third, the use of a validated nutrition risk screening tool also adds to the strength of our study, ensuring an accurate measure of nutrition risk. Finally, this study is the first to observe food parenting practices in a Canadian context, which allows us to better understand the mealtime environments in which Canadian preschoolers are fed.

Despite the many strengths, there are limitations that should be noted when interpreting our results. This study was cross-sectional, and thus, the bi-directional nature of parent-child feeding interactions could not be determined. For example, it is possible that more controlling feeding practices are used with picky eaters; parents may use these practices in an attempt to improve their child's nutritional intake. Prospective research is needed to understand the temporal order of the association between food parenting practices and children's dietary intake as well as the bi-directional nature of these feeding interactions. While families recorded three mealtimes, we only observed food parenting practices during the evening meal. It is possible that food parenting practices differ during less structured eating occasions such as snack time. The level of nutrition risk reported in this study was much lower than previous studies exploring NutriSTEP® risk scores in Canada. Results may differ among families with children who have higher nutrition risk. Similarly, the families in this study also had high levels of family functioning. Results may also differ among families with lower functioning. While we found a significant association between mothers' use of physical restriction and mothers' and fathers' positive comments about the target child's food with NutriSTEP® risk scores, it should be noted that the effect sizes of the associations were relatively small. We have NutriSTEP® data from just one parent (primarily mothers) which may impact our findings and explain the few associations between fathers' food parenting practices and NutriSTEP® scores. Parents may perceive their child's nutrition risk differently; future research should seek to understand differences in how mothers' and fathers' report their child's nutrition risk. We calculated 36 tests (Table 4) and did not account for multiple comparisons. However, of these tests, five were statistically significant at the $p < 0.05$ level, which is larger than the one test we would expect by chance. Finally, the families in this study were highly educated and the majority identified as "white"; our results may not be generalizable to more diverse populations.

5. Conclusions

Mothers' observed use of physical restriction was associated with increased nutrition risk and mothers' and fathers' use of positive comments about the target child's food was associated with lower nutrition risk among preschool aged children. Family functioning did not moderate or confound the associations between parental food parenting practices and children's nutrition risk. Results suggest that supporting parents to use more positive encouragement rather than restriction may help to reduce preschoolers' nutrition risk. Future research should test interventions aimed at changing food parenting practices among families with preschoolers at medium-high nutrition risk. While we found few associations between fathers' food parenting practices and preschoolers' nutrition risk, we found differences among the types and frequency of food parenting practices employed by mothers and fathers. This underscores the importance of including fathers in food parenting research. As this was the first Canadian study to observe food parenting practices, future research is needed among more diverse populations, including those with more socio-economic diversity, higher levels of nutrition risk, and lower levels of family functioning, to further elucidate the association between food parenting practices and children's nutrition risk in Canada.

Author Contributions: K.W., J.H., and E.H. developed study methods and sought funding. K.W. led the study, data analysis and manuscript preparation. E.H. was part of K.W.'s dissertation committee, developed the mealtime coding scheme, supported video coding and manuscript preparation. K.J. conducted study visits, coded videos and supported study analysis. A.B. was part of K.W.'s dissertation committee, assisted with study methods and manuscript preparation. J.R.S. supported manuscript preparation and assisted with interpretation of results. J.H. was K.W.'s PhD advisor and supported the study, analyses, manuscript preparation and interpretation of results.

Acknowledgments: The authors would like to thank the families that participated in FaMOS, who generously welcomed us into their homes to allow us to learn from their mealtimes.

Abbreviations

FaMOS	Family Mealtime Observation Study
FMCS	Family Mealtime Coding Scheme
BMI	Body Mass Index
NutriSTEP®	Nutrition Screening Tool for Every Preschooler
WHO	World Health Organization
FAD	Family Assessment Device

References

1. Nicklas, T.A.; Hayes, D.; Association, A.D. Position of the American Dietetic Association: Nutrition guidance for healthy children ages 2 to 11 years. *J. Am. Diet. Assoc.* **2008**, *108*, 1038–1044. [PubMed]
2. Savage, J.S.; Fisher, J.O.; Birch, L.L. Parental influence on eating behavior: Conception to adolescence. *J. Law Med. Ethics* **2007**, *35*, 22–34. [CrossRef] [PubMed]
3. Birch, L.L.; Fisher, J.O. Development of eating behaviors among children and adolescents. *Pediatrics* **1998**, *101*, 539–549. [PubMed]
4. Birch, L.L. Development of food preferences. *Annu. Rev. Nutr.* **1999**, *19*, 41–62. [CrossRef] [PubMed]
5. Skinner, J.D.; Carruth, B.R.; Wendy, B.; Ziegler, P.J. Children's food preferences: A longitudinal analysis. *J. Am. Diet. Assoc.* **2002**, *102*, 1638–1647. [CrossRef]

6. Freedman, D.S.; Khan, L.K.; Dietz, W.H.; Srinivasan, S.R.; Berenson, G.S. Relationship of childhood obesity to coronary heart disease risk factors in adulthood: The Bogalusa Heart Study. *Pediatrics* **2001**, *108*, 712–718. [CrossRef]
7. Rylatt, L.; Cartwright, T. Parental feeding behaviour and motivations regarding pre-school age children: A thematic synthesis of qualitative studies. *Appetite* **2016**, *99*, 285–297. [CrossRef]
8. Eyre, H.; Kahn, R.; Robertson, R.M.; Clark, N.G.; Doyle, C.; Hong, Y.; Gansler, T.; Glynn, T.; Smith, R.A.; Taubert, K.; et al. Preventing cancer, cardiovascular disease, and diabetes: A common agenda for the American Cancer Society, the American Diabetes Association, and the American Heart Association. *Stroke* **2004**, *35*, 1999–2010. [CrossRef] [PubMed]
9. Jessri, M.; Nishi, S.K.; L'Abbe, M.R. Assessing the nutritional quality of diets of Canadian children and adolescents using the 2014 Health Canada Surveillance Tool Tier System. *BMC Public Health* **2016**, *16*, 381. [CrossRef] [PubMed]
10. Garriguet, D. *Findings from the Canadian Community Health Survey: Overview of Canadians' Eating Habits*; Canada, S., Ed.; Statistics Canada: Ottawa, ON, Canada, 2004.
11. Randall Simpson, J.A.; Keller, H.H.; Rysdale, L.A.; Beyers, J.E. Nutrition Screening Tool for Every Preschooler (NutriSTEP): Validation and test-retest reliability of a parent-administered questionnaire assessing nutrition risk of preschoolers. *Eur. J. Clin. Nutr.* **2008**, *62*, 770–780. [CrossRef]
12. Watson-Jarvis, K.; McNeil, D.; Fenton, T.R.; Campbell, K. Implementing the Nutrition Screening Tool for Every Preschooler (NutriSTEP®) in community health centres. *Can. J. Diet. Pract. Res.* **2011**, *72*, 96–98. [CrossRef] [PubMed]
13. Watterworth, J.C.; Hutchinson, J.M.; Buchholz, A.C.; Darlington, G.; Randall Simpson, J.A.; Ma, D.W.L.; Haines, J.; Study, G.F.H. Food parenting practices and their association with child nutrition risk status: Comparing mothers and fathers. *Appl. Physiol. Nutr. Metab.* **2017**, *42*, 667–671. [CrossRef] [PubMed]
14. Birch, L.L.; Fisher, J.O.; Davison, K.K. Learning to overeat: Maternal use of restrictive feeding practices promotes girls' eating in the absence of hunger. *Am. J. Clin. Nutr.* **2003**, *78*, 215–220. [CrossRef] [PubMed]
15. Faith, M.S.; Berkowitz, R.I.; Stallings, V.A.; Kerns, J.; Storey, M.; Stunkard, A.J. Parental feeding attitudes and styles and child body mass index: Prospective analysis of a gene-environment interaction. *Pediatrics* **2004**, *114*, e429–e436. [CrossRef] [PubMed]
16. Blissett, J.; Meyer, C.; Haycraft, E. Maternal and paternal controlling feeding practices with male and female children. *Appetite* **2006**, *47*, 212–219. [CrossRef] [PubMed]
17. Johannsen, D.L.; Johannsen, N.M.; Specker, B.L. Influence of parents' eating behaviors and child feeding practices on children's weight status. *Obesity (Silver Spring)* **2006**, *14*, 431–439. [CrossRef]
18. Campbell, K.; Andrianopoulos, N.; Hesketh, K.; Ball, K.; Crawford, D.; Brennan, L.; Corsini, N.; Timperio, A. Parental use of restrictive feeding practices and child BMI z-score. A 3-year prospective cohort study. *Appetite* **2010**, *55*, 84–88. [CrossRef]
19. Ventura, A.K.; Birch, L.L. Does parenting affect children's eating and weight status? *Int. J. Behav. Nutr. Phys. Act.* **2008**, *5*, 15. [CrossRef]
20. Skouteris, H.; McCabe, M.; Ricciardelli, A.; Milgrom, J.; Baur, L.; Aksan, N.; Dell'Aquila, D. Parent-child interactions and obesity prevention: A systematic review of the literature. *Early Child Dev. Care* **2012**, *182*, 153–174. [CrossRef]
21. Bergmeier, H.; Skouteris, H.; Haycraft, E.; Haines, J.; Hooley, M. Reported and observed controlling feeding practices predict child eating behavior after 12 months. *J. Nutr.* **2015**, *145*, 1311–1316. [CrossRef]
22. Farrow, C.; Blissett, J.; Haycraft, E. Does child weight influence how mothers report their feeding practices? *Int. J. Pediatr. Obes.* **2011**, *6*, 306–313. [CrossRef] [PubMed]
23. Haycraft, E.L.; Blissett, J.M. Maternal and paternal controlling feeding practices: Reliability and relationships with BMI. *Obesity (Silver Spring)* **2008**, *16*, 1552–1558. [CrossRef] [PubMed]
24. Bergmeier, H.; Skouteris, H.; Hetherington, M. Systematic research review of observational approaches used to evaluate mother-child mealtime interactions during preschool years. *Am. J. Clin. Nutr.* **2015**, *101*, 7–15. [CrossRef] [PubMed]
25. Broderick, C. *Understanding Family Process: Basics of Family Systems Theory*; Sage: Thousand Oaks, CA, USA, 1993.
26. Rhee, K. Childhood overweight and the relationship between parent behaviours, parenting style and family functioning. *Ann. AAPSS* **2008**, *615*, 12–37. [CrossRef]

27. Haines, J.; Rifas-Shiman, S.L.; Horton, N.J.; Kleinman, K.; Bauer, K.W.; Davison, K.K.; Walton, K.; Austin, S.B.; Field, A.E.; Gillman, M.W. Family functioning and quality of parent-adolescent relationship: Cross-sectional associations with adolescent weight-related behaviors and weight status. *Int. J. Behav. Nutr. Phys. Act.* **2016**, *13*, 68. [CrossRef]
28. Khandpur, N.; Blaine, R.E.; Fisher, J.O.; Davison, K.K. Fathers' child feeding practices: A review of the evidence. *Appetite* **2014**, *78*, 110–121. [CrossRef]
29. Davison, K.K.; Kitos, N.; Aftosmes-Tobio, A.; Ash, T.; Agaronov, A.; Sepulveda, M.; Haines, J. The forgotten parent: Fathers' representation in family interventions to prevent childhood obesity. *Prev. Med.* **2018**, *111*, 170–176. [CrossRef]
30. Orrell-Valente, J.K.; Hill, L.G.; Brechwald, W.A.; Dodge, K.A.; Pettit, G.S.; Bates, J.E. "Just three more bites": An observational analysis of parents' socialization of children's eating at mealtime. *Appetite* **2007**, *48*, 37–45. [CrossRef]
31. Shea, C.; Dwyer, J.J.; Heeney, E.S.; Goy, R.; Simpson, J.R. The effect of parental feeding behaviours and participation of children in organized sports/activities on child body mass index. *Can. J. Diet. Pract. Res.* **2010**, *71*, e87–e93. [CrossRef]
32. Haycraft, E. Child Feeding Practices in Fathers and Mothers of Young Children. Ph.D. Thesis, University of Birmingham, Birmingham, UK, 2007.
33. Birch, L.L.; Fisher, J.O.; Grimm-Thomas, K.; Markey, C.N.; Sawyer, R.; Johnson, S.L. Confirmatory factor analysis of the Child Feeding Questionnaire: A measure of parental attitudes, beliefs and practices about child feeding and obesity proneness. *Appetite* **2001**, *36*, 201–210. [CrossRef]
34. Epstein, N.; Baldwin, L.; Bishop, D. The McMaster Family Assessment Device. *J. Marital Fam. Ther.* **1983**, *9*, 171–180. [CrossRef]
35. Miller, I.; Epstein, N.; Bishop, D.; Keitner, G. The McMaster Family Assessment Device: Reliability and validity. *J. Marital Fam. Ther.* **1985**, *11*, 345–356. [CrossRef]
36. Pesch, M.H.; Lumeng, J.C. Methodological considerations for observational coding of eating and feeding behaviors in children and their families. *Int. J. Behav. Nutr. Phys. Act.* **2017**, *14*, 170. [CrossRef] [PubMed]
37. Hallgren, K.A. Computing Inter-Rater Reliability for Observational Data: An Overview and Tutorial. *Tutor. Quant. Methods Psychol.* **2012**, *8*, 23–34. [CrossRef] [PubMed]
38. Shloim, N.; Edelson, L.R.; Martin, N.; Hetherington, M.M. Parenting styles, feeding styles, feeding practices and weight status in 4-12 year-old children: A systematic review of the literature. *Front. Psychol.* **2015**, *6*, 1–20. [CrossRef]
39. Vereecken, C.A.; Keukelier, E.; Maes, L. Influence of mother's educational level on food parenting practices and food habits of young children. *Appetite* **2004**, *43*, 93–103. [CrossRef]
40. Hughes, S.O.; Frazier-Wood, A.C. Satiety and the Self-Regulation of Food Take in Children: A Potential Role for Gene-Environment Interplay. *Curr. Obes. Rep.* **2016**, *5*, 81–87. [CrossRef]
41. Hughes, S.O.; Power, T.G.; Papaioannou, M.A.; Cross, M.B.; Nicklas, T.A.; Hall, S.K.; Shewchuk, R.M. Emotional climate, feeding practices, and feeding styles: An observational analysis of the dinner meal in Head Start families. *Int. J. Behav. Nutr. Phys. Act.* **2011**, *8*, 60. [CrossRef]
42. Farrow, C.V.; Haycraft, E.; Blissett, J.M. Observing Maternal Restriction of Food with 3–5-Year-Old Children: Relationships with Temperament and Later Body Mass Index (BMI). *Int. J. Environ. Res. Public Health* **2018**, *15*. [CrossRef]
43. Fisher, J.O.; Birch, L.L. Restricting access to palatable foods affects children's behavioral response, food selection, and intake. *Am. J. Clin. Nutr.* **1999**, *69*, 1264–1272. [CrossRef]
44. Holley, C.E.; Haycraft, E.; Farrow, C. 'Why don't you try it again?' A comparison of parent led, home based interventions aimed at increasing children's consumption of a disliked vegetable. *Appetite* **2015**, *87*, 215–222. [CrossRef] [PubMed]
45. Powell, F.; Farrow, C.; Meyer, C.; Haycraft, E. The Stability and Continuity of Maternally Reported and Observed Child Eating Behaviours and Feeding Practices across Early Childhood. *Int. J. Environ. Res. Public Health* **2018**, *15*, 1017. [CrossRef] [PubMed]
46. Berge, J.M.; Wall, M.; Larson, N.; Loth, K.A.; Neumark-Sztainer, D. Family functioning: Associations with weight status, eating behaviors, and physical activity in adolescents. *J. Adolesc. Health* **2013**, *52*, 351–357. [CrossRef] [PubMed]

47. Horton, N.J.; Fitzmaurice, G.M. Regression analysis of multiple source and multiple informant data from complex survey samples. *Stat. Med.* **2004**, *23*, 2911–2933. [CrossRef]
48. Harris, H.A.; Jansen, E.; Mallan, K.M.; Daniels, L.; Thorpe, K. Do Dads Make a Difference? Family Feeding Dynamics and Child Fussy Eating. *J. Dev. Behav. Pediatr.* **2018**, *39*, 415–423. [CrossRef] [PubMed]

14

Sugar-Sweetened Beverage Consumption and Associated Factors in School-Going Adolescents of New Caledonia

Guillaume Wattelez, Stéphane Frayon, Yolande Cavaloc, Sophie Cherrier, Yannick Lerrant and Olivier Galy *

Interdisciplinary Laboratory for Research in Education, EA 7483, University of New Caledonia, Noumea BP R4 98851, New Caledonia; guillaume.wattelez@unc.nc (G.W.); stephanefrayon@hotmail.com (S.F.); yolande.cavaloc@unc.nc (Y.C.); sophie.cherrier@unc.nc (S.C.); yannick.lerrant@unc.nc (Y.L.)

* Correspondence: olivier.galy@unc.nc

Abstract: This cross-sectional study assessed sugar-sweetened beverage (SSB) consumption and its associations with the sociodemographic and physical characteristics, behavior and knowledge of New Caledonian adolescents. The survey data of 447 adolescents from ages 11 to 16 years were collected in five secondary public schools of New Caledonia between July 2015 and April 2016. These data included measured height and weight, SSB consumption, sociodemographic characteristics, body weight perception, physical activity, and knowledge (sugar quantity/SSB unit; energy expenditure required to eliminate a unit) and opinions about the SSB-weight gain relationship. Ninety percent of these adolescents declared regularly drinking SSBs. Quantities were associated with living environment (1.94 L·week^{-1} in urban environment vs. 4.49 L·week^{-1} in rural environment, $p = 0.001$), ethnic community (4.77 L·week^{-1} in Melanesians vs. 2.46 L·week^{-1} in Caucasians, $p < 0.001$) and knowledge about energy expenditure (6.22 L·week^{-1} in unknowledgeable adolescents vs. 4.26 L·week^{-1} in adolescents who underestimated, 3.73 L·week^{-1} in adolescents who overestimated, and 3.64 L·week^{-1} in adolescents who correctly responded on the energy expenditure required to eliminate an SSB unit, $p = 0.033$). To conclude, community-based health promotion strategies should (1) focus on the physical effort needed to negate SSB consumption rather than the nutritional energy from SSB units and (2) highlight how to achieve sustainable lifestyles and provide tools for greater understanding and positive action.

Keywords: consumption behavior; knowledge; Melanesian; Pacific; physical activity; sugar-sweetened beverage; noncommunicable diseases; weight status; self-weight perception

---

1. Introduction

Adolescent overweight and obesity are associated with lifestyle factors like low physical activity (PA) and frequent consumption of energy-dense foods high in saturated fats and refined carbohydrates [1]. Sugar-sweetened beverages (SSBs), in particular, are a frequent source of refined carbohydrates in adolescent nutrition [2–4]. According to the 2010 Dietary Guidelines for Americans, SSBs are "liquids that are sweetened with various forms of sugars that add calories. These beverages include, but are not limited to, soda and fruit drinks, and sports and energy drinks" [5]. SSBs are the largest source of added sugars and major energy contributors to diet [6]. Harnack et al. [2] showed that US school children drinking an average of 265 mL or more of soft drinks daily consumed almost 835 kJ more total energy per day than those drinking no soft drinks. Moreover, epidemiological studies have quantified the positive relationships between SSB consumption and long-term weight gain, type 2 diabetes mellitus and cardiovascular diseases [6,7].

SSB consumption is also related to weight status [8], self-weight perception and body dissatisfaction [8], and PA [9,10]. It may also be related to knowledge or opinions about SSB [6,11]. For example, Park et al. [6] found that SSB consumption was higher among adults who disagreed that SSBs contribute to weight gain, whereas knowledge about the energy content of regular soda was not associated with SSB intake. Conversely, other authors found that adolescents or young adults (college students) with the poorest nutrition knowledge had the highest SSB consumption [11].

The Pacific Island Countries and Territories (PICTs) are also facing problems of obesity, overweight and changing nutrition patterns [4]. Kessaram et al. [10] reported the high prevalence of overweight and obesity in adolescents, likely explained by environmental mutations and shifts in nutrition and PA [12]. Traditional diets of root crops, vegetables, fruits and fresh fish and meat have been steadily replaced by imported, processed, energy-dense, low-nutrient foods [13], including SSBs. In six PICTs, 42% of 13- to 15-year-old students declared drinking SSBs daily [10]. Pak et al. [14] assessed soft drink consumption and reported 84 L/person in Palau in 2011.

Obesity and comorbidities are a health concern for young adults in Oceania, especially those in New Caledonia [15]. New Caledonia is a French archipelago in the South Pacific located between 162° E–169° E longitude and 19° S–23° S latitude. Melanesians were the first inhabitants of this archipelago, and consecutive arrivals of different populations since the era of colonization have now provided a multi-ethnic society with several "ethnic communities" that are representative of the Pacific populations. Melanesian (39%), European (or Caucasian) (27%), Polynesian (8%), Asian (2.5%) and other populations live together [16]. In 1989, New Caledonia was divided into three provinces: the Southern Province, the Northern Province and the Loyalty Islands Province. The capital city Noumea (Southern Province) is nevertheless the center for most economic activities. As a consequence, Noumea and its suburbs are the only areas that can be considered urban. The lifestyles of urban and rural areas differ greatly, and cultural and socioeconomic differences are also observed among the main ethnic groups, especially in rural areas. Indeed, New Caledonia's economy is overall on par with that of the Western world, especially in Noumea and other small towns, although half the population lives a traditional Pacific lifestyle. The traditional lifestyle is characterized by daily physical activities oriented toward agriculture, fishing or other activities to meet a family's daily needs. Disparities are seen in all age groups including school-going adolescents. Whereas an "equitable school system" exists—i.e., offering every adolescent the same access to school and a standardized academic curriculum, as well as a health education program [17]—the differences between the ethnic communities may lead to dramatic consequences for health in future generations [18]. Although few studies have focused on 11- to 16-year-old adolescents in New Caledonia [13,19,20], the prevalence of overweight or obesity was found to be three times greater in New Caledonian adolescents than in French adolescents in the same age range [21]. In addition, Frayon et al. [13] showed that in this multi-ethnic society, the risk of being overweight/obese was significantly greater in Polynesian and Melanesian adolescents. Adolescent overweight was also associated with rural lifestyles and low socioeconomic status (SES) for girls and breakfast skipping for boys [22]. Melanesian adolescents were more physically active and had a higher body mass percentage, mainly in rural girls compared with urban girls [20]. PA and food intake, and adolescent knowledge about and consumption of SSBs remain inadequately explored in the New Caledonian population, but research suggests that socio-environmental variables should be taken into account. We therefore hypothesized that SSB consumption would be associated with ethnicity (i.e., being Melanesian), living environment (i.e., rural) and knowledge about SSBs (i.e., sugar contained in SSBs, energy expenditure to eliminate consumed SSBs and association with weight gain).

This study aimed to broaden the vision on health among the 11- to 16-year-old adolescents in New Caledonia by assessing their SSB consumption behaviors and the associations with individual and socio-environmental factors.

2. Materials and Methods

2.1. Data Collection and Participants

Our study was part of a community-based obesity prevention project conducted in five selected representative school sites in the three provinces (Northern Province, Southern Province and Loyalty Islands) of New Caledonia. The schools were selected on the basis of the following criteria: (1) a representative repartition of the schools between rural and urban areas (respectively, 63% and 37% of the population), and (2) sufficient school size ($n > 200$). Eight schools were eligible in the Southern Province (urban), four in the Northern Province (rural) and only one in the Loyalty Islands (rural). Selected schools were then randomly drawn among these eligible schools: two in the Southern Province, two in the Northern Province and one in the Loyalty Islands. The school and participant selection process are further described elsewhere [19].

Data were collected between July 2015 and April 2016 from 696 school-going adolescents (11–16 years old) during class time. In each school, only 95% of the expected participants responded due to absences or parental refusal. Adolescents with missing data (no height, no weight, no PA, inconsistent or no response: $n = 221$) were then excluded from this study, as were adolescents from an ethnic community other than Caucasian or Melanesian (mostly Asian and Polynesian: $n = 28$), as these subsamples were too small. The final total sample was 447 adolescents.

Parents gave informed written consent prior to the children's participation in the study, in line with the legal requirements and the Declaration of Helsinki. The protocol was also approved by the Ethics Committee of the University of New Caledonia.

2.2. Measures

2.2.1. Anthropometric Parameters

All anthropometric data, including body mass index (BMI) and the International Obesity Task Force (IOTF) criteria [23], were collected by trained staff (the senior researcher) in the school nurse's office. Height was measured to the nearest 0.1 cm using a portable stadiometer (Leicester Tanita HR 001, Tanita Corporation, Tokyo, Japan). Weight was determined to the nearest 0.1 kg using a scale (Tanita HA 503, Tanita Corporation, Tokyo, Japan), with adolescents weighed in light clothing. Body mass index (BMI) was calculated by dividing weight in kilograms by height squared in meters.

The BMI standard deviation score (BMI-SDS) and percentile were calculated by the LMS method using the IOTF reference values. Weight status was defined according to the IOTF criteria, which are used to classify BMI values according to age and gender as thin (underweight), normal weight, overweight, or obese, based on adult BMI cutoffs at 18 years [23].

2.2.2. Sociodemographic Characteristics

Ethnicity was self-reported by the adolescents using an anonymous survey tool and categorized as recommended in the report on New Caledonia [24] from the *Institut National de la Santé Et de la Recherche Médicale* (INSERM; National Institute of Health and Medical Research). Three SES categories were generated according to the National Statistics Socio-Economic Classification [25]: managerial and professional occupations (high), intermediate occupations (medium), and routine and manual occupations (low). According to the latest census in New Caledonia [26] and a European standard for the degree of urbanization [27], Noumea and its suburbs were classified as urban and the other areas were classified as rural.

2.2.3. SSB Consumption

SSB consumption was assessed by first asking: "Do you drink SSBs?" Average amounts were then assessed with the question: "How many glasses (250 mL), cans (330 mL), small bottles (500 mL) or big bottles (1500 mL) do you drink per week on average?" The total SSB intake per week, converted to liters, was calculated by adding up the volumes of the total number of glasses, cans and bottles. Adolescents who answered "No" to the first question were considered as consuming 0 L per week.

2.2.4. Self-Weight Perception

Adolescents were asked about their self-weight perception with the following question: "Given your age and height, would you say that you are about the right weight, too big, or too skinny?" [28]

2.2.5. Physical Activity

The self-report International Physical Activity Questionnaire-Short Form (IPAQ-SF) was filled out on the research day with the researchers' assistance. The total number of days and minutes of PA was calculated for each participant [29]. Total PA time was converted to hours per week.

2.2.6. Knowledge and Opinion about SSBs

Three parameters assessed participants' knowledge about SSBs.

First, participants expressed their opinion about the effects of SSBs on weight by responding to this statement: "Drinking regular sodas, fruit drinks, sports or energy drinks, and other sugar-sweetened drinks can cause weight gain." Responses were categorized as: agree (strongly/somewhat agree) or disagree (disagree completely, strongly/somewhat disagree).

Second, participants answered the following question to assess their "knowledge about sugar": "How many sugar lumps does a regular can of, for example, non-diet cola contain?" Responses were categorized as: underestimated (<5 lumps), accurate (5–10 lumps), overestimated (>10 lumps), and don't know.

Last, participants answered the following question to assess their "knowledge about energy expenditure": "How much time do you need to run (at moderate speed) to eliminate the energy intake from drinking a regular can of, for example, non-diet cola?" The four response categories were: underestimated (<30 min), accurate (30–60 min), overestimated (>60 min), and don't know.

2.3. *Statistics*

All analyses were conducted using R 3.1.0. [30] with a significance level of $p = 0.05$.

First, differences between categories for each explanatory factor were tested one by one. Differences were tested with the χ^2 test or Fisher's exact test (according to implementation conditions) for categorical variables and with means equality tests (Student, Welch or Wilcoxon) for numerical variables with binary factors. One-way ANOVA and the Kruskal-Wallis test were coupled with a post-hoc t-test and Nemenyi's test, respectively, when needed for numerical variables with other factors. The PA-quantity of SSB consumption correlation was determined and tested with Spearman's test because Pearson's test was not applicable.

The adolescents' quantified SSB consumption was globally assessed by multiple regression and multifactorial ANOVA to detect associations, possible interactions and a confounding bias between factors. The significant pairwise interactions were included in the regression and ANOVA.

3. Results

Table 1 shows that socioeconomic factors were not discriminant for the "prevalence" of SSB consumption. Sex, living environment, ethnic community, SES and weight status were not significant factors and generally about 90% of the adolescents declared consuming SSBs. In addition, boys were significantly more physically active than girls (14.31 $h \cdot week^{-1}$ for boys vs. 12.18 $h \cdot week^{-1}$ for girls, $p = 0.01$), Melanesians were significantly more physically active than Caucasians (11.23 $h \cdot week^{-1}$ for Caucasians vs. 14.05 $h \cdot week^{-1}$ for Melanesians, $p < 0.01$), and adolescents were significantly more physically active in rural areas than in urban areas (13.64 $h \cdot week^{-1}$ in rural vs. 10.88 $h \cdot week^{-1}$ in urban, $p < 0.01$).

Table 1. Population: proportions of weight status, weight perception, SSB consumption (yes or no) and physical activity according to sex, living environment, ethnic community, socioeconomic status (SES) and weight status ($n = 447$).

			Weight Status (%)				Self-Weight Perception (%)				SSB Consumption (%)			Physical Activity (h·week^{-1})	
		Size	UnN *	Overweight	Obese	*p*-Value #	Too Skinny	Normal	Too Big	*p*-Value #	Yes	No	*p*-Value #	Mean ± SD	*p*-Value †
Sex	Boys	194	65.5	19.1	15.5	0.453	13.9	67.5	18.6	0.393	90.7	9.3	0.946	14.31 ± 9.31	0.011
	Girls	253	64.0	23.3	12.7		16.6	61.3	22.1		90.9	9.1		12.18 ± 7.81	
Living environment	Rural	361	60.9	23.0	16.1	0.002	15.2	63.7	21.1	0.873	91.7	8.3	0.278	13.64 ± 8.68	0.007
	Urban	86	80.2	15.1	4.7		16.3	65.1	18.6		87.2	12.8		10.88 ± 7.62	
Ethnic community	Caucasian	149	75.8	12.8	11.4	0.001	15.4	67.8	16.8	0.354	87.9	12.1	0.183	11.23 ± 8.67	0.001
	Melanesian	298	59.1	25.8	15.1		15.4	62.1	22.5		92.3	7.7		14.05 ± 8.34	
SES	Low	205	58.1	24.9	17.1	0.041	16.1	62.9	21.0	0.831	89.8	10.2	0.751	12.69 ± 8.03	0.586
	Medium	115	65.2	20.9	13.9		17.4	61.7	20.9		92.2	7.8		13.21 ± 8.94	
	High	127	74.8	16.5	8.7		12.6	67.7	19.7		91.3	8.7		13.68 ± 9.28	
Weight status	UnN *	289					23.5	71.6	4.8	<0.001	92.4	7.6	0.289	13.25 ± 8.62	0.731
	Overweight	96					1.0	56.3	42.7		88.5	11.5		13.18 ± 8.36	
	Obese	62					0.0	40.3	59.7		87.1	12.9		12.32 ± 8.56	

* UnN: underweight and normal. # χ^2 test or Fisher's exact test. † Binary factors: Student's or Welch's *t*-test. Other factors: one-way ANOVA.

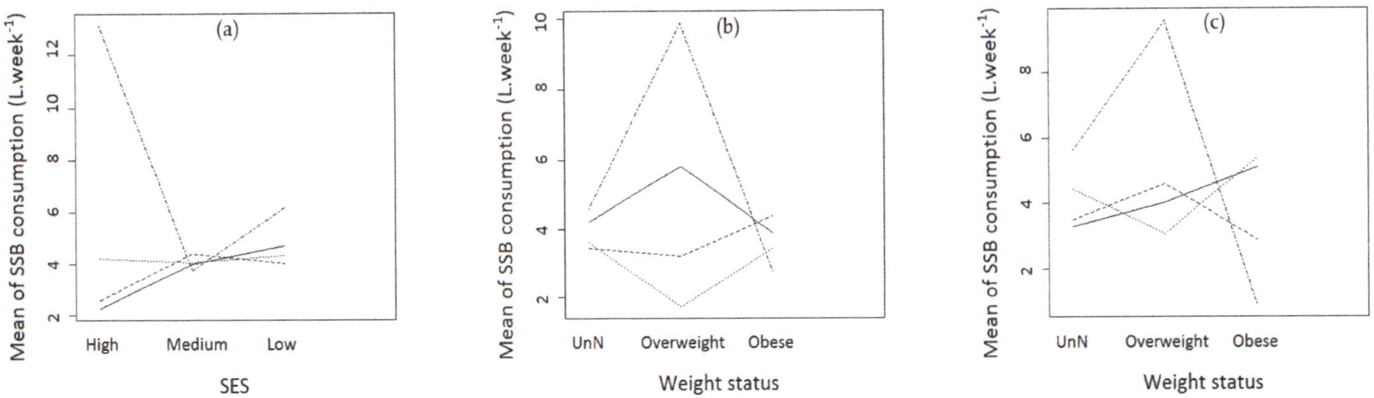

Figure 1. Pairwise factor interaction plots for SSB consumption: (**a**) Socioeconomic status (SES) vs. knowledge about energy expenditure, $p = 0.005$; (**b**) Weight status vs. knowledge about sugar, $p = 0.011$; (**c**) Weight status vs. knowledge about energy expenditure, $p = 0.002$. Type of line corresponds to knowledge. Solid line: adolescents who overestimated; dashed line: adolescents who gave accurate answers; dotted line: adolescents who underestimated; dotted-dashed line: adolescents who did not know.

The analysis of factor interactions revealed significant pairwise interactions between SES and knowledge about energy expenditure ($p < 0.01$), weight status and knowledge about sugar ($p = 0.01$), weight status and knowledge about energy expenditure ($p < 0.01$), and PA and knowledge about energy expenditure ($p = 0.02$). Figure 1 shows the significant pairwise interactions between these categorical factors.

Table 2 shows that sex, SES, weight status, self-weight perception, knowledge about sugar, opinion about SSBs and weight gain, and PA were not significantly associated with quantity of SSB consumption. Conversely, living environment, ethnic community and knowledge about energy expenditure were significantly related to the quantity of SSBs consumed. In this general model, only interactions between SES and knowledge about energy expenditure ($p = 0.01$) and between PA and knowledge about energy expenditure ($p = 0.02$) were significant.

SSB consumption was significantly higher in rural environments than in urban environments, with respective values of 4.49 $L \cdot week^{-1}$ and 1.94 $L \cdot week^{-1}$ ($p < 0.01$, Table 2).

Melanesian adolescents consumed many more SSBs than their Caucasian counterparts, with respective values of 4.77 $L \cdot week^{-1}$ and 2.46 $L \cdot week^{-1}$ ($p < 0.01$, Table 2).

Weight status and self-weight perception were not significant factors of SSB consumption ($p = 0.94$ and 0.59, respectively). However, weight status significantly interacted with knowledge about sugar (Figure 1b, $p = 0.01$) and knowledge about energy expenditure (Figure 1c, $p < 0.01$), but these interactions were not satisfactory factors in the general ANOVA model (Table 2, $p = 0.15$ and $p = 0.37$, respectively).

The correlation between PA and the quantity of SSB consumption was $\rho = 0.026$ and this was not significant ($p = 0.583$). However, PA has to be taken into account to explain SSB consumption (even if $p = 0.11$) because of the significant interactions between PA and knowledge about energy expenditure ($p = 0.02$).

Knowledge about sugar was not a significant factor for SSB consumption ($p = 0.12$, Table 2), but most of the adolescents (192 for "accurate" and 153 for "overestimated", i.e., 77%) reported knowing that there is a lot sugar in an SSB can. Conversely, knowledge about energy expenditure was a significant factor ($p = 0.03$), and the adolescents categorized as "don't know" for energy expenditure knowledge consumed significantly more SSBs (6.22 $L \cdot week^{-1}$) than the others did (4.26 $L \cdot week^{-1}$ for adolescents who underestimated, 3.64 $L \cdot week^{-1}$ for adolescents who gave an accurate answer, and 3.73 $L \cdot week^{-1}$ for adolescents who overestimated the energy expenditure required to eliminate a SSB unit). The multiple regression in Table 2 shows that the higher the estimated expenditure, the lower the SSB consumption (B = −6.18 for "underestimated", B = −7.75 for "accurate" and B = −8.29 for "overestimated").

Opinion about the SSB consumption—weight gain relationship was not a significant factor for SSB consumption (B = 0.57, $p = 0.20$) and most of the adolescents (349, i.e., 78%) agreed with the statement "consuming SSBs can cause weight gain."

Table 2. SSB consumption: quantity, multifactorial regression and ANOVA ($n = 447$).

			Quantity ($L \cdot week^{-1}$)		Multiple Regression [1] ($R^2 = 0.25$; $R^2_{adj} = 0.18$)		Multifactorial ANOVA [1]
		Size	Mean ± SD	*p*-Value *	B ± SE (95% CI)	*p*-Value	*p*-Value
Sex	**Boys**	194	4.25 ± 4.30	0.258	0.50 ± 0.38 (−0.24;1.24)	0.187	0.187
	Girls	253	3.81 ± 4.00				
Living environment	**Rural**	361	4.49 ± 4.31	<0.001			0.001
	Urban	86	1.94 ± 2.39		−1.67 ± 0.51 (−2.67;−0.66)	0.001	
Ethnic community	**Caucasian**	149	2.46 ± 3.23	<0.001			<0.001
	Melanesian	298	4.77 ± 4.32		1.91 ± 0.43 (1.07;2.75)	<0.001	
SES †	**Low**	205	4.44 ± 4.17^{a}	0.014	−11.08 ± 3.23 (−17.42;−4.74)	0.001	0.607
	Medium	115	$4.20 \pm 3.83^{a,b}$		−11.06 ± 3.19 (−17.34;−4.79)	0.001	
	High	127	3.11 ± 4.23^{b}				
Weight status	**Underweight and normal**	289	3.86 ± 3.91	0.392			0.943
	Overweight	96	4.51 ± 4.75		1.86 ± 2.62 (−3.28;7.01)	0.477	
	Obese	62	3.87 ± 4.09		−1.54 ± 3.09 (−7.61;4.53)	0.618	
Weight perception	**Too skinny**	69	4.31 ± 4.30	0.748			0.590
	Normal	286	3.99 ± 4.09		−0.35 ± 0.53 (−1.39;0.69)	0.511	
	Too big	92	3.81 ± 4.18		−0.75 ± 0.73 (−2.19;0.69)	0.305	
How many sugar lumps in a SSB can?	**Do not know**	24	5.23 ± 5.72	0.071			0.124
	Underestimate	78	3.25 ± 3.61		−0.52 ± 1.30 (−3.08;2.03)	0.689	
	Accurate	153	3.53 ± 3.59		−0.30 ± 1.26 (−2.77;2.16)	0.808	
	Overestimate	192	4.53 ± 4.42		−0.11 ± 1.23 (−2.53;2.32)	0.932	
How much running is needed to eliminate the sugar contained in a SSB can?	**Do not know**	27	6.22 ± 6.39	0.174			0.033
	Underestimate	137	4.26 ± 4.23		−6.18 ± 3.09 (−12.26;−0.10)	0.046	
	Accurate	201	3.64 ± 3.75		−7.75 ± 3.03 (−13.71;−1.79)	0.011	
	Overestimate	82	3.73 ± 3.74		−8.29 ± 3.15 (−14.47;−2.10)	0.009	
Consuming SSBs can cause weight gain	**Agree**	349	3.77 ± 4.06	0.027			0.204
	Disagree	98	4.82 ± 4.28		0.57 ± 0.45 (−0.31;1.46)	0.204	
Physical activity		447			0.29 ± 0.11 (0.08;0.50)	0.006	0.111

[1] Analyses adjusted by the significant pairwise interactions: SES and knowledge about energy expenditure ($p = 0.011$), weight status and knowledge about sugar ($p = 0.147$), weight status and knowledge about energy expenditure ($p = 0.367$), and physical activity and knowledge about energy expenditure ($p = 0.017$). * Binary factors: Student's, Welch's or Wilcoxon's test. Other factors: one-way ANOVA or Kruskal-Wallis' test. † One or several subscripted letters in a cell indicate a post-hoc pairwise t-test result. Similar letters: no significant difference between two groups. Post-hoc pairwise *t*-test *p*-values: $p = 0.604$ for low and medium, $p = 0.013$ for low and high and $p = 0.081$ for medium and high.

4. Discussion

The main result of this study was that 90% of the New Caledonian adolescents claimed to regularly drink SSBs. Moreover, the entire population was concerned since they reported regular consumption regardless of sex, living environment, ethnic community, socioeconomic status and weight status. Notably, the quantity of SSBs was strongly correlated with social factors like living environment and ethnic community but weight status and self-weight perception were surprisingly not linked to quantity.

Knowledge about sugar was not significantly linked to quantity of SSB consumption but knowledge about energy expenditure was.

4.1. Sociodemographic Factors

In New Caledonia, the living environment, ethnic community and SES are interconnected factors. For example, most of the people living in rural environments have tribal lifestyles and are Melanesian, and most of the people from other ethnic communities (such as Caucasians) live in the urban environments of Noumea and its suburbs. Moreover, rural inhabitants are usually classified as low SES since they generally live of food crops [4]. Therefore, it is unsurprising that the quantity of consumed SSBs presented in Table 2 was significantly higher in rural environments, Melanesian adolescents, and low-SES adolescents as these factors are very much intertwined. This also may explain why, although the high-SES adolescents consumed significantly fewer SSBs than the low-SES adolescents, this factor was not significant in the general regression model (Table 2).

Adolescents living in rural areas reported significantly higher SSB consumption than those living in urban areas (4.49 L·week^{-1} vs. 1.94 L·week^{-1}, respectively). This has also been observed in other countries. Indeed, Park et al. [6] reported that SSB intake differs significantly among US adults according to geographic region. They found that the proportion of adults who consumed SSBs $\geq$2 times per day, or more than 3.5 L·week^{-1}, was highest among adults living in the East South Central region of the US [6]. Sharkey et al., who studied eating behaviors among rural and urban adults, found that the prevalence and high level of SSB consumption ($\geq$3 cans or glasses of SSB per day, or more than 5 L·week^{-1}) were greater among rural adults (52.4% prevalence and 17.7% high consumption) compared with urban counterparts (43.7% prevalence and 10.5% high consumption) [31]. The differences were partially explained by cultural norms, SSB availability, and/or state and local obesity prevention programs [6,31]. In New Caledonia, SSBs are widely available near all schools before, during and after the school day, and health education programs are delivered to all areas of the archipelago. Media access is nevertheless easier in the urban environments, and the media often provide strong warnings about the sugar in industrial products and its impact on health [10]. Moreover, Hughes and Lawrence [12] pointed out some of the factors that have changed Pacific Islanders' behaviors, notably the acceptance and/or belief that foreign (imported) goods are superior. This may explain why Melanesian adolescents reported consuming significantly more SSBs than their Caucasian counterparts (4.77 L·week^{-1} and 2.46 L·week^{-1}, respectively). In addition, a recent review evaluated the interventions targeting the consumption of high-sugar products by Pacific Island adolescents [10]. The authors reported that school and community-based interventions have had little success in reducing the consumption of these products for the moment [10].

As studies have shown, SSBs may also replace water as the daily beverage [32], and access to potable water might explain our observation in parts of rural New Caledonia [33]. In particularly remote areas, the water comes from desalination plants and/or the treated water may be of poor bacteriological quality [33]. People living in environments where access to drinking water is a problem might become suspicious of this essential natural resource, especially as the taste can be unpleasant. This might explain the preference for SSBs among some rural populations.

Several factors and their mutual interactions may in fact explain the prevalence of SSB consumption in rural environments and should be considered in the future: (1) drinking tap water may be not safe, so it is better to drink something else; (2) drinking SSBs or giving money to children to buy SSBs may be a way to ostensibly show personal earning power (more than buying bottled water); and (3) adolescent eating habits are influenced by media campaigns that communicate health and nutrition warnings, especially in urban environments.

4.2. Weight Status and Self-Weight Perception

A previous study reported that weight status might be linked to SSB intake [10], although another study found no association [34]. Researchers have explained this non-significant finding as underreported intake [35] or reduced intake by overweight and obese adolescents wanting to lose weight [34]. Our study shows that neither weight status ($p = 0.94$) nor self-weight perception ($p = 0.59$) was a significant explanatory factor for the quantity of SSB consumption (Table 2).

Previous studies conducted in New Caledonia have shown that people are aware that obesity can exacerbate noncommunicable diseases but they may not know the actual definition of obesity [36] and thus whether they are concerned. Adolescents have also shown a mismatch between weight perception and reality [19]. It is therefore possible that some of the overweight adolescents in the current study were not aware of their own weight status. In addition, overweight is overall associated with unhealthy lifestyles—not only SSB consumption but also other energy-dense food consumption. The total energy intake was unfortunately not assessed in this study and this might explain why weight status was not a significant explanatory factor for quantity of SSB consumption.

However, weight status related to knowledge may be linked to SSB intake (Figure 1) although, as shown in Table 2, the interactions between weight status and knowledge were not significant in the multiple regression ($p = 0.15$ for interactions between weight status and knowledge about sugar; $p = 0.37$ for interactions between weight status and knowledge about energy expenditure). Jasti et al. [11] found that overweight status modified the effect of SSB knowledge on SSB consumption. In their study, less SSB knowledge was associated with higher SSB consumption (OR = 3.56) only among overweight students, with no association in non-overweight students [11]. Our analysis of pairwise interactions (Figure 1b,c) showed that among the adolescents categorized as "don't know" for sugar knowledge, those who were overweight had higher SSB intake than the others. Their overweight status may have been due in part to their lack of knowledge: they did not know how to behave healthily. On the contrary, the obese adolescents categorized as "don't know" consumed fewer SSBs. This might be explained by medical monitoring: these adolescents had undoubtedly been warned against excessive SSB consumption and thus they refrained from drinking "too much" even if they had little knowledge about SSBs (sugar content and energy expenditure). In addition, the more highly the overweight adolescents estimated the sugar quantity in a can, the higher their SSB intake was. This may be due to fatalistic feelings or enjoyment being prioritized over health, especially when friends also drink SSBs: "There's a lot of sugar in sweetened beverages, it's unhealthy and it may cause weight gain, but sweetened beverages are so good and my friends are drinking a can ... So, yes! I drink a can too!" [37]. But these observations should be carefully considered because of the small sample sizes in some subcategories.

4.3. Physical Activity

Bibiloni et al. [9] found that even though beverage intake and beverage total energy intake were positively associated with PA in Spanish adolescents, there was no association between PA and SSB intake (fruit drinks, soda or energy/sport beverages). In this study, inactive boys claimed that they drank more than 9 $L{\cdot}week^{-1}$ of SSBs (370.8 mL fruit drinks, 441.6 mL soda and 495.0 mL energy/sport beverages per day) and active boys claimed drinking more than 8 $L{\cdot}week^{-1}$ (338.3 mL fruit drinks, 474.0 mL soda and 337.1 mL energy/sport beverages per day). Inactive girls claimed drinking more than 6.5 $L{\cdot}week^{-1}$ of SSBs (312.6 mL fruit drinks, 400.4 mL soda and 233.3 mL energy/sport beverages per day) and active girls also claimed drinking more than 6.5 $L{\cdot}week^{-1}$ (269.7 mL fruit drinks, 365.4 mL soda and 330.0 mL energy/sport beverages per day) [9]. Our method differed from that of Bibiloni et al. Indeed, PA was not categorized but was processed as a continuous variable; for this reason, any comparisons must be cautiously made. However, when the active and inactive adolescents in New Caledonia were mixed, they reported drinking fewer SSBs than the Spaniards (4.25 L·week^{-1} in boys and 3.81 L·week^{-1} in girls, Table 2). In contrast to Bibiloni et al.'s study, our findings showed a positive correlation between PA and quantity of SSB consumption (B = 0.29, $p \leq 0.01$). To explain this result, we need to consider that being active at school in a year-round subtropical climate requires high levels of hydration [38] and adolescents may prefer drinking other drinks than tap water in some remote areas (see Section 4.1.). In addition, the adolescents were significantly more active when they were boys (14.31 h·week^{-1} in boys vs. 12.18 h·week^{-1} in girls, $p = 0.01$), Melanesian (14.05 h·week^{-1} for Melanesians vs. 11.23 h·week^{-1} for Caucasians, $p < 0.01$), and living in rural areas (13.64 h·week^{-1} for rural adolescents vs. 10.88 h·week^{-1} for urban adolescents, $p < 0.01$) (Table 1). These results are in accordance with Zongo et al.'s study [20] and they support the observation that the interactions between sociocultural factors and behavioral factors are mutual in New Caledonia.

4.4. *Knowledge and Opinion*

Interestingly, knowledge about sugar was not a satisfactory explanatory factor ($p = 0.12$). This finding lines up with Park et al.'s findings [6] but is opposed to those of Jasti et al. [11]. The non-explanatory nature of this factor seems to indicate that thinking SSBs contain a lot of sugar does not affect the New Caledonian adolescents' consumption. Notably, many of them gave an accurate answer or overestimated the quantity of sugar, and consequently they "knew"—or certainly thought they knew – that there was a lot of sugar, but that knowledge was not always totally accurate. In addition, despite this often vague knowledge, they consumed SSBs. However, knowledge about energy expenditure seemed to encourage the young people to consume less [39]. Indeed, the adolescents who were categorized as "don't know" claimed that they drank many more SSBs than the others (6.22 L·week^{-1} for the "don't know" vs. <4.3 L·week^{-1} for the others). Moreover, more than 78% reported agreeing with the statement "consuming SSBs can cause weight gain" and the adolescents who agreed that drinking SSBs can cause weight gain drank less than the others (3.77 L·week^{-1} for "agree" vs. 4.82 L·week^{-1} for "disagree", $p = 0.03$). Similarly, Park et al. found many more individuals ($\geq$29%) with high SSB consumption (more than 3.5 L·week^{-1}, $\geq$2 servings per day) among those who did not think that drinking SSBs contributes to weight gain, compared with those who agreed about the SSB-weight gain relationship (18.3% consumed 3.5L·week^{-1}, $\geq$2 times per day) [6]. Nevertheless, opinion about the SSB consumption–weight gain relationship was not a satisfactory predictive factor (B = 0.57, $p = 0.20$), i.e., statistically, the B coefficient can be assumed to be zero. This seems to suggest that thinking SSBs can cause weight does not influence the SSB consumption in the adolescents of New Caledonia.

Our findings suggest that the key factor is "the notion of effort" related to SSB intake rather than "accurately knowing." Indeed, the adjusted analyses showed that the "don't know" adolescents consumed many more SSBs than the others, and the adolescents who thought that high energy expenditure was needed to eliminate the content of a SSB unit—that is, the "overestimators"—claimed consuming fewer SSBs than those who "underestimated" or were "accurate" (Table 2). Having an accurate answer seemed to be not that important as long as the notion of the physical effort needed to negate SSB intake had been learned. Moreover, even though most of the New Caledonian adolescents thought consuming SSBs can cause weight gain, they nonetheless drank them. Further studies are now needed to explain this observation.

4.5. *Limitations and Strengths of the Study*

This cross-sectional study does not provide evidence of causal associations or trends in the long term. However, the data were directly collected in the schools of interest: anthropometric measures were obtained during medical examination, providing more reliable assessments [19], and the survey was filled out on research days in the presence of researchers.

Adolescents were asked about their SSB consumption, PA, and knowledge and opinions about SSBs. The questions seemed to be easily understood and produced straightforward answers [39]. Yet some adolescents still gave aberrant answers probably because of a misunderstanding about the weekly average and the container volumes, and these answers were removed from analysis. The significant results were nevertheless based on robust statistical tests and thus were not impacted. Moreover, some of the adolescents might have taken sips from the drinks of the regular consumers. We assume that they took these small quantities into account in their responses, even though such quantities were probably negligible compared to drinking from one's own container.

This study examined self-reported data, as well: SSB consumption, ethnic community and PA. These measures are subjective, especially PA quantification, but the associated surveys are commonly used to obtain this type of data [29,40]. This limitation might explain the non-significance of PA in explaining the quantity of SSB consumption. Future studies will therefore need to use objective data to assess PA.

As noted, the total energy intake was not assessed in this study even though weight status was introduced as an explanatory factor. It was therefore not possible to adjust the multiple regression with the total energy intake.

This study aimed to determine associations between SSB consumption and sociodemographic characteristics, including ethnic community, in adolescents of New Caledonia. However, for statistical reasons—that is, the sample size—only the two main ethnic communities were retained, i.e., Caucasian and Melanesian. This may have introduced a bias for comparisons with the general population of New Caledonia.

5. Conclusions

This study provides insight into the links between SSB consumption and socioeconomic factors, actual weight status and self-weight perception, PA, and knowledge and opinions about SSBs in New Caledonian adolescents.

First, this study showed that SSB consumption in New Caledonia is strongly associated with ethnic community and living environment. This result should contribute to developing community-based health promotion strategies.

Second, New Caledonian adolescents seem to have an inadequate understanding of the associations between PA, food consumption and health, which raises questions about health communication campaigns from an educational point of view [4,6]. Notably, knowing how much physical effort is needed to negate an SSB seems to have more influence than knowing the sugar quantity in an SSB can. As noted, the "notion of effort" related to SSB intake may best drive adolescents to moderate SSB consumption.

Yet more studies are needed on how New Caledonian youths relate to issues of health, nutrition and physical activity. Longitudinal and qualitative studies should examine why adolescents drink so many SSBs even when they "know"—that "knowledge" often being quite inexact—that there is too much sugar in them and they think SSBs can cause weight gain.

Author Contributions: S.F. and O.G. conceived and designed the study. S.F., S.C., Y.C. and Y.L. collected data. G.W. conducted the statistical analyses and drafted the manuscript. All the authors revised and approved the final submitted version of the manuscript.

Acknowledgments: We thank the school teaching teams and administrative staff for their help and support in our investigations, especially the Department 'Promotion de la santé en milieu scolaire' of the Vice-Rectorat of New Caledonia.

References

1. Stubbs, C.O.; Lee, A.J. The obesity epidemic: Both energy intake and physical activity contribute. *Med. J. Aust.* **2004**, *181*, 489–491. [PubMed]
2. Harnack, L.; Stang, J.; Story, M. Soft Drink Consumption Among US Children and Adolescents: Nutritional Consequences. *J. Am. Diet. Assoc.* **1999**, *99*, 436–441. [CrossRef]
3. Grimm, G.C.; Harnack, L.; Story, M. Factors associated with soft drink consumption in school-aged children. *J. Am. Diet. Assoc.* **2004**, *104*, 1244–1249. [CrossRef] [PubMed]
4. Aldwell, K.; Caillaud, C.; Galy, O.; Frayon, S.; Allman-Farinelli, M. Tackling the Consumption of High Sugar Products among Children and Adolescents in the Pacific Islands: Implications for Future Research. *Healthcare* **2018**, *6*, 81. [CrossRef] [PubMed]
5. United States Department of Agriculture. *Department of Health and Human Services Nutrition and your health: Dietary Guidelines for Americans, 2010*, 7th ed.; United States Department of Agriculture: Washington, DC, USA, 2010.
6. Park, S.; Onufrak, S.; Sherry, B.; Blanck, H.M. The relationship between health-related knowledge and sugar-sweetened beverage intake among US adults. *J. Acad. Nutr. Diet.* **2014**, *114*, 1059–1066. [CrossRef] [PubMed]
7. Malik, V.S.; Hu, F.B. Sweeteners and Risk of Obesity and Type 2 Diabetes: The Role of Sugar-Sweetened Beverages. *Curr. Diab. Rep.* **2012**, *12*, 195–203. [CrossRef] [PubMed]
8. Mardiyati, N.; Song, W.; Opoku-Acheampong, A.; Miller, C.; Kidd, T.; Wang, W. Effects of Body Weight Perception and Goals on Consumption Behaviour among College Students. *FASEB J.* **2015**, *29*, 900.22.
9. Bibiloni, M.D.; Özen, A.E.; Pons, A.; González-Gross, M.; Tur, J.A. Physical Activity and Beverage Consumption among Adolescents. *Nutrients* **2016**, *8*, 389. [CrossRef]
10. Kessaram, T.; McKenzie, J.; Girin, N.; Merilles, O.E.A.; Pullar, J.; Roth, A.; White, P.; Hoy, D. Overweight, obesity, physical activity and sugar-sweetened beverage consumption in adolescents of Pacific islands: Results from the Global School-Based Student Health Survey and the Youth Risk Behavior Surveillance System. *BMC Obes.* **2015**, *2*, 34. [CrossRef]
11. Jasti, S.; Rubin, R.; Doak, C.M. Sugar-sweetened Beverage Knowledge and Consumption in College Students. *Health Behav. Policy Rev.* **2017**, *4*, 37–45. [CrossRef]
12. Hughes, R.G.; Lawrence, M.A. Globalization, food and health in Pacific Island countries. *Asia Pac. J. Clin. Nutr* **2005**, *14*, 298–306. [PubMed]
13. Frayon, S.; Cherrier, S.; Cavaloc, Y.; Wattelez, G.; Lerrant, Y.; Galy, O. Relationship of body fat and body mass index in young Pacific Islanders: A cross-sectional study in European, Melanesian and Polynesian groups. *Pediatric Obes.* **2018**, *13*, 357–364. [CrossRef] [PubMed]
14. Pak, N.; Mcdonald, A.M.; McKenzie, J.; Tukuitonga, C. Soft drink consumption in Pacific Island countries and territories: A review of trade data. *Pac. Health Dialog* **2014**, *20*, 59–66. [PubMed]
15. Corsenac, P.; Annesi-Maesano, I.; Hoy, D.; Roth, A.; Rouchon, B.; Capart, I.; Taylor, R. Overweight and obesity in New Caledonian adults: Results from measured and adjusted self-reported anthropometric data. *Diabetes Res. Clin. Pract.* **2017**, *133*, 193–203. [CrossRef] [PubMed]
16. ISEE – Communautés. Available online: http://www.isee.nc/population/recensement/communautes (accessed on 16 November 2017).
17. Congrès de la Nouvelle-Calédonie. *Délibération n°106 du 15 janvier 2016 relative à l'avenir de l'école calédonienne*; Congrès de la Nouvelle-Calédonie: Nouméa, Nouvelle-Calédonie, 2016; Available online: https://www.ac-noumea.nc/IMG/pdf/de_libe_ration_no106_du_15.01.16_relative_a_l_avenir_de_l_e_cole_cale_donienne.pdf (accessed on 31 January 2019).
18. Eurisouke, V.; Gambey, C.; Welepa, P.; Bedon, P.; Berthou, L.; Demaneuf, T.; Eyherabide, M.; Poncet, E.; Bazenet, F.; Thomas, O.; et al. *Do Kamo Plan de Santé Calédonien 2018–2028*; Gouvernement de la Nouvelle-Calédonie: Nouméa, Nouvelle-Calédonie, 2018; p. 140. Available online: https://gouv.nc/sites/default/files/atoms/files/brochure_do_kamo_etre_epanoui_0.pdf (accessed on 31 January 2019).
19. Frayon, S.; Cherrier, S.; Cavaloc, Y.; Wattelez, G.; Touitou, A.; Zongo, P.; Yacef, K.; Caillaud, C.; Lerrant, Y.; Galy, O. Misperception of weight status in the pacific: Preliminary findings in rural and urban 11- to 16-year-olds of New Caledonia. *BMC Public Health* **2017**, *17*, 25. [CrossRef]

20. Zongo, P.; Frayon, S.; Antoine-Jonville, S.; Wattelez, G.; Le Roux, P.-Y.; Hue, O.; Galy, O. Anthropometric Characteristics and Physical Fitness in Rural and Urban 11- to 16-Year-Old Melanesian Adolescents: A Cross-sectional Study in New Caledonian Schools. *Asia Pac. J. Public Health* **2017**, *29*, 589–598. [CrossRef] [PubMed]
21. Tassié, J.; Papoz, L.; Barny, S.; Simon, D. Nutritional status in adults in the pluri-ethnic population of New Caledonia. *Int. J. Obes.* **1997**, *21*, 61–66. [CrossRef]
22. Frayon, S.; Cherrier, S.; Touitou, A.; Zongo, P.; Wattelez, G.; Yacef, K.; Caillaud, C.; Galy, O. Nutrition behaviors and sociodemographic factors associated with overweight in the multi-ethnic adolescents of New Caledonia. *Ethn. Health* **2017**, *24*, 194–210. [CrossRef]
23. Cole, T.J.; Lobstein, T. Extended international (IOTF) body mass index cut-offs for thinness, overweight and obesity. *Pediatric Obes.* **2012**, *7*, 284–294. [CrossRef]
24. Institut national de la santé et de la recherche médicale. *687 Situation sociale et comportements de santé des jeunes en Nouvelle-Calédonie. Premiers résultats*; Institut national de la santé et de la recherche médicale: Villejuif, France, 2008; p. 112.
25. Krieger, N.; Rose, D.; Pevalin, D.J. A Researcher's Guide to the National Statistics Socio-Economic Classification. *J. Public Health Policy* **2003**, *24*, 467. [CrossRef]
26. ISEE—Structure de la population et évolutions. Available online: http://www.isee.nc/population/recensement/structure-de-la-population-et-evolutions (accessed on 16 November 2017).
27. The European Union Labour Force Survey—Methods and Definitions—2001 (Eurostat, Guidelines, Labour Statistics, Survey). Available online: https://unstats.un.org/unsd/EconStatKB/KnowledgebaseArticle10230.aspx (accessed on 16 November 2017).
28. Jackson, S.E.; Johnson, F.; Croker, H.; Wardle, J. Weight perceptions in a population sample of English adolescents: Cause for celebration or concern? *Int. J. Obes.* **2015**, *39*, ijo2015126. [CrossRef] [PubMed]
29. *IPAQ Research Committee Guidelines for Data Processing and Analysis of the International Physical Activity Questionnaire (IPAQ)—Short and Long Forms.* The IPAQ group (www.ipaq.ki.se). 2005. Available online: https://docs.google.com/viewer?a=v&pid=sites&srcid=ZGVmYXVsdGRvbWFpbnx0aGVpcGFxfGd4OjE0NDgxMDk3NDU1YWRlZTM (accessed on 31 January 2019).
30. R Core Team. *A Language and Environment for Statistical Computing*; R Foundation for Statistical Computing: Vienna, Austria, 2014.
31. Sharkey, J.; Johnson, C.; Dean, W. Less-healthy eating behaviors have a greater association with a high level of sugar-sweetened beverage consumption among rural adults than among urban adults. *Food Nutr. Res.* **2011**, *55*, 5819. [CrossRef] [PubMed]
32. Lee, H.-S.; Park, S.; Kim, M.-H. Factors associated with low water intake among South Korean adolescents - Korea National Health and Nutrition Examination Survey, 2007–2010. *Nutr. Res. Pract.* **2014**, *8*, 74–80. [CrossRef] [PubMed]
33. Chavroche, J. *Contribution à l'élaboration d'un cadre réglementaire visant la distribution publique de l'eau en Nouvelle-Calédonie: Fondements sanitaires et propositions*; ENGEES, ENSP, DASS-NC: DASS Nouvelle-Calédonie; Ecole Nationale de Génie de l'eau et de l'environnement de Strasbourg: Strasbourg, France, 2005; p. 82. Available online: http://fulltext.bdsp.ehesp.fr/Ensp/Memoires/2005/igs/chavroche.pdf (accessed on 31 January 2019).
34. Park, S.; Sherry, B.; Foti, K.; Blanck, H.M. Self-Reported Academic Grades and Other Correlates of Sugar-Sweetened Soda Intake among US Adolescents. *J. Acad. Nutr. Diet.* **2012**, *112*, 125–131. [CrossRef] [PubMed]
35. Lioret, S.; Touvier, M.; Balin, M.; Huybrechts, I.; Dubuisson, C.; Dufour, A.; Bertin, M.; Maire, B.; Lafay, L. Characteristics of energy under-reporting in children and adolescents. *Br. J. Nutr.* **2011**, *105*, 1671–1680. [CrossRef] [PubMed]
36. ASS NC. *L'équilibre alimentaire: Rapport d'étude omnibus, Novembre 2011*; Agence Sanitaire et Sociale de la Nouvelle-Calédonie: Nouméa, Nouvelle-Calédonie, 2011.
37. Lawrence, H.; Nathan Reynolds, A.; Joseph Venn, B. Perceptions of the Healthfulness of Foods of New Zealand Adults Living with Prediabetes and Type 2 Diabetes: A Pilot Study. *J. Nutr. Educ. Behav.* **2017**, *49*, 339–345. [CrossRef] [PubMed]

38. Galy, O.; Antoine-jonville, S.; Reuillard, E.; Hue, O. Free hydration and well-being during physical education in tropical climate. In *Educ. St. Sociétés*; Editions des archives contemporaines: Paris, France, 2016; Volume 2, pp. 79–92.
39. Francis, J.; Martin, K.; Costa, B.; Christian, H.; Kaur, S.; Harray, A.; Barblett, A.; Oddy, W.H.; Ambrosini, G.; Allen, K.; et al. Informing Intervention Strategies to Reduce Energy Drink Consumption in Young People: Findings From Qualitative Research. *J. Nutr. Educ. Behav.* **2017**, *49*, 724–733. [CrossRef]
40. Lee, P.H.; Macfarlane, D.J.; Lam, T.; Stewart, S.M. Validity of the international physical activity questionnaire short form (IPAQ-SF): A systematic review. *Int. J. Behav. Nutr. Phys. Act.* **2011**, *8*, 115. [CrossRef]

Permissions

All chapters in this book were first published by MDPI; hereby published with permission under the Creative Commons Attribution License or equivalent. Every chapter published in this book has been scrutinized by our experts. Their significance has been extensively debated. The topics covered herein carry significant findings which will fuel the growth of the discipline. They may even be implemented as practical applications or may be referred to as a beginning point for another development.

The contributors of this book come from diverse backgrounds, making this book a truly international effort. This book will bring forth new frontiers with its revolutionizing research information and detailed analysis of the nascent developments around the world.

We would like to thank all the contributing authors for lending their expertise to make the book truly unique. They have played a crucial role in the development of this book. Without their invaluable contributions this book wouldn't have been possible. They have made vital efforts to compile up to date information on the varied aspects of this subject to make this book a valuable addition to the collection of many professionals and students.

This book was conceptualized with the vision of imparting up-to-date information and advanced data in this field. To ensure the same, a matchless editorial board was set up. Every individual on the board went through rigorous rounds of assessment to prove their worth. After which they invested a large part of their time researching and compiling the most relevant data for our readers.

The editorial board has been involved in producing this book since its inception. They have spent rigorous hours researching and exploring the diverse topics which have resulted in the successful publishing of this book. They have passed on their knowledge of decades through this book. To expedite this challenging task, the publisher supported the team at every step. A small team of assistant editors was also appointed to further simplify the editing procedure and attain best results for the readers.

Apart from the editorial board, the designing team has also invested a significant amount of their time in understanding the subject and creating the most relevant covers. They scrutinized every image to scout for the most suitable representation of the subject and create an appropriate cover for the book.

The publishing team has been an ardent support to the editorial, designing and production team. Their endless efforts to recruit the best for this project, has resulted in the accomplishment of this book. They are a veteran in the field of academics and their pool of knowledge is as vast as their experience in printing. Their expertise and guidance has proved useful at every step. Their uncompromising quality standards have made this book an exceptional effort. Their encouragement from time to time has been an inspiration for everyone.

The publisher and the editorial board hope that this book will prove to be a valuable piece of knowledge for researchers, students, practitioners and scholars across the globe.

List of Contributors

Vassiliki Benetou and Philippos Orfanos
Department of Hygiene, Epidemiology and Medical Statistics, School of Medicine, National and Kapodistrian University of Athens, 115-27 Athens, Greece

Afroditi Kanellopoulou
Department of Hygiene, Epidemiology and Medical Statistics, School of Medicine, National and Kapodistrian University of Athens, 115-27 Athens, Greece
Department of Hygiene and Epidemiology, School of Medicine, University of Ioannina, 451-10 Ioannina, Greece

Eleftheria Kanavou, Anastasios Fotiou, Myrto Stavrou and Anna Kokkevi
University Mental Health, Neurosciences, & Precision Medicine Research Institute "Costas Stefanis" (UMHRI), 115-27 Athens, Greece

Clive Richardson
Department of Economic and Regional Development, Panteion University of Social and Political Sciences, 176-71 Athens, Greece

Elida Sina, Christoph Buck and Antje Hebestreit
Leibniz Institute for Prevention Research and Epidemiology—BIPS, Achterstr. 30, 28359 Bremen, Germany

Hannah Jilani
Leibniz Institute for Prevention Research and Epidemiology—BIPS, Achterstr. 30, 28359 Bremen, Germany
Institute for Public Health and Nursing Research—IPP, University of Bremen, 28359 Bremen, Germany

Michael Tornaritis
Research and Education Institute of Child Health, 2035 Lefcosia, Cyprus

Toomas Veidebaum
Department of Chronic Diseases, National Institute for Health Development, 11619 Tallin, Estonia

Paola Russo
Institute of Food Sciences, National Research Council, 83100 Avellino, Italy

Luis A. Moreno
GENUD (Growth, Exercise, Nutrition and Development) Research Group, Instituto Agroalimentario de Aragón (IA2), Instituto de Investigación Sanitaria Aragón (IIS Aragón), Centro de Investigación Biomédica en Red Fisiopatología de la Obesidad y Nutrición (CIBERObn), University of Zaragoza, 50009 Zaragoza, Spain

Denes Molnar
Department of Pediatrics, Medical School, University of Pécs, 7623 Pécs, Hungary

Gabriele Eiben
Department of Biomedicine and Public Health, School of Health and Education, University of Skovde, 54128 Skovde, Sweden

Staffan Marild
Department. of Pediatrics, Institute of Clinical Sciences, Sahlgrenska Academy at University of Gothenburg, 40530 Gothenburg, Sweden

Valeria Pala
Department of Preventive and Predictive Medicine, Fondazione IRCCS, Istituto Nazionale dei Tumori, 20133 Milan, Italy

Wolfgang Ahrens
Leibniz Institute for Prevention Research and Epidemiology—BIPS, Achterstr. 30, 28359 Bremen, Germany
Faculty of Mathematics/Computer Science, University of Bremen, 28359 Bremen, Germany

Sarah K. Hibbs-Shipp, Morgan L. McCloskey, Savannah Hobbs and Laura L. Bellows
Department of Food Science and Human Nutrition, Colorado State University, Fort Collins, CO 80523, USA

Richard E. Boles and Susan L. Johnson
Department of Pediatrics, University of Colorado Anschutz Medical Campus, Aurora, CO 80045, USA

Manon Rouche and Lucille Desbouys
Research Center in Epidemiology, Biostatistics and Clinical Research, School of Public Health, Université libre de Bruxelles (ULB), 1040 Brussels, Belgium

Bart de Clercq and Maxim Dierckens
Department of Public Health and Primary Care, Ghent University (UGent), 9000 Ghent, Belgium

Thérésa Lebacq, Nathalie Moreau and Katia Castetbon
Research Center in Epidemiology, Biostatistics and Clinical Research, School of Public Health, Université libre de Bruxelles (ULB), 1040 Brussels, Belgium
Service d'Information Promotion Education Santé (SIPES), School of Public Health, Université libre de Bruxelles (ULB), 1040 Brussels, Belgium

Isabelle Godin
Research Centre in Social Approaches to Health, School of Public Health, Université libre de Bruxelles (ULB), 1040 Brussels, Belgium

Liisa Korkalo, Henna Vepsalainen, Essi Skaffari and Maijaliisa Erkkola
Department of Food and Nutrition, University of Helsinki, 00014 Helsinki, Finland

Carola Ray and Reetta Lehto
Folkhalsan Research Center, Topeliuksenkatu 20, 00250 Helsinki, Finland

Helena Henrietta Hauta-alus
Children's Hospital, Pediatric Research Center, University of Helsinki and Helsinki University Hospital, Biomedicum 2 C, 00020 HUS Helsinki, Finland

Kaija Nissinen
Seinajoki University of Applied Sciences, Kampusranta 11, 60101 Seinajoki, Finland

Jelena Meinila
Folkhalsan Research Center, Topeliuksenkatu 20, 00250 Helsinki, Finland
Department of Obstetrics and Gynecology, University of Helsinki and Helsinki University Hospital, 00014 Helsinki, Finland

Eva Roos
Folkhalsan Research Center, Topeliuksenkatu 20, 00250 Helsinki, Finland
Department of Public Health, University of Helsinki, 00014 Helsinki, Finland

Antje Hebestreit, Timm Intemann, Claudia Bornhorst and Iris Pigeot
Leibniz-Institute for Prevention Research and Epidemiology—BIPS, 28359 Bremen, Germany

Alfonso Siani
Institute of Food Sciences, National Research Council, 83100 Avellino, Italy

Stefaan De Henauw
Department of Public Health, Ghent University, 9000 Ghent, Belgium

Gabriele Eiben and Monica Hunsberger
Department of Public Health and Community Medicine, University of Gothenburg, 40530 Gothenburg, Sweden

Yiannis A. Kourides
Research and Education Institute of Child Health, 2035 Strovolos, Cyprus

Eva Kovacs
Institute for Medical Information Processing, Biometrics and Epidemiology, Ludwig-Maximilians-Universität München, 81377 Munich, Germany
German Center for Vertigo and Balance Disorders, Ludwig-Maximilians-Universität München, 81377 Munich, Germany

Vittorio Krogh and Valeria Pala
Department of Preventive and Predictive Medicine, Fondazione IRCCS Istituto Nazionale dei Tumori, 20133 Milan, Italy

Leonie H. Bogl
Leibniz-Institute for Prevention Research and Epidemiology—BIPS, 28359 Bremen, Germany
Department of Public Health, University of Helsinki, 00014 Helsinki, Finland
Finnish Institute of Molecular Medicine, University of Helsinki, 00014 Helsinki, Finland

Liya Denney, Myriam C. Afeiche and Alison L. Eldridge
Nestlé Research Center, Lausanne 1000, Switzerland

Salvador Villalpando-Carrión
Children's Hospital of Mexico Federico Gómez, National Institute of Health, Mexico City 06720, Mexico
Nestlé Infant Nutrition, Mexico City 11520, Mexico

Patricia Jane Lucas
School for Policy Studies, University of Bristol, Bristol BS8 1TZ, UK

Emma Patterson
Department of Public Health Sciences, Karolinska Institutet, SE-171 77 Stockholm, Sweden
Centre for Epidemiology and Community Medicine, Stockholm County Council, SE-113 65 Stockholm, Sweden

Gary Sacks and Natassja Billich
Global Obesity Centre, School of Health and Social Development, Deakin University, Geelong VIC 3220, Australia

Charlotte Elizabeth Louise Evans
Nutritional Epidemiology Group, School of Food Science and Nutrition, University of Leeds, Leeds LS2 9JT, UK

Maike Wolters and Wolfgang Ahrens
Leibniz Institute for Prevention Research and Epidemiology—BIPS, Department: Epidemiological Methods and Etiologic Research, Achterstr. 30, 28359 Bremen, Germany

Gesa Joslowski
IEL—Nutritional Epidemiology, University of Bonn, DONALD Study, Heinstuck 11, 44225 Dortmund, Germany

Sandra Plachta-Danielzik and Manfred J. Muller
Institute of Human Nutrition and Food Science, Christian-Albrechts University, 24118 Kiel, Germany

Marie Standl
Institute of Epidemiology I, Helmholtz Zentrum Munchen—German Research Center for Environmental Health, D-85764 Neuherberg, Germany

Anette E. Buyken
IEL—Nutritional Epidemiology, University of Bonn, DONALD Study, Heinstuck 11, 44225 Dortmund, Germany
Institute of Nutrition, Consumption and Health, Faculty of Natural Science, University Paderborn, 33098 Paderborn, Germany

Peter T. Katzmarzyk and Gang Hu
Pennington Biomedical Research Center, 6400 Perkins Road, Baton Rouge, LA 70808, USA

Jean-Philippe Chaput and Mark S. Tremblay
Children's Hospital of Eastern Ontario Research Institute, Ottawa, ON K1H 8L1, Canada

Mikael Fogelholm
Department of Food and Environmental Sciences, University of Helsinki, 00014 Helsinki, Finland

Carol Maher and Timothy Olds
School of Health Sciences, Sansom Institute, University of South Australia, Adelaide, SA 5001, Australia

Jose Maia
Faculdade de Desporto, University of Porto, Rua Dr. Plácido Costa, 91, 4200-450 Porto, Portugal

Olga L. Sarmiento
School of Medicine, Universidad de los Andes, Bogota 11001000, Colombia

Martyn Standage
Department for Health, University of Bath, Bath BA2 7AY, UK

Catrine Tudor-Locke
Department of Kinesiology, University of Massachusetts, Amherst, MA 01003, USA

Sibylle Kranz
Centre for Exercise, Nutrition and Health Sciences, University of Bristol, Bristol BS8 1TH, UK

Nicholas R. V. Jones and Pablo Monsivais
UKCRC Centre for Diet and Activity Research (CEDAR), Cambridge CB2 0QQ, UK

Brittany Davison, Pouya Saeedi, Katherine Black, Harriet Harrex, Jillian Haszard Sheila Skeaff and Paula Skidmore
Department of Human Nutrition, University of Otago, Dunedin 9054, New Zealand

Kim Meredith-Jones
Department of Medicine, University of Otago, Dunedin 9054, New Zealand

Robin Quigg
Cancer Society Social and Behavioural Research Unit, Department of Preventive and Social Medicine, Dunedin School of Medicine, University of Otago, Dunedin 9054, New Zealand

Lee Stoner
Department of Exercise and Sports Science, University of North Carolina, Chapel Hill, NC 27519, USA

Jyh Eiin Wong
School of Healthcare Sciences, Faculty of Health Sciences, Universiti Kebangsaan Malaysia, Kuala Lumpur 50300, Malaysia

Kathryn Walton
Department of Translational Medicine, The Hospital for Sick Children, Toronto, ON M5G 0A4, Canada

Emma Haycraft
School of Sport, Exercise and Health Sciences, Loughborough University, Loughborough, Leicestershire LE11 3TU, UK

Kira Jewell, Andrea Breen, Janis Randall Simpson and Jess Haines
Department of Family Relations & Applied Nutrition, University of Guelph, Guelph, ON N1G 2W1, Canada

Guillaume Wattelez, Stéphane Frayon, Yolande Cavaloc, Sophie Cherrier, Yannick Lerrant and Olivier Galy
Interdisciplinary Laboratory for Research in Education, EA 7483, University of New Caledonia, Noumea BP R4 98851, New Caledonia

Index

Printed in the USA
CPSIA information can be obtained
at www.ICGtesting.com
LVHW080047211023
761596LV00010BA/1955

9 781646 466221